Harper College Library

3 2158 00509 7215

FEB - - 2015

P9-DMU-958

DATE DUE

			PRINTED IN U.S.A.

Diseases *of the* Human Body

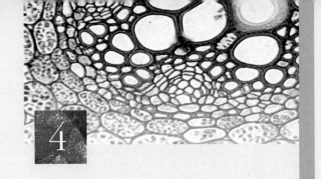

Diseases *of the* Human Body

FOURTH EDITION

Carol D. Tamparo, PhD, CMA
Formerly Dean of Business and Allied Health
Lake Washington Technical College
Kirkland, Washington

Marcia A. Lewis, EdD, RN, CMA
Associate Dean of Nursing Programs
Adjunct Professer, Medical Assisting
Formerly Associate Dean, Mathematics,
Engineering Sciences, and Health
Olympic College
Bremerton, Washington

FA Davis Company • Philadelphia

F. A. Davis Company
1915 Arch Street
Philadelphia, PA 19103
www.fadavis.com

Copyright © 2005 by F. A. Davis Company

Copyright © 2005 by F. A. Davis Company. All rights reserved. This book is protected by copyright. No part of it may be reproduced, stored in a retrieval system, or transmitted in any form or by any means, electronic, mechanical, photocopying, recording, or otherwise, without written permission from the publisher.

Printed in the United States of America

Last digit indicates print number: 10 9 8 7 6

Acquisitions Editor: Andy McPhee
Developmental Editor: Tom Robinson, Melissa Reed
Design and Illustration Manager: Joan Wendt

As new scientific information becomes available through basic and clinical research, recommended treatments and drug therapies undergo changes. The author(s) and publisher have done everything possible to make this book accurate, up to date, and in accord with accepted standards at the time of publication. The author(s), editors, and publisher are not responsible for errors or omissions or for consequences from application of the book, and make no warranty, expressed or implied, in regard to the contents of the book. Any practice described in this book should be applied by the reader in accordance with professional standards of care used in regard to the unique circumstances that may apply in each situation. The reader is advised always to check product information (package inserts) for changes and new information regarding dose and contraindications before administering any drug. Caution is especially urged when using new or infrequently ordered drugs.

Library of Congress Cataloging-in-Publication Data

ISBN 10: 0-8036-1245-1   ISBN 13: 978-0-8036-1245-7

Library of Congress Cataloging-in-Publication data

Tamparo, Carol D., 1940-
  Diseases of the human body/Carol D. Tamparo, Marcia A. Lewis. --4th ed. p. ; cm.
  Includes bibliographical references and index.
  ISBN 0-8036-1245-1 (pbk. : alk. paper)
  1. Diseases. 2. Pathology.
  [DNLM: 1. Disease--Handbooks. 2. Pathology--Handbooks. 3. Internal Medicine--Handbooks.]
  l. Lewis, Marcia A. ll. Title.
  RC46. T27 2005
  616--dc22

                    2005002186

Authorization to photocopy items for internal or personal use, or the internal or personal use of specific clients, is granted by F. A. Davis Company for users registered with the Copyright Clearance Center (CCC) Transactional Reporting Service, provided that the fee of $.25 per copy is paid directly to CCC, 222 Rosewood Drive, Danvers, MA 01923. For those organizations that have been granted a photocopy license by CCC, a separate system of payment has been arranged. The fee code for users of the Transactional Reporting Service is: 8036-1245-1/05 0 + $.25.

HARPER COLLEGE LIBRARY
PALATINE, ILLINOIS 60067

Dedications

Tom and Les,

Not everyone gets a "second chance" at love. Anyone who does knows that it is always better the second time around. We have been especially blessed to have Tom Tamparo and Les Lewis in our lives. Both of them are …

- Great friends, husbands, and dads
- 100% supporters of our projects
- Engineers who love to "fix" and "tinker"
- Historians and naturalists
- Humorists
- Master gardeners
- Tender, thoughtful, and understanding
- Great encouragers of our friendship.

To you, Tom, and to you, Les, we dedicate the Fourth Edition of this book. Thank you so much for being who you are.

LOVE,
CAROL AND MARTI

Martiann, daughter of Marti and Les Lewis, served as a very special partner in this edition. Martiann was responsible for much of the up-to-date Internet research. She handled the word processing of almost all the new material, and that meant deciphering atrocious handwritten notes filled with private abbreviations. She kept our three computers on track and skillfully folded everything into our final files. As a graduate student in Counseling Psychology focusing on addictions, she provided valuable insight to the new chapter *Mental Health Diseases and Disorders*. Martiann also served as gourmet chef during our two week-long writing marathons at the beach condo. Our Chef and Administrative Assistant prepared nutritious snacks, high-energy and low-carbohydrate meals, and an occasional truly special dessert. Martiann kept the music playing and the chocolates available and pushed us out on the beach when the tension was high.

Without you, Martiann, this edition would have been much more difficult and taken twice as long to complete. You can be our "shrink" any time so long as we always have a table at your restaurant.

LOVE,
MOM AND CAROL

Preface

This text provides clear, succinct, and basic information about common medical conditions. *Diseases of the Human Body*, Fourth Edition, is carefully designed to meet the unique educational and professional needs of health-care personnel. The book focuses on human diseases and disorders that are frequently first diagnosed or treated in ambulatory health care. Each entry considers what the disease or disorder is, how it might be diagnosed and treated, and the likely consequences of the disease or disorder for the person experiencing it.

The first seven chapters—the disease process, integrative medicine and alternative therapies, pain and its management, infectious diseases, neoplasms, congenital diseases and disorders, and mental health diseases and disorders—provide a solid foundation for subsequent chapters. The coverage of major conditions is organized by body system. This pattern of organization is easily integrated with medical terminology or anatomy and physiology courses that health-care professional students often take concurrently with their study of human disease. Within the body system chapters, each disease condition is highlighted by means of a logical, seven-part format consisting of:

- Description
- Etiology
- Signs and Symptoms
- Diagnostic Procedures
- Treatment
  - Alternative Therapies
  - Teaching Tips
- Prognosis
- Prevention

The balance of information in each of these subsections varies according to the relative frequency and severity of the condition. In every case, however, the information selected is chosen to reflect the health-care professional's need for thorough yet concise information about the condition in question.

Research for this text indicated to the authors that alternative therapies and treatments were used far more often by clients than originally suspected. In fact, there is a strong movement toward "integrative medicine" that uses the best of both traditional or allopathic and alternative therapies to treat clients. Only when documentation was found indicating a viable alternative therapy is the therapy included; therefore, not all disease entries include alternative therapy.

The organization of the text is thoroughly contemporary and designed to help students retain and understand basic concepts within the context of their professions. Color in the interior further enhances its appeal. Features include clear chapter outlines, chapter learning objectives, pronunciation of key terms, and study questions and case studies to encourage critical thinking. Teaching tips and childhood and elder notes are included as appropriate. Special Focus sections present detailed coverage of important concerns related to the body system under discussion. Answers to case study questions can be found in the Instructor's Guide to this textbook. The comprehensive glossary appears at the end of the text. The authors used *Taber's Cyclopedic Medical Dictionary*, 19th Edition, as their reference. Throughout the text, carefully chosen illustrations help students visualize body structures and conditions. The appendices—which include succinct descriptions of most of the diagnostic procedures mentioned in the text, organizations and associations related to the disease entities, a comprehensive reference list that includes Web sites, and an exhaustive listing of normal laboratory values—help make *Diseases of the Human Body*, Fourth Edition, a valuable and useful reference after students have begun their professional career. Finally, in addition to a general subject index, a specialized index of diseases covered in this text directs the reader to the seven-part presentation of each disease covered.

The study of human disease is never easy. We have, however, attempted in every instance to make it clear and accessible by presenting information that will benefit both students and health-care professionals. To assist instructors, we have developed an Instructor's Guide, an Electronic Test Bank, and a PowerPoint presentation, which are available to adopters. The authors will note updated information on diseases and disorders on a Web page provided by F. A. Davis that also will allow e-mail access to the authors.

CAROL D. TAMPARO

MARCIA A. LEWIS

Acknowledgments

We are colleagues in the medical assistant profession. We are educators, administrators, and volunteers in community and technical colleges and in the health-care arena. We write as a team. We share our homes and meals, good times of laughter, and play. We write to the accompaniment of great music. We share sad times and tedious times. We agree and we disagree. Always we are friends and mentors of one another. We are co-authors.

We could not exist as such without the support of many individuals, including our publishers at F. A. Davis Company, especially Andy McPhee, Acquisitions Editor; Margaret Biblis, Publisher of Health Professions/Medicine; and Susan Rhyner, Manager of Creative Development. They have been encouraging and supporting and always believed in our goals for this project. Thomas Robinson, Freelance Development Editor, and Melissa Reed, Assistant Editor, made certain that this revision was produced in a readable manuscript. Still others, behind the scenes but no less important, provided their wisdom and knowledge.

They include Kimberly Harris, Administrative Assistant; Jack Brandt, Illustration Coordinator; Robert Butler, Production Manager; Joan Wendt, Design and Illustration Manager; and Kirk Pedrick, Senior Developmental Editor for Electronic Publishing.

No writing project could be undertaken without the support of our families, who allowed us time to work and gave us the moral support and encouragement that is so vital. Thank you, Tom, Les, Jayne, Duuana, and Martiann.

We also owe a debt of gratitude to students and peers who continually challenge us. They remind us that their desire for knowledge is the most important reason for this textbook.

Finally, we acknowledge all the authors of the many reference resources we used in this edition. The content of this text cannot be entirely new because it is based on the work of a community of researchers, clinicians, and authors; it is our hope that we have presented it in a manner that is unique and in a style that is useful to all readers.

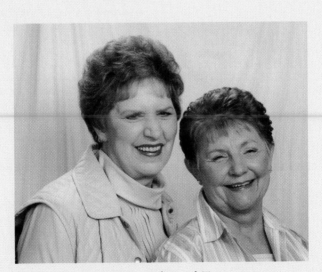

Marti Lewis and Carol Tamparo

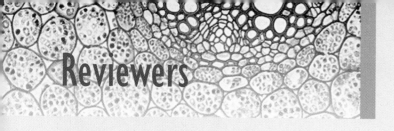

Reviewers

Anina Beaman, MS, RNC, CMA
Program Area Coordinator
Allied Health Department
Bryant and Stratton College
Richmond, Virginia

Wendy D. Bircher, PT, EdD
Director, PTA Program
Physical Therapy
San Juan College
Farmington, New Mexico

Sue Boulden, BSN, CMA
Director, Medical Assisting Program
Allied Health Department
Mount Hood Community College
Aloha, Oregon

Cindi Brassington, MS, CMA
Assistant Professor
Allied Health Department
Quinebaug Valley Community Technical College
Danielson, Connecticut

Michael Lewis Decker, BS, MA
Instructor and Director, Medical Assisting Program
Omaha College of Health Careers
Omaha, Nebraska

Sharon Eagle, RN, MSN
Nursing Educator
Nursing Program
Wenatchee Valley College
Wenatchee, Washington

Nancy Gardner, CMA, CPC
Adjunct Instructor
Des Moines Area Community College
Ankeny, Iowa

Cheri Goretti, MA, MT(ASCP), CMA
Program Coordinator, Medical Assisting Program, and
    Associate Professor
Medical Assisting, Phlebotomy and Health Information
    Management Programs
Allied Health Department
Quinebaug Valley Community Technical College
Danielson, Connecticut

Glenda Hart Hatcher, BSN, RN, CMA
Director, Medical Assisting Program
Department of Allied Health
Southwest Georgia Technical College
Thomasville, Georgia

Beulah Ann Hofmann, RN, BSN, MSN, CMA
Director, Medical Assisting Program
Health Sciences Department

Ivy Tech State College
Terre Haute, Indiana

Marie L. Kotter, PhD, MS, BS
Professor and Chairperson
Health Sciences
Weber State University
West Ogden, Utah

Suzanne Moe, RN
Instructor
Health Division
Northland Community and Technical College
East Grand Forks, Minnesota

Kay A. Nave, CMA/MRT
Program Director, Medical Assisting Program
Medical Department
Hagerstown Business College
Hagerstown, Maryland

Linda Platt, EdD, ATC
Assistant Professor, Athletic Training
Health Sciences Department
Duquesne University
Pittsburgh, Pennsylvania

Robin Snider-Flohr, EdD, RN, CMA
Associate Professor
Department of Health and Biological Sciences
Jefferson Community College
Watertown, New York

Marilyn M. Turner, RN, CMA
Director, Medical Assisting Program
Chair, Health Sciences Department
Ogeechee Technical College
Statesboro, Georgia

Cheryl A. Vineyard, CMA
Director, Medical Assisting Program
Eastern New Mexico University—Roswell Campus
Roswell, New Mexico

Deborah L. White, CMA, MS/HPE
Coordinator, Medical Assisting Program
Patient Care Services
Trident Technical College
Charleston, South Carolina

Marge Zerbe, RN, BS
Adjunct Instructor
Allied Health Department
Lake Sumter Community College
Leesburg, Florida

Note to Instructors

Every reasonable effort has been made to ensure the information in *Diseases of the Human Body*, Fourth Edition, is accurate, up to date, and in accord with accepted standards. Not all authorities agree, however, on the etiologies, signs and symptoms, diagnostic and treatment procedures, and prognosis/prevention for many of the medical conditions presented here. There may not be agreement on the alternative therapies or teaching tips we've included. In cases in which conflicting information was noted, we've attempted to present a consensus from among the authorities consulted.

Contents

Contents

Chapter 7

Mental Health Diseases and Disorders   120

Chapter 8

Urinary System Diseases and Disorders   144

Chapter 9

Reproductive System Diseases and Disorders   166

Chapter 10

Digestive System Diseases and Disorders   200

Chapter 11

Respiratory System Diseases and Disorders   232

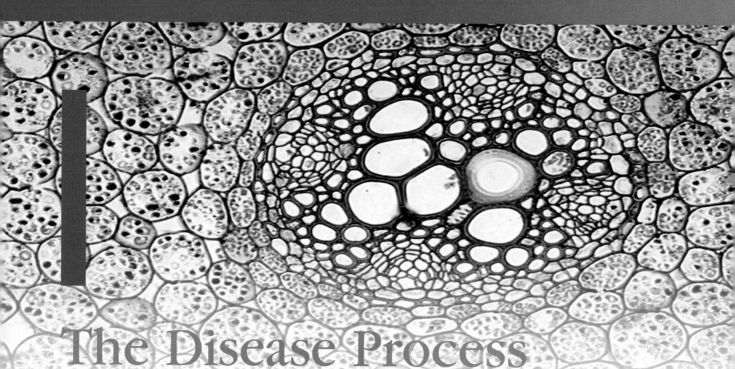

The Disease Process

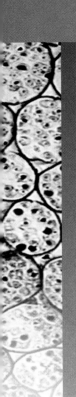

KEY WORDS

Amino acid (ă•mē′nō•ă•sĭd)
Analgesic (ăn•ăl•jē′sĭk)
Anaphylaxis (ăn•ă•fī•lăk′sĭs)
Antibody (ăn′tĭ•bŏd•ē)
Antiemetic (ăn•tĭ•ē•mĕt′ĭk)
Antigen (ăn′tĭ•jĕn)
Chromosome (krō′mō•sōm)
Diuretic (dī•ū•rĕt′yk)
Dyspnea (dĭsp•nē′ă)
Edema (ĕ•dē′mă)
Erythema (ĕr•ĭ•the′mă)
Exocrine (ĕks′ō•krĭn)
Genotype (jĕn′ō•tīp)
Heterozygous (hĕt•ĕr•ō•zī′gŭs)
Homeostasis (ho•mē•ō•stă′sĭs)
Homozygous (hōm•ō•zī′gŭs)
Hypovolemic shock (hī•pō•vō•lē′mĭk shŏk)
Hypoxemia (hī•pŏks•ē′mē•ă)
Incontinence (ĭn•kŏn′tĭ•nĕns)
Lymphadenopathy
   (lĭm•făd•ĕ•nŏp′ă•thē)
Macrophage (măk′rō•fāj)
Metastasis (mĕ•tăs′tă•sĭs)
Pathogenic (păth•ō•jĕn′ĭk)
Phagocytosis (făg•ō•sī•tō′sĭs)
Phenotype (fē′nō•tīp)
Polymorphonuclear leukocyte (pŏl•ē•mō
   r•fō•nū′klē•ăr loo′kō•sīt)
Pruritus (proo•rī′tŭs)
Stridor (strī′dōr)
Syncope (sĭn′kō•pē)
Tachycardia (tăk•ē•kăr′dē•ă)
Urticaria (ŭr•tĭ•kā′rē•ă)
Wheal (hwēl)

> *All interest in disease and death is only another expression of interest in life.*
>
> —THOMAS MANN

LEARNING OBJECTIVES

Upon successful completion of this chapter, you will be able to:

- Define *disease.*
- Contrast illness and disease.
- Restate at least three predisposing factors of disease.
- Identify the three classifications of hereditary diseases.
- Describe the genetic activity of DNA.
- Distinguish between genotype and phenotype.
- Identify the process of inflammation.
- Describe how infections are transmitted.
- Name at least four groups of microorganisms.
- Identify the most likely anatomic sites for traumatic injuries.
- Recall at least six physical and chemical agents that may cause disease.
- Contrast neoplasm and cancer.
- Define *benign* and *malignant* tumors.
- Identify three means of protection afforded by the immune system.
- Differentiate between:
  a. Natural and acquired immunity
  b. Humoral and cell-mediated immunity
  c. B-cell and T-cell immunity
- Name three classifications of immune-related diseases.
- Identify allergic reactions.
- Describe how anaphylactic shock can occur in any of the allergic reactions.
- Name four categories of immunodeficiency diseases.
- Give three examples of nutritional imbalance.
- Define *idiopathic* and *iatrogenic* causes of disease.

Even though a rapid growth in medical research and a phenomenal development in technology have been accompanied by society's increased awareness of wellness and health, we have not been able to eradicate disease from our lives. Disease is a pathologic condition of the body in response to an alteration in the normal body harmony. Disease is usually tangible or measurable. It may be the direct result of trauma, physical agents, and poisons or the indirect result of genetic anomalies and metabolic and nutritional disturbances.

Keep in mind that there is a difference between illness and disease. *Illness* describes the condition of a person who is experiencing a disease. It encompasses the way in which individuals perceive themselves as suffering from a disease. Illness is highly individual and personal. A *disease*, on the other hand, is known by its medical classification and distinguishing features. For most health-care providers, a disease is easier to treat than an illness. Proper and effective medical management should deal with both the disease and the illness.

Fear, anxiety, embarrassment, and concern about the cost of treatment or about possible disfigurement may be some of the troubling emotions persons feel when faced with an illness. Some desire to know everything about their particular disease; others choose complete ignorance. Most expect the medical community to have a "cure," few fully understand the importance of their participation in the "getting well" process.

This chapter provides a brief synopsis of the causes of disease and disorders. When considering the disharmony that occurs in the body in the form of disease, remember the harmony that exists most of the time.

PREDISPOSING FACTORS

A *predisposing factor* is a condition or situation that may make a person more susceptible to disease. Some predisposing factors include age, sex, heredity, environment, and lifestyle. For example, an infant's immune system is not fully developed and functioning at birth. Consequently, any undue exposure to disease-producing agents could cause serious illness. For a short time, a newborn does have residual immunity provided by its mother, but the infant needs to be protected by immunization shortly after birth.

Elderly persons have unique problems that arise from the aging process itself. Physiologic changes occur in the body systems, and some of these changes can cause functional impairment. Elderly persons experience problems with temperature extremes, have lowered resistance to disease as the result of decreased immunity, and have less physical activity

tolerance. Certain conditions and diseases are more common in the elderly population, including degenerative arthritis, presbyopia, atrophy of the ovaries and testes, hyperplasia of the prostate, osteoporosis, senile dementia, and Alzheimer's disease.

Men have gout more frequently than do women, whereas osteoporosis is more common in women. However, sex is a predisposing factor only when the disease is physiologically based—for example, prostate cancer occurs only in men; ovarian cancer occurs only in women, and lung cancer is as prevalent in women as in men. Also, women experience heart disease as often as do men.

Hereditary influences are discussed later in this chapter. If hereditary risks are known, individuals can be better prepared to prevent, treat, or cope with possible problems.

Environmental hazards may have an effect on health. Exposure to air, noise, and other environmental pollutants may predispose individuals to disease. For example, living close to a heavily traveled thoroughfare in a city may be a predisposition to respiratory disease. Some geographical locations have a higher incidence of insect bites and exposure to venom. Living in rural areas where fertilizers and pesticides are commonly used can predispose one to disease. Conditions and diseases once endemic to only one area of the world are crossing borders to invade an unsuspecting and unprepared society. This invasion is due largely to the increased mobility of the world's inhabitants and population density. Even the office employee may be affected by environmental or occupational health problems; for instance, carpal tunnel syndrome and eye problems can be the result of heavy use of computer technology.

Lifestyle choice may predispose some diseases. Smoking is known to be a major cause of lung cancer. Poor nutritional choices and lack of exercise are often cited as predispositions to diseases and disorders.

HEREDITARY DISEASES

The problem with the gene pool is there is no lifeguard.

—STEVEN WRIGHT

Hereditary diseases are the result of a person's genetic makeup. It is uncertain to what extent environmental factors influence the course of a hereditary disease, but the two do interact. Hereditary diseases do not always appear at birth. Mild hemophilia and muscular dystrophy may go undetected until adolescence or adulthood.

Genetic diseases are the result of monogenic (Mendelian) alterations, chromosome aberrations, and multifactorial errors. There are thousands of genetic diseases identified in humans—some are fatal. All genetic information is contained in deoxyribonucleic acid (DNA), a complex molecular structure found in the nucleus of cells. The DNA itself is incorporated into structures called **chromosomes**. The normal number of chromosomes in humans is 46 (23 pairs). In the formation of the ovum and sperm cells (sex cells, or gametes), this number is reduced by half, with each gamete having 23 chromosomes. When the two sex cells unite at the time of fertilization, the 23 chromosomes from the ovum combine at random with the 23 chromosomes from the sperm, producing a cell with a full complement of 46 chromosomes. Two of these chromosomes are responsible for our sex (Y = male, X = female).

A gene is the basic unit of heredity. Each gene consists of a fixed segment of the DNA on a specific chromosome. Our physical traits result from the expression of pairs of genes. Gene pairs are **homozygous** when they possess identical genes from each parent for a particular trait and when they are both dominant or both recessive in their expression of a trait. Gene pairs are **heterozygous** when they possess different genes from each parent for a particular trait and if one gene is dominant and one is recessive. Recessive genes are expressed only when the gene pair is homozygous, whereas dominant genes are expressed whether the gene pair is homozygous or heterozygous. When trying to determine genetic makeup, a family history is taken to determine a person's **genotype,** which is a description of the combination of a person's genes, either with respect to a single trait or with respect to a larger set of traits. Genotype includes all of the genes you have inherited from your parents. Your **phenotype** consists of the observable physical characteristics, determined by the combined influences of your genetic makeup and the effects of environmental factors. Phenotype is revealed in your appearance—the color and texture of your hair, the shape of your nose, your height, and so on.

A sex-linked hereditary disease can occur when one of the parents contributes a defective gene from the sex chromosome. In color blindness, the inability to distinguish reds from greens is the result of a recessive gene located on the X chromosome. The trait shows up when there is no dominant gene for normal color vision to override the recessive gene.

Changes in the structure of genes, called *mutations,* may cause disturbances in body functions. Mutations occur when the normal sequence of DNA units is disrupted. How such a disruption is manifested depends on whether the affected gene is dominant or recessive and on whether it is homozygous or heterozygous. The causes of mutations are largely unknown, but they could be the result of environmental factors, such as exposure to certain chemicals or radiation.

Classification of Hereditary Diseases

The conventional method of classifying hereditary diseases is to group them into monogenic or Mendelian alterations, chromosomal alterations, and multifactorial errors.

Monogenic (Mendelian) Disorders

Monogenic disorders are those caused by mutation in a single gene. The way in which the disorder is passed on to succeeding generations (the pattern of inheritance) is determined by whether the gene is dominant, recessive, or sex-linked. (A sex-linked gene is carried on the X chromosome. Because males have only one X chromosome, a sex-linked gene will be expressed in males whether it is dominant or recessive.) Figure 1.1 illustrates the three most common patterns of inheritance of monogenic disorders.

Autosomal Recessive

- Cystic fibrosis: A chronic, generalized disease of the glands that release their secretions into the digestive tract or to the outer surface of the body, or **exocrine** glands, primarily affecting the pancreas, respiratory system, and sweat glands (see Chapter 6, Congenital Diseases and Disorders).
- Tay-Sachs disease: A rare lipid abnormality distinguished by progressive neurologic deterioration and a cherry-red spot with a gray border on both retinas. It chiefly affects infants of eastern European Jewish (Ashkenazi) ancestry, resulting in deafness, blindness, and paralysis. Recurrent bronchopneumonia is a

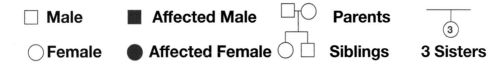

Index of Symbols

☐ **Male**   ■ **Affected Male**   **Parents**

○ **Female**   ● **Affected Female**   **Siblings**   **3 Sisters**

Figure 1.1 Patterns of inheritance. *(A)* Pedigree illustrating inheritance of autosomal dominant character. Individual is a male heterozygous for the mutant trait; if he were homozygous, all of the progeny in generation II would show the trait. None of the individuals in generation II or III can be homozygotes, because each has received a normal recessive allele from one parent. Note the large number of affected individuals (50% in generation II). *(B)* Pedigree illustrating inheritance of an autosomal recessive character. If the trait were dominant rather than recessive, then either III-3 or III-4 would have to show the trait for IV-2 and IV-6 to have inherited it. There is no indication of sex linkage. *(C)* Pedigree illustrating inheritance of sex-linked recessive character. The affected individuals (II-1, III-4, and IV-4) are all males. Individuals II-2 (and her mother), III-2, and the wife of II-1 must all be carriers. (Adapted from Purves, WK: Life: The Science of Biology, ed 2. Sinauer Associates, Sutherland, MA, 1987, p 284, with permission.)

problem after age 2. Death usually occurs by the age of 5.

- Cretinism (or hypothyroidism): An undersecretion of hormones from the thyroid gland causing retarded growth and delay in the development of secondary sexual characteristics (see Chapter 14).
- Phenylketonuria (PKU): An inability to metabolize phenylalanine, an essential **amino acid**. Amino acids are organic compounds that constitute the primary building blocks of proteins. Mental retardation results unless a special diet is followed (see Chapter 6).
- Sickle cell anemia: A disease affecting mostly black populations around the world. It occurs because the body produces a defective form of hemoglobin that causes red blood cells to roughen and become sickle shaped (see Chapter 12).

Autosomal Dominant

- Diabetes insipidus: A condition that results from insufficient secretion of vasopressin by the posterior portion of the pituitary gland, characterized by excessive and dilute urination (see Chapter 14).
- Retinoblastoma: A rare eye tumor usually present at birth (see Chapter 5).

X- or Sex-Linked

- Hemophilia: A rare group of bleeding disorders caused by a deficiency of specific types of serum proteins called clotting factors.
- Duchenne-type muscular dystrophy: A progressive bilateral wasting of skeletal muscles (see Chapter 15).

Chromosomal Disorders

Chromosomal disorders are caused by abnormalities in the number of chromosomes or by changes in chromosomal structure, such as *additions (more than necessary), deletions* (missing genes) or *translocations* (genes shifted from one chromosome to another or to a different location on the same chromosome).

Diseases caused by chromosomal alterations include:

- Klinefelter's syndrome: A condition that occurs when there is an additional X chromo-

some in males. The body shape is elongated, the testes are small, the mammary glands are abnormally large, and mental retardation is common.
- Turner's syndrome: A condition caused by the loss of the X chromosome in either the ovum or the sperm. This syndrome is often characterized by shortened stature, swollen hands and feet, and coarse, enlarged, prominent ears.
- Trisomy 21 or Down syndrome: A condition in which an individual has three No. 21 chromosomes instead of the normal two. The condition is more likely to occur in babies born to parents of advanced age (35 to 50 years old). Infants with this condition typically have a sloping forehead, folds of skin over the inner corners of their eyes, and other physical abnormalities. They generally become moderately to severely retarded.

Multifactorial Disorders

Multifactorial disorders result from the interaction of many factors, both hereditary and environmental. Among the multifactorial diseases are:

- Diabetes mellitus: A disorder of carbohydrate, fat, and protein metabolism. The disease is due primarily to insufficient insulin production by the pancreas (see Chapter 14).
- Congenital heart anomalies: This category includes six major anatomic defects that cause circulatory problems (see Chapter 6).

INFLAMMATION AND INFECTIONS

Inflammation is the body's response to trauma, physical agents (temperature extremes, radiation) or chemical agents (poisons, venoms), allergens, and disease-producing, or **pathogenic,** organisms (bacteria, viruses, fungi). It is a process that begins with the physical irritant and ends with healing. How well the body responds to inflammation depends on (1) an individual's general health, nutritional state, and age, (2) tissue factors, and (3) type of physical irritant.

Inflammation may be acute or chronic. In its acute phase, there is redness, swelling, pain, heat, and loss of function. At the site of injury, there are a large number of **polymorphonuclear leukocytes,** which are white blood cells that possess a nucleus composed of 200 or more lobes or parts. Examples of acute inflammation include insect bites, mild burns, and minor abrasions and cuts. The inflammation may persist, spread to adjacent or distant tissue, and become chronic. In chronic inflammation, there is an increase in the number of lymphocytes, monocytes, and plasma cells.

Inflammation occurs when microorganisms gain entry through a break in the skin. The microorganisms release a toxin that causes the capillaries of the host to become permeable and allow access to white blood cells—hence, the redness, swelling, heat, and pain. Factors that help in abating the inflammatory response include adequate nutrition, rest, and good blood supply.

Inflammation is a beneficial biological response in most instances; however, if it becomes chronic, inflammation can be debilitating, as is the case, for example, in rheumatoid arthritis. Whatever the cause of inflammation, it is the body's protective response.

Infection is the invasion and multiplication of **pathogenic** microorganisms in the body. Most microorganisms in our bodies are nonpathogenic and, in fact, are often necessary to maintain **homeostasis,** a state of stability that the body tries to maintain even though it is exposed to continually changing outside forces. When one or more of the requisite factors in the infectious process are present, a microorganism can become a potential pathogen.

People serve as hosts for organisms, as do animals. A host does not necessarily have to be "diseased" or "sick" but simply serves as a reservoir for the microorganisms. Transmission can be through coughing, sneezing, or touching something contaminated from the infected host, as well as through direct contact with the microorganism. If the receiving host is not susceptible, then the microorganism has little chance of becoming a pathogen. The susceptible host, however, may have low resistance or provide the microorganism with an unusual means of entry, such as an open wound.

Whenever a pathogenic microorganism finds a suitable environment for growth in an appropriate host, disease may result. Growth factors for microorganisms vary and include the presence or absence of oxygen, a ready source of food, an optimal temperature, moisture, darkness, and a specific pH.

Microorganisms, including those that cause disease, can be classified into six general groups.

■ **FUNGI** This group includes yeasts and molds that may be present in the soil, air, and water. Only a few species cause disease (Fig. 1.2). Fungal diseases, called mycoses, usually develop slowly, are resistant

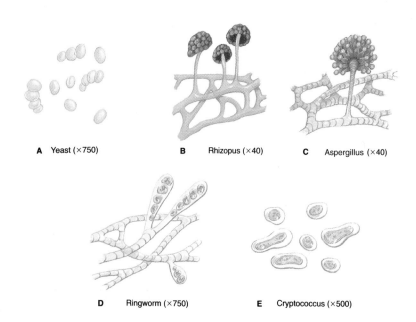

A Yeast (×750) **B** Rhizopus (×40) **C** Aspergillus (×40)

D Ringworm (×750) **E** Cryptococcus (×500)

Figure 1.2 Fungi. (From Scanlon, VC, and Sanders, T: Essentials of Anatomy and Physiology, ed. 4. FA Davis, Philadelphia, 2003, with permission.)

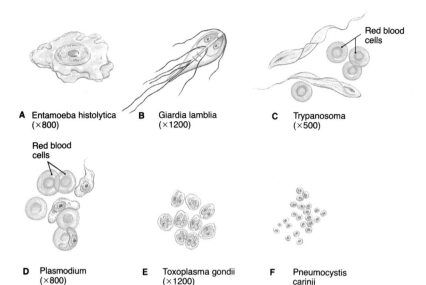

A   Entamoeba histolytica
    (×800)

B   Giardia lamblia
    (×1200)

C   Trypanosoma
    (×500)

Red blood cells

D   Plasmodium
    (×800)

E   Toxoplasma gondii
    (×1200)

F   Pneumocystis carinii
    (×1200)

Figure 1.3 Protozoa. (From Scanlon, VC, and Sanders, T: Essentials of Anatomy and Physiology, ed. 4. FA Davis, Philadelphia, 2003, with permission.)

to treatment, and are rarely fatal. The more common mycoses include histoplasmosis, coccidioidomycosis (see Chapter 11), ringworm, athlete's foot, and thrush.

■ **RICKETTSIAE** This group of bacteria-like organisms live parasitically inside living cells. They are transmitted through bites from infected lice, fleas, ticks, mosquitoes, and mites. Rickettsial diseases include Rocky Mountain spotted fever, typhus, and trench fever. These diseases are more likely to occur where unsanitary conditions prevail.

■ **PROTOZOA** These single-celled organisms have animal-like characteristics (Fig. 1.3). Malaria, amebic dysentery, and African sleeping sickness are examples of protozoan diseases. *Trichomonas vaginalis* is a protozoon that causes trichomoniasis or vaginitis, a disease fairly common among women.

■ **VIRUSES** These are the smallest microorganisms, visible only through the use of electron microscopy. Figure 1.4 illustrates three common viruses and compares their size with that of the

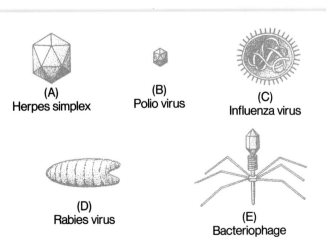

(A) Herpes simplex

(B) Polio virus

(C) Influenza virus

(D) Rabies virus

(E) Bacteriophage

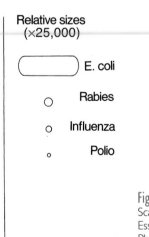

Relative sizes
(×25,000)

E. coli

Rabies

Influenza

Polio

Figure 1.4 Viruses. (From Scanlon, VC, and Sanders, T: Essentials of Anatomy and Physiology, ed 3. FA Davis, Philadelphia, 1999, p 496, with permission.)

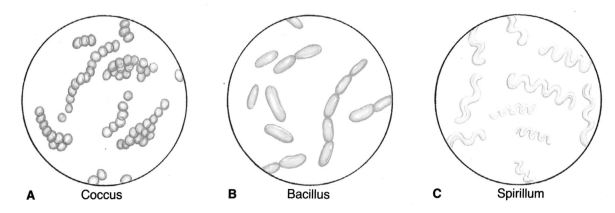

A Coccus **B** Bacillus **C** Spirillum

Figure 1.5 Bacteria. (From Scanlon, VC, and Sanders, T: Essentials of Anatomy and Physiology, ed. 3. FA Davis, Philadelphia, 1999, p 494, with permission.)

Escherichia coli bacillus. They are independent of host cells, they are difficult to isolate, and few are susceptible to drug therapy. Viruses may remain dormant in a host for long periods before becoming active. Viral infections include the common cold, yellow fever, measles, mumps, rabies, chickenpox, herpes, poliomyelitis, hepatitis, influenza, and certain types of pneumonia and encephalitis.

■ **BACTERIA** There are many varieties of these single-celled organisms. Most are nonpathogenic and useful. Bacteria, including those that cause disease, are classified according to their shape (Fig. 1.5)

- Bacilli are rod-shaped bacteria. Diseases caused by bacilli include tuberculosis, whooping cough, tetanus, typhoid fever, and diphtheria.
- Spirilla are spiral-shaped bacteria. Diseases caused by spirilla include syphilis and cholera.
- Cocci are dot-shaped bacteria. Diseases caused by cocci include gonorrhea, meningitis, tonsillitis, bacterial pneumonia, boils, scarlet fever, sore throats, and certain skin and urinary infections.

■ **PARASITES** A group of host-requiring organisms that include external and internal parasites. External parasites include lice and mites (insects) and are discussed in Chapter 16. Helminthes are wormlike internal parasites that are typically transmitted from person to person via fecal contamination of food, water, or soil. Three classes of helminthes may infect humans (Fig. 1.6):

- Roundworms resemble earthworms in appear-

ance. Those most frequently affecting humans are pinworms.
- Tapeworms are long and narrow, as their name indicates, and they depend on two hosts, one human and one animal, from the development of the egg to the larva to the adult. The easiest way to remember their names is by the name of the animal that acts as the second host: that is, beef tapeworm, pork tapeworm, fish tapeworm, and dog tapeworm.
- Flukes are small, leaf-shaped, flat, nonsegmented worms.

TRAUMA

The leading cause of death in the United States for persons younger than 35 is physical trauma, an injury or a wound caused by external force or violence. Overall, it is the third leading cause of death in the United States, following cardiovascular disease and cancer.

Head Trauma

Injuries to the head include concussion; cerebral contusion; skull, nose, and jaw fractures; and perforated eardrum.

Cerebral contusions and concussions cause the brain to be jostled inside the skull. Cerebral contusions are more serious than concussions because contusions bruise the brain tissue and disrupt normal nerve function. Contusions may cause loss of consciousness, hemorrhage, and even death. Concussions

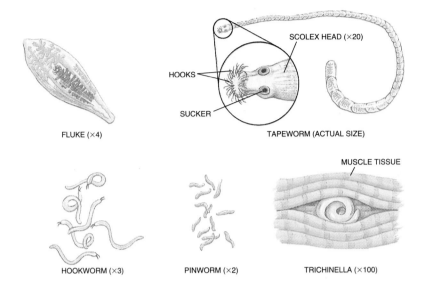

Figure 1.6 Worms. (From Scanlon, VC, and Sanders, T: Essentials of Anatomy and Physiology, ed. 4. FA Davis, Philadelphia, 2003, with permission.)

cause temporary neural dysfunction but are not severe enough to cause a contusion. This kind of trauma is normally the result of a fall, a severe blow to the head area, or an automobile accident. If unconsciousness, convulsions, forceful and persistent vomiting, blurred vision, staggering walk, or hemorrhage occurs, the person should be taken to a hospital immediately. A physician should determine the seriousness of the event and the proper treatment needed.

Skull fractures often are accompanied by scalp wounds and profuse bleeding. The concern in the individual with a skull fracture is possible damage to the brain. Fractures generally are accompanied by pain, tenderness, and swelling of the affected areas. Surgery may be required to remove foreign bodies or bone fragments. The person is closely monitored in a hospital.

Perforated eardrums normally result from the insertion of sharp objects into the ear canal or from a severe blow to the side of the head. Sudden and excessive changes in air pressure can cause perforation. Children who have acute otitis media (earache) may experience a perforated eardrum as a complication of this disease.

Chest Trauma

Penetrating chest injuries are often caused by knife and gunshot wounds. Penetrating chest wounds typically cause a sucking sound as air enters the chest cavity through the chest wall opening. The person may be in severe pain. An abnormally rapid heartbeat, or **tachycardia,** is apt to occur. There may be a weak pulse, blood loss, and possible **hypovolemic shock**, a condition of severe physiologic distress. Hypovolemic shock is caused by a decrease in the circulating blood volume so great that the body's metabolic needs cannot be met. It is important to control blood loss in penetration wounds.

Nonpenetrating chest injuries such as rib fractures usually result from an automobile accident in which the driver is thrown against the steering wheel. There is a sensation of tenderness and pain that worsens with deep breathing or exertion. A potential complication of rib fractures is the penetration of a rib into the pleura, lung tissue, or myocardium.

X-ray examination is necessary to determine the extent and location of the damage. An electrocardiogram (ECG) and blood studies help assess cardiac damage. Immediate assessment and attendance by a physician are paramount. Surgical repair is often necessary.

Abdominopelvic Trauma

Injuries to the abdominopelvic region may cause hemorrhages within the liver, spleen, pancreas, and kidneys and/or rupture of the stomach, intestine, gallbladder, and urinary bladder. Rupture of the organs results in the spilling of the contents of the organs (including bacteria) into the abdominopelvic cavity.

This is a major cause of infection. Blood loss and hypovolemic shock are also a concern. Emergency attention is necessary to determine the extent of the damage and the necessary treatment. Most abdominal injuries require surgical repair. The prognosis depends on the extent of the injury, but prompt attention generally improves the outcome.

Neck and Spine Trauma

Neck and spine injuries include fractures, contusions, and compressions of the vertebral column. The greatest concern with this type of trauma is damage to the spinal cord and paralysis. Spinal cord injuries are discussed in connection with the nervous system (see Chapter 13).

Extremities Trauma

Sprains, strains, and fractures to the arms and legs are common. They are discussed with musculoskeletal diseases in Chapter 15.

EFFECTS OF PHYSICAL AND CHEMICAL AGENTS

Physical and chemical agents can adversely affect the body; the degree to which this occurs depends on many factors. If the exposure to the irritant is short in duration and frequency and is fairly localized and the person is healthy, the damage may be unnoticed or reversible; however, the irritant may cause irreversible systemic damage if the person is debilitated, diseased, very young, or elderly; has lowered resistance; or is on some medication.

Some of the more common physical and chemical agents include extreme heat and cold, ionizing radiation, extremes of atmospheric pressure, electric shock, poisoning, near-drowning, bites of insects, spiders, and snakes, asphyxiation, and burns.

Extreme Heat and Cold

Extreme heat may result in **syncope** (a transient loss of consciousness), heat exhaustion, heat cramps, and heatstroke. Causes of these heat disorders include overexertion in heat, prolonged heat exposure, salt depletion, dehydration, failure of the body's heat-regulating mechanisms, or a combination of these causes. Heat exhaustion, sometimes resulting in syn-

cope, is caused by overexposure to heat, insufficient water intake, insufficient salt intake, and deficiency of sweat production. Heat cramps in the legs and abdomen result from heavy salt loss. The person is usually pale and clammy, with a rapid, weak pulse and shallow breathing. Individuals treated at this stage generally respond promptly to rest, cooling, and weak salty liquids administered orally. If the person does not respond or is not treated, heat exhaustion may lead to heatstroke when the body's temperature-control mechanism malfunctions. Sweating ceases and the body temperature rises. The skin becomes hot, dry, and flushed. This is a life-threatening condition that may require hospitalization with intravenous therapy, cooling therapy, increased fluid intake, temperature monitoring, and muscle massaging. Hypersensitivity to heat may remain for some time. Any of these heat disorders can be fatal.

Extreme cold may occasion disorders such as chilblain, frostbite, and hypothermia. Causes include overexposure to cold air, wind, or water. Chilblain, a mild frostbite, produces red, itching skin lesions, usually on the extremities, whereas frostbite, the freezing of exposed areas, causes tingling and redness followed by paleness and numbness of the affected areas. Untreated, either condition can lead to gangrene and may necessitate amputation. Hypothermia is a systemic reaction; it can be fatal. Treatment of any of the cold disorders includes gradually warming the person, monitoring body temperature, protecting the affected part, preventing infection, and administering pain relievers, or **analgesics,** as necessary.

Ionizing Radiation

Depending on the duration and intensity of exposure and the form of the irradiating agent, the effects of ionizing radiation range from mild skin burns to fatal tissue destruction. The exposure to radiation may be via ingestion, inhalation, or direct contact. Causes include (1) occupational or accidental exposure and (2) the misuse of radiation for diagnostic or treatment purposes. Persons at risk include those with cancer who are receiving radiation therapy and employees in nuclear power plants. The harmful effects of radiation may be immediate or delayed, acute or chronic. Treatment is symptomatic and supportive and may include drugs used to prevent or stop vomiting, or **antiemetics**; simple and palatable foods; blood transfusions; and emotional support.

Extremes of Atmospheric Pressure

Extremes of atmospheric pressure result from changing too rapidly from a high-pressure to a low-pressure environment or from a low-pressure to a high-pressure environment. Decompression sickness is an occupational hazard for deep-sea divers and airplane pilots who descend or ascend too quickly and for hospital personnel who work in hyperbaric chambers. Systemic damage occurs following rapid decompression when gases dissolved in the blood and other tissues escape faster than they can be diffused through respiration. Nitrogen gas bubbles form in the blood and tissue, causing respiratory problems and pain. Treatment consists of emergency oxygen until the person can be transported to a hyperbaric chamber, where recompression is followed by slow decompression. Supportive measures are also used.

Electric Shock

Electric shock can occur anywhere there is electricity—home, work, or school. The causes of electric shock can be natural (as from lightning) or contrived (due to carelessness or ignorance, or from faulty equipment). The victim must be freed from the source of electric current without the rescuer contacting the current, and treatment must begin immediately. Cardiopulmonary resuscitation (CPR) may be necessary. If the damage is severe, hospitalization may be required to observe the individual, treat any burns, and prevent infection.

Poisoning

Poisoning is a common occurrence, especially among curious children. In addition, society has become increasingly aware of poisonous chemicals that have been dumped or buried. Such chemicals cause soil and water contamination that result in ecologic and personal damage.

Poisons may be accidentally ingested, inhaled, injected, or absorbed through the skin, but poisoning can also be the result of occupational exposure when working with toxic chemicals; of improper cooking, storage, and canning of food; and of drug overdoses or abuse. Treatment consists of first aid measures, identifying and providing the correct antidote if one exists, and instituting supportive measures. The local poison control center offers valuable help. Prompt, correct treatment can save a life.

Near-drowning

Near-drowning is a common occurrence during the warm summer months and could be prevented in many cases by following water safety precautions. In near-drowning, the person generally aspirates fluid, or the person may have an obstructed airway caused by a spasm of the larynx when gasping under water, resulting in insufficient oxygenation of the arterial blood, or **hypoxemia**. Later, within minutes or possibly days of near-drowning, the person may experience respiratory distress. Emergency treatment is critical. Hospitalization may be required for oxygenation, airway maintenance, observation of the cardiovascular status of the patient, and prevention of further complications.

Bites of Insects, Spiders, and Snakes

Insect, spider, and snake bites occur most often during the warm summer months. Bee, yellow jacket, wasp, and hornet stings may cause localized pain, but they usually require little more than symptomatic treatment. Allergic reactions and multiple stings or bites, however, are a more serious matter and should be treated as a medical emergency. Poisonous bites require quick emergency measures to prevent venom absorption and life-threatening symptoms from occurring. The victim should be immobilized and transported immediately to a hospital, where the specific antidote can be administered. Whether the bite is considered serious or mild, close observation of the victim is essential.

Asphyxiation

Asphyxiation, which is the lack of oxygen coupled with accumulating carbon dioxide in the blood, may result from near-drowning, hypoventilation, airway obstruction, or inhalation of toxic substances. Emergency treatment is generally required, and it may involve removal of any obstruction, CPR, oxygenation, and intubation. Hospitalization may be necessary to stabilize the victim's vital signs. Obviously, any breathing difficulty is frightening to the victim, so reassurance and encouragement are needed.

Burns

Tragically, burns are a leading cause of death among children. They usually are preventable by following fire safety guidelines. Burns are classified by extent, depth, person's age, and associated illness and injury. The *rule of nines* is useful for assessing the extent of burns. Figure 1.7 illustrates the rule of nines and burn classification criteria. Emergency measures may be necessary to maintain the burn victim's airway, cool the wound, and prevent serious loss of body fluids. Once the victim has been transported to a hospital, frequently a special burn center, the focus is on maintaining fluid balance, preventing infection, and providing patient support. Severe burns can be extremely painful and require a lengthy rehabilitation period, including possible skin grafting and plastic surgery. Emotional support is essential.

NEOPLASIA AND CANCER

Neoplasia means "new formation" or "new growth." The terms *tumor* and *neoplasm* are commonly used synonymously and are thus used herein. Specific neoplastic diseases are discussed in Chapter 5; here we discuss etiologic factors and their results.

The actual cause of neoplasms is not known, but an alteration in genes does occur, allowing independent and uncontrollable growth. As was discussed earlier under "Hereditary Diseases," an alteration in a gene on a chromosome is a mutation. The mutant cell differs from the normal cell in that the abnormal cell is no longer subject to normal control mechanisms. Apparently, mutations such as this occur relatively frequently, but the body usually is able to destroy the resulting mutant cells as soon as they appear. Therefore, a tumor may represent a failure on the part of the body's immune system. The harmful effects of the neoplastic growth may be from the growth itself or from the destruction of surrounding tissue.

The neoplasm may be benign or malignant, depending on its growth pattern. A *benign* tumor is one that remains circumscribed, although it may vary in size from small to large. A *malignant* tumor, or cancer, is one that spreads to other cells, tissues, and parts of the body through the bloodstream or lymphatic system. The spreading process is called **metastasis**.

Cancer is a general term for numerous diseases, all of which are characterized by the uncontrollable growth of cells. The diagnosis, treatment, prognosis, and prevention of cancer are discussed in Chapter 5.

IMMUNE-RELATED FACTORS IN DISEASE

The Immune Response

An ideally designed body would be free of disease. A careful study of body chemistry and cellular function reveals a blueprint for maintaining a disease-free state. The body is protected in three ways:

1. Normal body structures function to block the entry of germs through the use of tears, mucous membranes, intact skin, cilia, and body pH.
2. Inflammatory response rushes leukocytes to a site of infection, where invading organisms are engulfed in a process called **phagocytosis**.
3. Specific immune response causes a protective reaction to a foreign antigen.

The body's immune system is both natural and acquired. Natural immunity is a genetic feature spe-

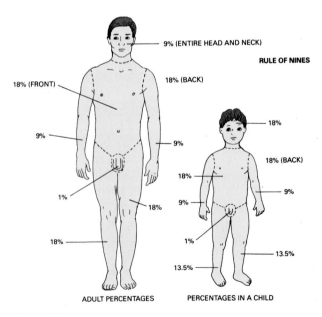

Figure 1.7 Rule of nines and burn classification. (From Thomas, CL [ed]: Taber's Cyclopedic Medical Dictionary, ed. 19. FA Davis, Philadelphia, 1985, p 1827, with permission.)

cific to race, sex, and the individual's ability to respond. The body's normal structure and function are natural defenses. For example, the skin is a barrier to invading organisms, the gastric juices destroy swallowed organisms, and the white blood cells, through phagocytosis, destroy bacteria. The term *acquired immunity* indicates that the body has developed the ability to defend itself against a specific agent. This can occur after actually having a disease or after receiving immunization against a disease. Although the human body does not begin developing protein substances produced by the body's immune system in response to and interacting with specific antigens, or **antibodies,** until 3 to 6 weeks of age, an infant has temporary immunity, because it receives antibodies produced by its mother's immune system in utero.

There are two types of acquired immunity:

1. *Humoral immunity* is the body's major defense against bacteria. Here the body produces antibodies or immunoglobulins that combine with and eliminate the foreign substance, or **antigen**. An antigen is any substance that, when produced into the body, causes the production of a specific antibody by the immune system. These antibodies are formed by white blood cells called B-cell lymphocytes. The humoral response is rapid, beginning immediately, or within 48 hours of antigen contact. Humoral immunity, in the presence of an antigen, causes an antibody to be released, which in turn reacts exclusively with that antigen. This binding of antibody to antigen encourages phagocytosis of the antigen and activates the complement system. The complement system is responsible for enzyme development, which helps remove the antigen from the body.

2. *Cell-mediated immunity* is action by another group of white blood cells, called T-cell lymphocytes. These provide the main protection against viruses, fungi, parasites, some bacteria, and tumors. The T cells mature in the thymus and are stored in the lymphatic system and spleen. Cell-mediated immunity is initiated when a T lymphocyte becomes sensitized by contact with a specific antigen. In response to additional contacts with the antigen, the T lymphocyte releases sensitized

lymphocytes, which migrate to the inflammation site. These lymphocytes help to transform local cells within the body tissues having the ability to engulf particular substances and microorganisms, or **macrophages,** into "killer" T lymphocytes that are highly phagocytic. The migration of antigens also is prohibited. Some normal tissue can be destroyed during this process, which is very intense.

The ability to generate an immune response is controlled by genetics. Immune response genes regulate B-cell and T-cell proliferation; therefore, they influence resistance to infection and tumors. The immune response normally recognizes its own body cells, thereby preventing damage to tissue.

Although this complex system to protect the body is an example of the disease-free design of the body, the immune response can malfunction. Immunologic malfunctions are classified as (1) *allergy*, when the immune response is inappropriate; (2) *autoimmunity,* when the immune response is misdirected; and (3) *immunodeficiency,* when the immune response is inadequate.

Allergy

Allergic reactions that reflect malfunctioning immunity commonly include **urticaria**, or hives (Fig. 1.8). The symptoms include generally round, transient elevations of the skin, or **wheals,** surrounded by a reddened area that may cover a small region or the entire body. Causative factors include foods (especially milk, fish, and strawberries), the presence of pets, insect bites, certain fabrics, inhalants, and cosmetics. Familial history, stress, and general physical condition may predispose to allergies.

Another allergic reaction results from transfusion of the wrong type of blood or blood components, which become toxic to the body's cells. Transfusion reactions may be mild or severe, depending on the amount of transfused fluid and the person's condition. Symptoms of transfusion reaction range from chills and fever, pain, nausea, and vomiting to a sudden, unusually severe, and possibly life-threatening allergic reaction, or **anaphylaxis,** and congestive heart failure. Blood and laboratory tests have to be performed to confirm the type and severity of reaction. The attention of a physician is necessary to prevent complications.

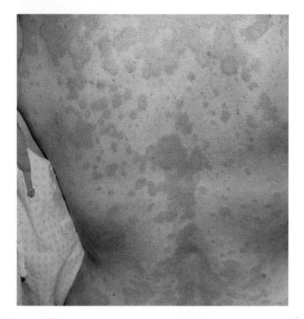

Figure 1.8 Urticaria (hives). (From Goldsmith, L, Lazarus, G. and Tharp, M: Adult and Pediatric Dermatology. FA Davis, Philadelphia, 1997, p 209, with permission.)

Allergy is also seen in hypersensitivity reactions to drugs. In some people, certain drugs can act as antigens, stimulating the formation of sensitizing antibodies. Although any drug can be the offender, common ones include penicillin, sulfa drugs, and aspirin. The degree of hypersensitivity depends on the extent and duration of exposure to the drug; the person's genetic background, age, and sex; and the presence of underlying disease. Symptoms range from a local rash, severe itching, or **pruritus**, flulike symptoms, and diffuse redness of the skin, or **erythema,** to more severe conditions such as asthma, anemia, or anaphylaxis.

Anaphylactic shock is considered by some authorities to be an allergic reaction. This reaction is acute and potentially life-threatening. It may be caused by drug hypersensitivity, foods (the most likely offenders are nuts, legumes, berries, and seafood), and insect stings (honeybees, wasps, yellow jackets, mosquitoes, ants, and certain spiders). Anaphylaxis may occur after a single exposure to an antigen or after repeated exposures. For this reason, it is important to be alert for an allergic reaction in any person at any time. In some cases, the reaction may occur within seconds, but it is usually no later than 40 to 50 minutes after contact with the allergen.

Cardiovascular symptoms can include hypotension, shock, and cardiac irregularities. Respiratory symptoms can include nasal congestion, profuse watery rhinorrhea, itching, and sudden sneezing. **Edema,** or excessive accumulation of fluid in bodily tissues, of the nose or throat can cause a high-pitched sound during respiration, or **stridor**, labored and difficult breathing, or **dyspnea**, or acute respiratory failure. Gastrointestinal and genitourinary symptoms include stomach cramping, nausea, diarrhea, and urinary urgency and the inability to control the passage of urine, or **incontinence**.

Anaphylactic shock is an emergency. It requires immediate countermeasures, which may include injection of epinephrine. It is important to maintain the individual's airway and to administer CPR in the event of cardiac arrest.

Autoimmunity

In autoimmune disease, self-antigens, or abnormal immune cells develop that incite the immune response into abnormal or excessive activity of T cells or B cells.

In this text, most of the autoimmune diseases are discussed in conjunction with the specific organ systems affected; however, a brief summary of five types follows:

- Gastrointestinal: Primary biliary cirrhosis, ulcerative colitis, and atrophic gastritis (see Chapter 10)
- Cardiovascular: Pernicious anemia, hemolytic anemia, idiopathic thrombocytopenia, and leukopenia (see Chapter 12)
- Endocrine: Insulin-dependent diabetes, thyrotoxicosis, and Hashimoto's thyroiditis (see Chapter 14)
- Musculoskeletal: Mixed connective-tissue diseases, rheumatoid arthritis, systemic lupus erythematosus (SLE), and myasthenia gravis (see Chapter 12)
- Dermatologic: Dermatomyositis and scleroderma (see Chapter 16)

Immunodeficiency

The immunodeficiency diseases are a result of B-cell or T-cell deficiency, or both, or some unknown immunodeficient factor. The majority of immunodeficient diseases are diagnosed by immunologic analyses, as many persons are asymptomatic except for recurrent infections. Most immunodeficient persons have impaired resistance to infections, and it is these infectious conditions that may cause death.

Acquired immunodeficiency syndrome (AIDS) (see Chapter 4) is a severe form of acquired immunodeficiency. Another immunodeficiency disease is Hodgkin's disease, a neoplastic malignancy of the lymph system. The immunodeficiency is thought to be due to impaired T-cell function, which leaves the person more susceptible to infections. Once a fatal disease, it is now potentially curable, even in advanced stages. Hodgkin's disease is discussed in detail in Chapter 12.

Malignant lymphomas, also known as non-Hodgkin's lymphomas, and sometimes lymphosarcomas, are malignant neoplasms of the lymphoreticular system. Persons with genetic, or acquired, immunodeficiency disorders clearly are predisposed to these malignant neoplasms. A symptom is swelling of lymph glands. Diagnosis is chiefly by lymph node biopsy to differentiate lymphoma from Hodgkin's disease and other causes of **lymphadenopathy** or diseases of the lymph nodes. Identification of the disease is necessary for proper treatment, and chemotherapy and radiation are used with some success. Non-Hodgkin's lymphomas cause more deaths than does Hodgkin's disease.

NUTRITIONAL IMBALANCE

Nutritional imbalance can cause growth problems, specific diseases, and even death. Nutritional imbalances, deficiencies, and excesses are becoming more apparent as causes of health problems. Nutritional deficiencies can cause grave intellectual and physical impairments, as well as affecting an individual's overall well-being. Causes of nutritional imbalances include malnourishment, vitamin and mineral deficiencies and excesses, obesity, and starvation.

Malnourishment

Malnourishment may be due to:

- Improper intake of foodstuffs in both quality and quantity, as seen in people with alcoholism, anorexia nervosa, and bulimia or in those who engage in diet faddism.

- Improper intake of foodstuffs because of gastrointestinal problems, as exhibited in the person who has no taste or smell, the postoperative anorexic, or the person who has a lesion in the throat.
- Malabsorption or poor utilization of foodstuffs, as seen when an individual is unable to absorb nutrients properly.
- Increased need for food or certain nutrients, as seen in a marathon runner, a person in a febrile state, and a person with cancer.
- Impaired metabolism of foodstuffs, as in both hereditary and acquired biochemical disorders.
- Food and drug interactions, as seen in those taking corticosteroid medications, which are known to deplete muscle protein, lower glucose tolerance, and induce osteoporosis.

Vitamin Deficiencies and Excesses

Early signs of vitamin deficiency are generally vague and nonspecific. Vitamin deficiency diseases include scurvy, which is caused by a lack of vitamin C and is characterized by abnormal bone formation and hemorrhages of mucous membranes; rickets, which is due to a lack of vitamin D, and beriberi, in which a lack of vitamin B_1 causes neurologic damage. Treatment typically consists of a diet high in protein and the required vitamin. Vitamin excess may occur when people take vitamins in an attempt to cover missed or inadequate meals, when they hope to prevent some disease (e.g., the common cold), or when they self-treat a condition. Large doses of some vitamins are toxic and may cause illness, especially when taken over a long period of time.

Mineral Deficiencies and Excesses

Minerals are a vital component of a balanced diet. Mineral deficiencies of chloride, potassium, sodium, calcium, and magnesium are the more common deficiencies. Causes include dietary deficiencies and metabolic disorders. Treatment may involve increasing the intake of a deficient mineral through foodstuffs or medication, or addressing any underlying metabolic disorder. Mineral excess also may be caused by diet, medication, or a metabolic error. Treatment consists of locating the cause and correcting the problem.

Obesity

Obesity has been defined as a condition where body weight is 10% to 20% above the ideal. Of course, "ideal" is difficult to determine, and factors such as family history and body build need to be considered. The cause of obesity may be too many calories, too little activity, or, less frequently, an endocrine and metabolic problem. In addition, fluid retention may cause an increase in weight. Treatment may include lowering caloric intake, increasing physical activity, or, in the case of metabolic disorders, correcting the error. If fluid retention is a problem, drugs that promote the secretion of urine, or **diuretics,** may be prescribed, and any underlying cause of the retention should be detected and treated. The prognosis for obesity is not good. Although a small percentage of obese individuals are able to lose weight, an even smaller percentage are able to maintain permanent weight reduction. Obesity poses a serious risk for the development of diabetes mellitus, hypertension, gallbladder disease, and heart disease.

Starvation

Causes of starvation include lack of food or an unbalanced diet over a long period of time, causing metabolic and physiologic body changes. A starved person generally is one who does not have adequate food, whereas someone who is malnourished generally has adequate food available but the food is of inadequate nutritive value. Starvation can be the result of illness, poverty, and poor dietary planning. Starvation is seen at any age; however, infants and children aged 1 to 3 years suffer more severely than do adults. Pregnant women and elderly people are also vulnerable.

IDIOPATHIC AND IATROGENIC DISEASES

Some diseases, having no known cause, are described as *idiopathic*. Of course, when the cause is unknown, the disease can be treated only symptomatically.

Some diseases are *iatrogenic*—that is, they are caused by medical treatment and its effects. This can be seen in the treatment of some cancers, where the chemotherapy drugs used can cause severe anemia, or when hepatitis develops as a result of a contaminated blood transfusion.

Summary

The disease process is varied, complex, and sometimes unknown. When the body is out of harmony, there is a need for care and treatment. Only when the disease process is understood are the best care and treatment possible. The body's disharmony affects each individual differently and for many different reasons. Health-care professionals will always want to remember the person with the illness who is affected by the disease or disorder.

CASE STUDIES

■ Case Study 1

Just off the Oregon coast, a fishing boat filled with eager tourists pulled out of the harbor on a beautiful, sunny, cool day. The tide was unusually low as the boat was crossing the bar. This was the third boat to go out that morning, and the first two encountered no problems. This boat, however, hit a wave broadside and capsized. About half of the passengers were wearing lifejackets. Some of the passengers were trapped below deck in the overturned boat and attempted to break through the glass barriers to swim to the surface of the water. Hypothermia set in within minutes, and 10 of the 17 passengers drowned. Two persons were not recovered.

Case Study Questions

1. Describe the physiologic effects of hypothermia.
2. What preventative measures could the tourists have taken?
3. What preventative measures could the captain of the boat have taken?

■ Case Study 2

Jayne and Brandon have three active children, who are 7, 9, and 11 years old. Tonight they have to take the two boys, Jason and Kyle, to a baseball game and their daughter, Miranda, to karate practice. Both Jayne and Brandon leave work a bit early to allow time to take the family to the local fast food drive-through. Everyone orders "super size." Jayne drops the boys and Brandon off at the baseball game and drives the van to karate practice with Miranda. Jayne and Miranda return to the baseball game as the coach is giving his winning players candy bars, soda, and chips. The family leaves for home, and Miranda is wanting candy and chips from the boys. Mom ponders the nutritional value of the evening's meal, activities, and snacks.

Case Study Questions

1. Identify the nutritional implications of the meal.
2. What are the negative and positive effects of tonight's activities and the family habits?

REVIEW QUESTIONS

True/False

Circle the correct answer:

T F 1. Some of the disorders caused by exposure to extreme cold are chilblain, frostbite, and hypothermia.

T F 2. Burns are a leading cause of death in children.

T F 3. *Neoplasia* is defined as "cancer."

T F 4. Humoral immunity is the body's major defense against bacteria.

T F 5. Allergy is an example of an inappropriate immune response.

Matching

Match each of the following definitions with its correct term:

_____ 1. Genes inherited from parents

_____ 2. Describes condition of a sick person

_____ 3. DNA sequence is disrupted

_____ 4. Smallest microorganism

_____ 5. Not in harmony

_____ 6. Contains all hereditary information

_____ 7. Worms

_____ 8. Process of engulfing invading organisms at the site of infection

_____ 9. Caused by treatment

_____ 10. Helps assess extent of burns

a. Disease

b. Illness

c. Genotype

d. DNA

e. Mutation

f. Virus

g. Helminthes

h. "Rule of nines"

i. Phagocytosis

j. Iatrogenic

k. Homeostasis

l. Phenotype

Short Answer

1. List nine causes of diseases and/or disorders.

   a.

   b.

   c.

   d.

   e.

   f.

g.

h.

i.

2. The leading cause of death in the United States for those younger than 35 years is

_____.

3. Predisposing factors in disease are

a.

b.

c.

d.

e.

Multiple Choice

Place a check next to the correct answers:

1. Trauma may include

   a. Heat exhaustion, heatstroke, and dehydration.

   b. Accidental exposure to radiation.

   c. Injury or wound from external force or violence.

   d. Decompression sickness and near-drowning.

2. B-cell lymphocytes

   a. Provide cell-mediated immunity.

   b. Are responsible for acquired humoral immunity.

   c. Are the slowest and least aggressive response of antigen contact.

   d. Are processed in the thymus.

3. Cell-mediated immunity

   a. Is both natural and acquired immunity.

   b. Is formed by B-cell lymphocytes.

   c. Is initiated when a T-cell lymphocyte is sensitized by contact with a specific antigen.

   d. Is not effective against fungal and viral invasion.

4. Malignant tumors

   a. Are circumscribed.

   b. Are not cancerous.

   c. Do not spread through the lymphatic system.

   d. Are characterized by uncontrollable growth cells.

Discussion Questions/Personal Reflection

1. Compare and contrast the two situations as follows. What potential causes of disease would you think either or both persons would have?

   Jim Hofmann lives in Los Angeles, California, and Sandi Smith lives in rural western Nebraska. Jim commutes to work via an automobile for about $1\frac{1}{2}$ hours to a high-rise building, whereas Sandi works outdoors much of the time managing her wheat farm.

2. Discuss malnourishment and vitamin/mineral deficiencies and the influence of poverty.

Notes

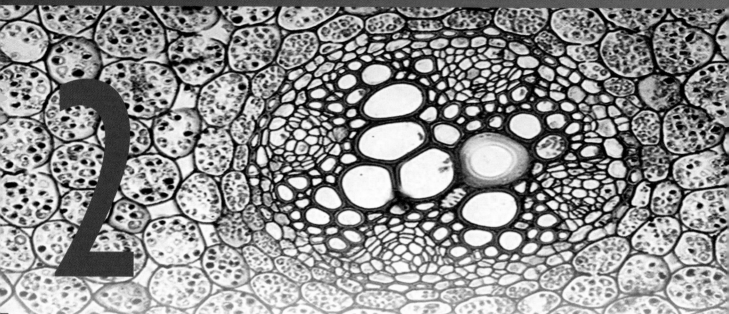

2

Integrative Medicine and Alternative Therapies

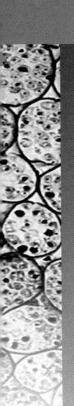

Endorphin (ĕn•dŏr′fin)
Enkephalin (in′ke•fa•lan)

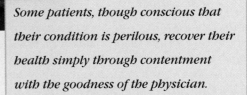

Some patients, though conscious that their condition is perilous, recover their health simply through contentment with the goodness of the physician.

—HIPPOCRATES, 460–400 B.C.

LEARNING OBJECTIVES

Upon successful completion of this chapter, you will be able to:

- Compare the growth of alternative forms of treatment between 1993 and 1997.
- Identify the growth in the number of alternative physicians compared with conventional physicians.
- List at least six terms for "alternative medicine."
- Recall the history of conventional medicine.
- Describe the history of integrative medicine.
- Identify a minimum of five hurdles to clear as society moves toward integrative health care.
- Define the role of the National Center for Complementary and Alternative Medicine (NCCAM).
- Name a minimum of five alternative health-care providers licensed to practice.
- Describe the connection of mind and body in relation to the disease process.
- Discuss personal responsibility in relation to our health.
- Identify at least two external and two internal environmental factors that influence our health and well-being.
- List at least four influences of personal lifestyle on our health.
- Describe the effects of unexpressed negative emotions on our bodies.
- Define *stress* and *distress*.
- Identify at least three dietary goals for the population of the United States.
- Discuss the importance of laughter and play in our health.
- Compare and contrast conditional and unconditional love.
- Discuss the effects of a personal faith on a healthy lifestyle.

From Carol and Marti

*When the first edition of this book was written, we felt the need for the chapter called The Holistic Approach to Disease. This need grew out of our personal experiences with the health-care system and a doctoral dissertation. We were already personally embracing the use of laughter and play in our lives to increase our **endorphins**, those wonderful chemicals in our brain that act to lessen our pain. We use music as therapy, and even today we rarely work without the accompaniment of music, and have intervals of laughter and play. Our editors, reviewers, colleagues, and peers, however, thought the topic was inappropriate for a text called Diseases of the Human Body. Finally, our personal wishes prevailed, but the chapter was placed toward the end of the book. Reviews and suggestions for this current edition tell us that some of you do not use this chapter, either because of lack of time or lack of awareness or because you share the same belief as our early readers. Today's climate identifying how individuals seek attention for their medical problems, however, dictates that this topic, along with the chapter on pain management, move from the back of the book to a prominent place in the early pages of this book. What does the future hold? We have taken a bold step in this text. Significant alternative therapies have been included with conventional or allopathic therapies for the management of diseases and disorders of the human body.*

—CAROL AND MARTI

THE CHANGING CLIMATE FOR ALTERNATIVE THERAPIES

The first serious documentation of the use of alternative medicine in the United States came from a 1993 study published by *The New England Journal of Medicine* indicating that more than one-third of the adult population chose alternative over conventional forms of treatment. In 1997, $27 billion was spent by individuals for alternative health care in the United States. Most of this amount was out-of-pocket expense; health insurance still does not cover many of these treatments. In 2001, the World Health Organization estimated that 65% to 80% of the world's population relied on alternative medicine as their primary health care. One third of U.S. medical schools now have courses in alternative medicine, and 74% of Americans desire a more natural approach to health care.

Perhaps the most startling statistic related to alternative medicine's increasing popularity is a study estimating that by 2010 there will be a 124% increase in the per capita supply of alternative physicians compared with only 16% for conventional physicians. By 2010, it is expected that there will be a 230% increase in the number of classical acupuncturists (excluding those who are already medical doctors) and the number of naturopaths will triple.

DEFINITION OF TERMS

Many terms are used to refer to alternative medicine: *integrative, complementary,* and *alternative* are increasingly popular. Other terms include *holistic* (or *wholistic*), *natural,* and *accommodative*. The U.S. Congress established the National Center for Complementary and Alternative Medicine (NCCAM) in 1998. Practitioners in the field are not totally satisfied with either term used in the name for this center. "Alternative" can imply that one medical treatment is to be used instead of another. "Complementary" medicine can imply that it is being used alongside traditional medicine, but many times the term is misspelled and "Complimentary" is used instead—there is no desire among any practitioners for this form of treatment to be seen as something "nice." The term *integrative,* introduced by Andrew Weil, MD, promotes the blending of the best of both conventional and nonconventional therapies.

The authors use *integrative* to refer to the model of care and *alternative* to refer to the therapies themselves.

HISTORY OF CONVENTIONAL MEDICINE

Conventional medicine can be traced back to René Descartes (1596–1650), a scientist and philosopher characterized by his rationalistic and dualistic world view. Whether or not intended, his philosophy eventually led to the separation of the "mind" from the "body." Ultimately, today's specialization of various branches of medicine and treatment by body systems is partly a result of this separation. During the mid-nineteenth century, the discovery of disease-producing microbes and Louis Pasteur's (1822–1895) theory that germs caused illness opposed the earlier theory and approach to medicine that such microbes became infectious only if conditions inside the body were out of balance. Modern medicine went on to expand its role in the treatment of illness.

The development of microscopy, bacterial cultures, radiography, vaccines, and antibiotics led medical science more into the germ theory of disease and away from the idea that an individual had an important role to play in his or her own health. Medical schools organized into various departments, forcing students to focus their studies on one organ at a time independent of all other organs. Even today we identify our diseases by a specific organ or system—gallbladder disease, colitis (inflammation of the large intestine), prostatitis (inflammation of the prostate gland). We even name cancers by the organ it affects. This terminology diverts attention away from the interrelatedness of all parts of the body into one whole person. This system-based approach to medicine was coined "allopathic medicine" by the German physician and chemist Samuel Hahnemann, who questioned the inherent limitations of this form of treatment.

HISTORY OF INTEGRATIVE MEDICINE

As early as 5,000 B.C., healing traditions from Chinese medicine and Ayurvedic medicine, which is practiced in India, were based on the belief that health represented a balance and harmony that included body, mind, and spirit. Health was linked to harmony, whereas disease was linked to disharmony or imbalance. Even Hippocrates (477–360 B.C.), the father of Western medicine, recognized and taught that health depended on living in harmony with life forces.

Although conventional medicine is unsurpassed in its treatment of acute life-threatening illness and injuries, alternative medicine practitioners recognize that the most effective form of health care treats a person's entire being and educates and empowers individuals to take personal responsibility for their health.

INTEGRATION OF BOTH WORLDS

Acceptance of the conventional and the alternative methods of treatment of diseases and disorders by practitioners in both worlds may offer the wisest form of health care for individuals seeking treatment. There are a number of hurdles to clear as society moves toward this integration:

1. Spiraling health-care costs led by the need for and use of increased technology.
2. Spending "little" to treat the cause of chronic disease but spending "much" when major illness results.
3. Spending huge sums on heroic measures, especially at both ends of life.
4. Ignoring lifestyle causes of diseases and disorders.
5. Integrating preventive medicine with rescue medicine.
6. Learning not to rely on only drug-based therapies to bring relief.
7. Seeking answers that address the root causes of health problems.
8. Obtaining insurance coverage for alternative therapies.

SEPARATING FACT FROM FALLACY

An individual seeking to embrace a particular alternative method of care has to rely on word of mouth in most instances to determine who are legitimate providers and to separate those who would do no harm from those whose particular treatment protocol has little or no value. Although the number of providers of alternative care has greatly increased, not all are licensed or regulated in their practice by the states in which they work. Osteopaths and chiropractors are licensed in every state. Naturopaths are licensed in Alaska, Arizona, Connecticut, Hawaii, Maine, Missouri, New Hampshire, Oregon, Utah, Vermont, and Washington. Kansas registers only naturopaths. Acupuncturists are licensed in 36 states, but homeopaths are not licensed in any state. Midwives and massage therapists are licensed in all states. Many licensed practitioners incorporate one or more of the alternative methods of treatment identified in their practices.

NCCAM, one of the 27 institutes and centers that make up the National Institutes of Health (NIH), was charged with studying the various forms of alternative therapies to separate fact from fallacy and to present their findings to the public. Four main categories are included in this text when appropriate as alternative treatment methods. Those categories and a brief definition of each are listed here.

Alternative Systems of Medical Practice

Ayurveda is based on an 8,000-year-old system from India. In Ayurveda, humans are classified into one of three basic body types. This system stresses mind-body practices such as yoga and meditation. Proper nutrition, herbal medicines, and massage also are involved.

Traditional Chinese medicine (TCM) is as ancient as Ayurveda. TCM refers to the five elements of fire, earth, metal, water, and wood. The feminine aspect of life, or *Yin*, and the male element of life, or *Yang*, are considered. TCM considers *Qi* (pronounced "chee") to be the life force or energy that flows in channels or meridians to all parts of the body to nourish, protect, and heal.

Homeopathy is a system of healing developed and published by Samuel Hahnemann in 1796. He believed that low doses of certain substances, prescribed in miniscule doses, could bring about a cure. The idea is that highly diluted substances leave an "energy imprint" in the body and stimulate the immune system, thereby helping to cure an illness. This system is generally accepted in England, parts of Europe, and India. Homeopathy is increasingly known in the United States, but there is much controversy surrounding it.

Naturopathy is a system of medicine that stresses prevention and the use of nontoxic, natural therapies. Naturopathy treats the whole person and stresses a positive mental attitude and a healthy lifestyle that includes exercise, sleep, and a healthy diet. Nutritional supplements, vitamins, and minerals, and physical modifications in breathing and posture may be emphasized.

Additional Therapies Referred to as Alternative

Bioelectromagnetic or *bioenergetic therapies* concentrate on modifying the disease processes by directing energy (electrical or magnetic) within or through the body. Drugs or surgery are not used. Healing touch and therapeutic touch are also included. Bioelectromagnetic therapy encourages you to be aware of your own body's signals or energy field and strives to help you create a more healthy or positive energy force.

Diet and nutrition therapies emphasize general dietary goals, in particular, ensuring sufficient amounts of essential fatty acids, amino acids and enzymes, and minerals and vitamins. Most conventional physicians stress diet and nutrition as well.

Herbal medicine therapies use any number of herbs to assist in the healing process. The practice of herbal medicine is considered mainstream in many cultures. Much of modern traditional medications are based on the use of herbs. Although herbal medicines do not go through the rigor of approval by the U.S. Food and Drug Administration (FDA), the World Health Organization (WHO) has indicated that the historical use of herbal preparations is evidence of safety unless there is scientific evidence to the contrary.

Manual healing methods include osteopathic medicine, chiropractic, and massage therapy. *Osteopathy* was founded in 1874 by Dr. Andrew Taylor Still, who believed the musculoskeletal system played a more significant role than is usually believed in allopathic medicine. Osteopathic manipulation is often used to deal with the body's dysfunction. Many osteopaths also practice conventional medicine. *Chiropractic* officially began in 1895. Much like osteopathy, chiropractic principles involve spinal biomechanics and musculoskeletal, neurologic, vascular, and nutritional relationships. *Massage* therapy is well known and has been increasingly popular in the past decade, especially in sports medicine arenas. There are a number of different techniques, but all apply therapy with gliding strokes, kneading, rubbing, percussion, and sometimes vibration. Thai massage uses the elbows, knees, and feet as well as the hands in application of the massage and provides therapeutic relief.

Mind-body medicine integrates the mind and body and teaches that each system is equally significant medically. Biofeedback may be used to help train individuals to become more aware of the body's signals. Psychoneuroimmunology is another concept used in mind-body medicine; it is derived from *logy* ("study of"), *psych* ("mind"), *neuro* ("brain"), and *immuno* ("immune system"). This system promotes a strong interrelatedness between emotions, stress, and the body's reaction through the immune system. Participants are taught how to use relaxation and visualization to reduce stress in their lives. Deep breathing from the diaphragm, meditation, repetitive exercise and/or prayer, progressive muscle relaxation, yoga or Tai Chi, and imagery may be used as a part of this therapy. Hypnotherapy may be suggested.

The use of humor and laughter, journaling exercises, music, dance, and art also may be used as therapy.

NCCAM has an excellent Website (http://nccam.nih.gov) that disseminates up-to-date information to the public on which complementary and alternative modalities work and why. One of the goals of the NCCAM is to promote the integration of scientifically proved complementary and alternative modalities into conventional medicine. Fact sheets are available that cover general information about complementary and alternative medicine (CAM) on specific topics and treatments.

Whether you embrace only traditional medicine or only alternative medicine or you integrate the two, there are a number of general themes that run through all three possibilities. Those themes are identified here.

MIND'S CONNECTION WITH HEALTH AND DISEASE

It is difficult to identify or even define the mind. The mind has been described by the writer Candace Pert, PhD, as "an enlivening energy in the information realm throughout the brain and body that enables the cells to talk to each other, and the outside to talk to the whole organism." The mind has everything to do with our health. Moods and attitudes embodied in our emotions are part of the mind's physical expression. Our emotions affect all of our organs and tissues. Negative emotions have a negative effect on health, especially over a long period of time; positive emotions have a positive effect on health.

It appears that sustained negative emotions over a long period of time can seriously hinder the body's immune system and keep it from functioning at an optimal level. Such links between our psychological state and the body's biological processes call on the medical community and each of us to pay closer attention to our emotions and levels of stress.

PERSONAL RESPONSIBILITY

Because our body is not indestructible, we need to be taught self-care and responsibility from birth. Often, however, it is not until we see someone become disabled or die that we gain a proper appreciation for our body. From the moment of birth, the road to death begins. And during the period of life, we continually make choices about our body's well-being. Early in life, we are taught and learn by observation of those close to us either to respect or to ignore our bodies.

If we accept ourselves, feel self-worth, and have been taught well, we ought to listen to our body's signals and seek necessary attention. There is little or nothing even the most influential medical practitioner can do when our body breaks down if we do not want help or are unwilling to ask for it.

Andrew Weil, MD, says that the most common correlation between mind and healing in people with chronic illness is total acceptance of the circumstances of one's life, including illness. This acceptance seems to allow and encourage a profound internal relaxation that enhances a person's spirit and immune system.

INFLUENCE OF LIFESTYLE

Lifestyle is the consistent, integrated way of life of an individual, as typified by mannerisms, attitudes, and possessions. From the time one is born, choices are made that influence lifestyle. These influences come from the following: (1) modeling of family members and peers, (2) education and knowledge, (3) personal attitudes, (4) degree of self-confidence, (5) individual responsibilities, (6) where we are in life, and (7) life's opportunities. From this list, we can see that individuals have a great deal of control over their own lifestyles. These lifestyle choices have great influence, whether positive or negative, on our own health and that of others. Parents who provide a model of healthful living influence their children toward a healthy lifestyle.

Personal responsibility requires a person to act safely in a potentially dangerous situation. Conversely, being responsible for oneself requires that the individual avoid potentially harmful behaviors and attitudes, such as smoking, failing to exercise, driving without a seatbelt, or disregarding treatments prescribed by health-care providers. It requires that we listen to our bodies.

If you are seeking an integrative approach to your health care, you will want to remember that you have a personal responsibility to share *all* of your treatment methods with your health-care provider. Your traditional or allopathic physician should be a part of your decision to seek alternative therapies. Likewise, an alternative practitioner must be aware of any treatment you are receiving from your allopathic physician.

ENVIRONMENTAL INFLUENCES—INTERNAL AND EXTERNAL

Personal health and well-being are greatly influenced by environment, both internal and external. Internal environmental factors include the genetic traits, familial tendencies, and physical and psychological characteristics inherent in each person. External environmental factors may be more easily defined; they include the air we breathe, the water we drink, the food we eat, and the surroundings in which we live and work.

Unfortunately, internal environmental factors are not easily controlled, changed, or altered. We are unable to change our genetic makeup; however, through genetic engineering, it is possible that we may alter the genetic makeup of our offspring. Familial tendencies are almost as difficult to influence as genetics, and we know that children often reflect the traits of their parents. Physical and psychological characteristics and attitudes can be altered; but deliberate, consistent, and continuous efforts must be instituted before change occurs.

Some, but not all, external environmental influences are more easily managed. A conscious effort may be made to refrain from smoking, but can you leave your job working in a coal mine? The air is cleaner in Portland, Oregon, than in New York City, but can you move? Food may be purer with no preservatives or additives, but what about the risk of food poisoning? Should the government control the spraying of fruits and vegetables with pesticides, or should we take our chances in the market?

In the final analysis, we must recognize the influences that lifestyle and both internal and external environment have on health. It is important to understand that these factors also greatly affect our body's disorders and diseases.

Value of Good Nutrition

Gluttony is not a secret vice.

—Orson Wells

"You are what you eat"—how many times have you heard that? We understand the logic of advice such as, "Beware of saturated fats," "Avoid refined sugar," and "Low salt, or no salt," so why does eating often get out of control? Perhaps it comes from the philosophy that we should clean all the food from our plates. It may occur because food is used to relieve emotions or physical pain and as a reward.

Improper nutrition may result in body disorders or diseases. Bowel cancer is more common among groups of people who consume high amounts of animal fat and little fiber. There also is evidence that breast cancer may be linked to a high-fat/low-fiber dietary pattern and that where there is high meat consumption, cancer mortality rates are correspondingly high.

The *Dietary Goals for Americans*, adapted from the U.S. Department of Agriculture, includes the ABCs with the following suggestions:

A Aim for Fitness

- Aim for healthy weight.
- Be physically active each day.

B Build a Healthy Base

- Let the Food Pyramid guide your choices.
- Choose a variety of whole grains daily.
- Choose a variety of fruits and vegetables daily.
- Keep food safe for eating.

C Choose Sensibly

- Choose a diet low in saturated fat and cholesterol and moderate in total fat.
- Choose beverages and foods to moderate intake of sugars.
- Choose and prepare foods with less salt.
- If you drink alcoholic beverages, do so in moderation.

It is important to realize that we have the power to improve our lifestyle by eating properly each and every day. Good nutrition can make a difference—if not in prolonging life, at least in enabling us to face life's stresses with greater ease.

Stress and Distress

It is generally believed that biological organisms require a certain amount of stress in order to maintain their well-being. Stress is always present. "Good" stress enables the body to meet the challenges of everyday activity. For example, stress keeps us alert when driving in heavy traffic or helps us respond to needs of family members in crises. Without a correct balance of stress, people would be unable to respond to any stimuli.

Distress, however, tends to be a negative influence. When stress occurs in quantities that the system cannot handle, it may produce pathological changes. These stressors can be either a person or a condition; some examples are, children, spouses, bosses, the weather, traffic, noise, money, school, environment, retirement, divorce, death, disease—any change that occurs in our lives. The amount of distress experienced depends a great deal on how we respond to these stressors.

The recognition of stressors in life and their subsequent management constitute one of the keys to a healthy lifestyle. It has been shown that good nutrition, proper exercise, and a quality support system help alleviate distress.

MANAGING NEGATIVE EMOTIONS

Humans are emotional creatures. Feelings of joy, sorrow, anger, jealousy, love, resentment, fear, and hate are part of existence. How we deal with our emotions has much to do with our physical health.

Emotions may be categorized as positive or negative. Fear is a negative emotion if, for instance, it keeps us from functioning as normal human beings; it is a positive emotion if it cautions us to be safe. A sense of joy may warm the body, cleanse the spirit, relax muscles, lighten air passages, and generally make people feel "good all over." Anger or resentment may cause the fist to clench, breathing to accelerate, the heart to pound, the head to ache, and muscles to tighten. Feelings of despair, panic, depression, fear, and frustration cause the healing resources of the human brain to be underutilized.

When we have a great will to live and expect the best in life, the brain has a greater ability to produce chemicals, such as endorphins and **enkephalins,** more wonderful brain chemicals that have a very positive effect on our bodies.

Some individuals may be sensitive to and recognize the physical signals given by the body. All too often, however, we have "buried" somewhere in our inner consciousness the negative impact emotions may have. Buried emotions later may exhibit themselves during an illness. Even then, illness may not be attributed to a negative emotion long since unexpressed. The kind of disease that results from unexpressed negative emotion is called psychosomatic illness. The symptoms of the disease are very real, but

Table 2.1
SOME POSITIVE WAYS OF WORKING OUT NEGATIVE EMOTIONS
Chop wood.
Scrub and wax a floor.
Run a mile—or several.
Ride a bike.
Beat up a pillow.
Relax in a hot tub.
See a counselor.
Wash the car.
Knead bread.
Lift weights.
Cry, weep.
Accept yourself.
Read a funny book or go to a funny movie. Laugh!
Roll up the car windows, scream a little or a lot.
Make certain there is someone who loves you unconditionally.

are likely the result of one or more unexpressed negative emotions.

It can be helpful to realize that negative emotions that are not dealt with in a wholesome manner probably express themselves physically in the body. We must learn how to express negative feelings without destroying ourselves or others if we wish to live a healthy life.

The next time anger or emotions have a negative effect, check the body to see which part is most affected. If you can feel a headache coming on, can feel the fire in your "gut," or feel your heart pounding, remember that you may need an emotional release.

LAUGHTER AND PLAY

Laughter has been described as "internal jogging." We are unable to experience despair and joy at the same time. Therefore, it is important for individuals to allow, even plan for, laughter and play in their lives.

There are several examples of the use of laughter and play in today's health care. Dr. O. Carl Simonton, noted radiation oncologist, tells of his work with teaching cancer patients how to juggle. On his first visit with patients, he gives them a set of juggling bags and one or two simple instructions. He juggles for them and tells them to practice every day and that they will do some juggling together each time they meet. Simonton reports that this activity (1) enables him and his patients to develop a relationship outside of "doctor-patient," (2) encourages a lot of laughing together, and (3) gives the patient something other than an illness to think about.

David Bresler, PhD, director of the Bresler Center for Allied Therapeutics in Los Angeles and Professor in the UCLA Department of Anesthesiology, Grathology/Occlusion, and Psychology, uses long, slender balloons blown up and shaped into all kinds of animal forms to help children cope with chronic pain. This activity takes their minds off the pain and may stimulate the release of endorphins in the body.

Norman Cousins reported in *Anatomy of an Illness* about the validity of laughter in healing his illness. He watched old Marx Brothers movies several times a day, laughing to near tears. Following this time of laughter, he was always able to function without pain medication.

It seems obvious that play and laughter ought to be a more important and deliberate part of our daily lives. All too frequently we forget to play as we become adults.

LOVE, FRIENDSHIP, AND FAITH

We learn in most psychology classes that we must love ourselves before we can love another. But what is love? Leo Buscaglia, in his book, *Love*, defines love as "a learned, emotional reaction. If we wish to know love, we must live love, in action." Love is spontaneous. If we love someone, we need to share that love now. Love must be given unconditionally. (Striking evidence of the positive effects of uncondi-

tional love comes from the successful use of pets in various kinds of therapy.) If we expect something in return for love, we are in error. We love because we feel it and want to share it. And we never "run out of" love.

Friendship is one part of love. Each of us needs at least one friend/mentor with whom we can share anything at any time. Our friend must love us as we are and not expect anything from us. Your authors hope you have a friendship as cherished as ours.

Not every person embraces religion or senses a strong spiritual influence in their lives, but at one time or another, we all have witnessed its influence in the life of someone. Some call it worship. Others refer to it as prayer. For your neighbor, it may be meditation. Yoga has been very helpful for many; for others, it is a mental discipline. The experience is a devotion, a setting aside, an adoration, a refreshing, or an enlightening. It may include service, witnessing, sharing, and a sense of community and belonging. Whatever it is, it is a very personal experience.

Practitioners of integrative health recognize the worth of such experiences in a person's life. A faith in something or someone greater and more powerful than ourselves can make the most desolate of times a little less frustrating.

Summary

Alternative therapies and integrative medicine play an important role in the treatment of diseases and disorders in today's climate. The greatest success in treatment will come from clients cared for by health-care practitioners who are able to integrate the traditional and alternative modalities, from practitioners who are effective in encouraging their clients to be open and honest about their choices, and from practitioners who are unafraid to take a bold step forward in uncharted waters.

CASE STUDIES

■ Case Study 1

Joyce Garcia, a 64-year-old surgical nurse, is diagnosed with breast cancer. After consultation with her primary care physician, undergoing mammography and ultrasonography, and seeing a specialist, a treatment protocol is determined. Joyce undergoes a lumpectomy. The lymph nodes are found to be clear of the cancer. Radiation treatment follows. Joyce notifies her closest friends and the women in her Bible study group. She asks for prayer and support. She uses visualization in her healing. She visualizes the cancer as a black, nasty-looking glob being removed in its entirety from her breast. Joyce's recovery is uneventful and she regularly returns to her physician for evaluation. She is so grateful that breast self-examination helped her find the lump.

Case Study Questions

1. Identify the conventional and traditional methods of treatment that Joyce sought.
2. Are there any alternative therapies that might have helped in Joyce's recovery?

■ Case Study 2

Robert Busabarger is the only physician in a small rural east coast village. He is all things to all people—physician, counselor, surgeon, obstetrician, pediatrician, and psychiatrist. He works 10-hour days and is rarely away from his practice unless on the ocean in his fishing vessel. He is frustrated that all he seems to have time for is to conduct minimal screening and to prescribe medications.

Case Study Questions

1. How might Dr. Busabarger use alternative therapies with his clients and decrease his work load?
2. Discuss how clients in this kind of setting might be able to help Dr. Busabarger and each other obtain medical treatment that treats the "whole" person.

REVIEW QUESTIONS

True/False

Circle the correct answer:

T   F   1. In 1997, $14 billion was spent for alternative health care in the United States.

T   F   2. By 2010, a 16% increase will occur in the number of conventional physicians.

T   F   3. Half of all medical schools offer courses in alternative medicine.

T   F   4. Norman Cousins coined the term "integrative medicine."

T   F   5. It is common to identify certain diseases by the organ(s) affected.

Matching

Match each of the following definitions with its correct term:

_____ 1. Father of Western medicine

_____ 2. OAM

_____ 3. Licensed in every state

_____ 4. Philosopher of conventional medicine

_____ 5. Medicine from India

a. René Descartes

b. Ayurvedic medicine

c. Hippocrates

d. Osteopaths and chiropractors

e. Office of Alternative Medicine

Short Answer

1. Internal environmental factors that influence health and well-being include

   a.

   b.

   c.

   d.

2. External environmental factors that influence health and well-being include

   a.

   b.

   c.

   d.

3. Personal lifestyle may be influenced by

   a.

   b.

c.

d.

e.

f.

4. The kind of disease that results from unexpressed negative emotion is called

_____ .

5. List at least four constructive outlets for expression of negative feelings beneficial to you.

6. Describe situations that cause stress to have a positive or a negative impact on our lives.

7. Create a day's eating plan to allow for four servings of fruits and vegetables.

Multiple Choice

Place a checkmark next to the correct answer.

1. Andrew Weil, MD, used the following term for nontraditional medicine:

   a. Complementary

   b. Holistic

   c. Alternative

   d. Integrative

2. Which of the following statements is true concerning conventional medicine?

   a. It can be traced back to Rene Descartes.

   b. It was strongly influenced by Chinese and Ayurvedic medicine.

   c. It treats a person's entire bearing and empowers an individual to take personal responsibility.

   d. It does not include specialization as various branches of medicine.

3. Identify the one group of alternative practitioners who are not licensed in any state.

   a. Naturopaths

   b. Homeopaths

   c. Midwives

   d. Acupuncturists

4. Norman Cousins in his book *Anatomy of an Illness*

   a. Teaches patients how to juggle bags to give them something else to think about besides the pain.

b. Blows up balloons to help children cope with pain.

c. Dresses up like a clown to bring laughter and play to patients.

d. Watches old Marx Brothers movies to bring laughter and decrease pain.

5. From the following list, select your four favorite stress relievers. Explain your choices.

a. Find a beach, take off your shoes, and let the sand squiggle through your toes.

b. Be a good jokester.

c. Laugh at yourself—then share it!

d. Dance.

e. Fly a kite or model airplane.

f. Go to the zoo.

g. Finger paint.

h. Play in the water while everyone thinks you are watering the lawn.

Discussion Questions/Personal Reflection

1. Identify a negative emotion you have difficulty expressing. Discuss with a friend what may be the consequences of such activity.

2. Share a cartoon, joke, or funny story with a classmate. Describe how you felt after sharing a laugh.

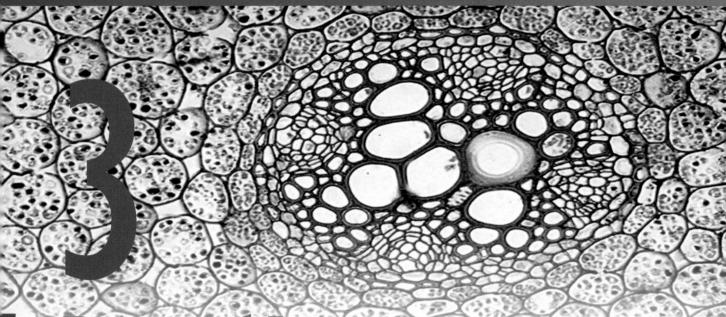

3

Pain and Its Management

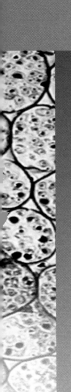

KEY WORDS

Acetylcholine (ăs•ĕ•tĭl•kō′lēn)
Adjuvant analgesics (ă′jĕ•vĕnt ăn•ăl•jē•sĭks)
Cordotomy (kŏr•dŏt′ō•mē)
Endorphin (ĕn•dŏr′fĭn)
Histamine (hĭs′tă•mĭn)
Hypophysectomy (hī•pŏf•ĭ•sĕk′tō•mē)
Neuromodulator (nū•rō•mŏd′u•lā•tŏr)
Neurotransmitter (nū•rō•trăns′mĭ•tĕr)
Neurotomy (nū•rŏt′ō•mē)
Nociception pain process (nō•sĭ′sĕp•shŭn pān pră•sĕs)
Nonopioids (năn•o′pē•oids)
Opioids (ō′pē•oids)
Synapse (sĭ′năps)

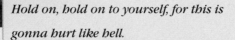

Hold on, hold on to yourself, for this is gonna hurt like hell.

—SARAH MCLACHLAN

LEARNING OBJECTIVES

Upon successful completion of this chapter, you will be able to:

- Define *pain*.
- List at least four factors that influence how we experience pain.
- Discuss the purpose of pain.
- Explain the gate control theory of pain.
- Describe the nociception pain process.
- Describe at least two pain assessment tools.
- Compare and contrast acute, chronic, and cancer-related pain.
- List and describe at least two types of traditional and at least five types of alternative therapies for the treatment of pain.

Pain affects each of us during our lifetime. Many diseases and disorders of the human body are accompanied by pain. It is feared by many people, as much as or more than the disease itself. What is pain? What purpose, if any, does it serve? What happens in the body when a person feels pain? How does the health professional assess pain? What are the different types of pain? Can pain be treated? If so, how? These are some of the questions that are addressed in this chapter. Pain is an expanding science and an increasing number of specialty clinics are emerging. Two of the earliest multidisciplinary pain centers were the University of Washington in Seattle and the City of Hope Medical Center in Duarte, California. Others slowly followed their lead. Today, numerous pain clinics address the treatment of acute, chronic, and cancer pain.

According to the Agency for Healthcare Research and Quality (AHRQ; formerly the Agency for Health Care Policy and Research [AHCPR]), a federal agency established in 1989, there are three major barriers to effective pain management: (1) the health-care system,

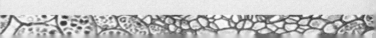

(2) health-care professionals, and (3) clients. The health-care system rarely holds itself accountable for assessing and relieving pain. Many suggest that assessment of pain be included with the measurement of taking vital signs such as temperature, pulse, respiration, and blood pressure. Pain assessment would be the fifth vital sign. Some believe that routinely assessing and relieving pain would prove more cost effective than ignoring the issue. Health professionals are not always educated about the meaning of and assessment of pain management and are often overly concerned about the use of **opioids** (narcotics), mainly due to possible addiction. Clients and their families also have grave concerns about any analgesic use and their potential addiction. Many clients believe that physicians tend to overprescribe pain medication and that chronic pain cannot be effectively treated. In all situations, education is a key element, for health-care professionals, and for clients and their families.

Physiologic pain accompanies many diseases and disorders of the body potentially causing tissue damage. Psychological pain often is expressed as sorrow over loss such as death or divorce. Psychological pain may become physiologic pain, or the two may be concurrent. Although pain may be sensed as having a negative effect on the body, it may also be positive. For instance, if pain could not be felt, you might not know you were burning your flesh on a hot stove. It also can be a symptom of a few more serious problems, diseases, and conditions.

Health professionals can be frustrated in their attempt to treat individuals who experience pain, especially when the cause of pain is not readily identifiable. Clients in pain may be frustrated and confused, too, especially if the pain is unbearable.

WHAT IS PAIN?

Definition of Pain

In dictionaries, *pain* is defined as a sensation of hurting or of strong discomfort in some part of the body, caused by an injury, a disease, or a functional disorder and transmitted through the nervous system. *Pain* also may be defined as the distress or suffering (mental or physical) that is caused by great anxiety, anguish, grief, disappointment, or other psychological or emotional stimuli. A nurse, Margo McCaffery, who has worked for years with clients in pain and has done extensive research in the field of pain, defines *pain* as whatever the experiencing person says it is, existing when he or she says it does. This definition is perhaps the most useful because it acknowledges the client's complaint, recognizes the subjective nature of pain, and implicitly suggests that diverse measures may be undertaken to relieve pain.

McCaffery states that The International Association for the Study of Pain (IASP) and the American Pain Society (APS) define *pain* as an unpleasant sensory and emotional experience associated with actual or potential tissue damage, or described in terms of such damage. Again, this definition further confirms the multiple components of pain in a person's psychological and physiologic existence.

How we experience pain is based, in part, on several different variables:

1. *Early Experiences of Pain.* Did the person experiencing pain in the past have a positive or negative experience in the management of the pain? Generally, a person's fear of pain increases with each pain experience.

2. *Cultural Backgrounds.* Recent research shows that culture generally does not influence how a person perceives pain but does have an influence on how a person responds to pain. Early in life, children learn from those around them. For example, children may learn that a sport's injury does not hurt as much as trauma from an automobile accident. Further, they learn what behaviors are acceptable or unacceptable. These behaviors vary from culture to culture. Rarely are these expectations changed; in fact, these perceptions are believed to be normal and acceptable.

3. *Anxiety and Depression.* Does anxiety increase or decrease pain? Is depression the cause or result of pain? Some research shows a relationship between anxiety and depression, and pain, and some do not. An effective way to relieve pain is by directing the treatment at the pain rather than at the anxiety or depression. The longer the duration of pain, the greater is the occurrence of depression. A person's anxiety and depression need to be addressed when treating pain.

4. *Age.* Pain perception does not change significantly with age, yet the way an elderly person responds to pain may differ from that of a

younger person. For example, as a person ages, they have a slower metabolism and greater ratio of body fat to muscle mass. Hence, they may require a smaller dosage of analgesics.

5. *Sex*. Recent research suggests that females and males experience pain differently. In fact, females demonstrate a greater frequency of pain-related symptoms than do males. In addition, when pain-free individuals were exposed to a variety of stimulus modalities and assessment methods, females exhibited greater sensitivity to the experimentally induced pain than did males.

As health-care professionals, we, too, are influenced by our past experience, our attitudes, cultures, and our beliefs regarding pain. Must there be an organic reason before pain is "real?" Who understands pain better—the person experiencing the pain or the health professional? Research suggests that health-care professionals may be overly concerned about the client's possible addiction to pain medication or they may believe that the person is merely malingering.

Purpose of Pain

Pain is a warning that something is wrong in normal body functioning. It is one of the most common complaints of a person seeking medical attention. It warns of inflammation, tissue damage, infection, bodily injury, or trauma—physical or emotional—somewhere in the body. Each disease or disorder produces characteristic patterns of tissue damage; hence, the quality, time, course, and location of a person's pain complaint and the location of tenderness provide important diagnostic clues.

Pathophysiology of Pain

The discussion of the pathophysiology of pain requires an understanding of the anatomy and physiology of the nervous system. Readers should refer to Chapter 13, or review an anatomy and physiology text. Two of the numerous theories and mechanisms of pain are discussed in this chapter: the gate control theory and the nociception pain process.

GATE CONTROL THEORY OF PAIN

What occurs at the cellular level when we experience pain? The gate control theory of pain, by P. D. Wall,

offers a useful model of the physiologic process of pain (Fig. 3.1). Some definitions will provide a background for an explanation of the actual theory. A **neurotransmitter** is a substance produced and released by one neuron (a nerve cell) that travels across the synapse, exciting or inhibiting the next neuron in the neural pathway. A **synapse** is the narrow gap between two neurons in a neural pathway where the termination (axon) of one neuron comes in close proximity with the beginning (dendrite) or cell body of another neuron. A **neuromodulator** is the alteration in function or status in response to a stimulus of a nerve. **Histamine** and **acetylcholine** are neurotransmitters, and **endorphins** are neuromodulators.

According to the gate control theory, "the experience of pain is the result of the summation of the action of both neurotransmitters and neuromodulators at each neural receptor site from the site of injury to the cortex. At each neuron synapse, if the amount of neurotransmitter (histamine, acetylcholine, etc.) exceeds the amount of neuromodulators (endorphins, etc.), then the impulse continues to the next synapse where similar interactions are in operation."

In other words, we experience pain whenever the substances that tend to propagate a pain impulse across each "gate" in a nerve pathway overpower the substances that tend to block such an impulse. Amid controversy and minor evolution, the gate control theory is recognized as a major basis of pain theory.

Studies of coping factors support a wider version of the gate control theory. These factors need to be considered before determining treatment for pain, and they raise a number of questions.

1. How well is the client coping with life?
2. Does the client have pain and if so, does he or she think that it is under control?
3. Does the client feel adequately informed about the painful condition?
4. Is the client occupied? How does the individual fill his or her time?
5. Does the client have other problems to cope with?
6. Does the client feel dissatisfied with his or her past life, or does he or she have any substantial regrets?
7. Are there any reasons why the client may not be coping?

These factors may help determine the best treatment for pain.

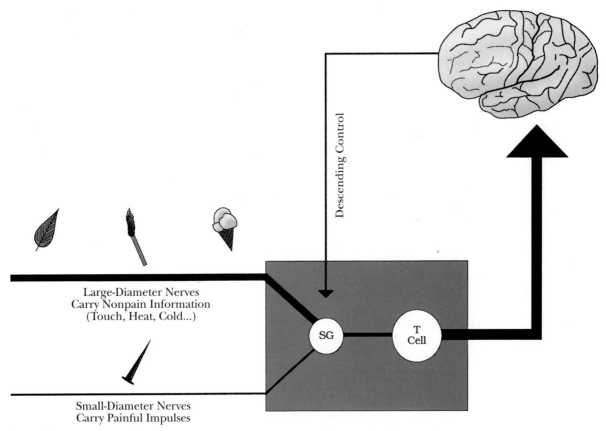

Figure 3.1 The gate control theory of pain transmission. The substantia gelatinosa (SG) accepts input both from large-diameter (nonpain) and small-diameter (pain) nerves. Based on the rate of input, the SG allows either the pain or nonpain stimulus to be passed on to the transmission cell (T cell) and up to the brain. Because nonpain impulses travel faster than pain impulses, stimulation of nonpain fibers can override the transmission of pain. In addition, the brain has an inhibiting influence both on the SG and the spinal cord that can work to limit the perception and reaction to pain. (From Starkey, C: Therapeutic Modalities for Athletic Trainers. FA Davis, Philadelphia, 1993, p 28, with permission.)

NOCICEPTION PAIN PROCESS

Another concept that incorporates some aspects of the gate control theory is the **nociception pain process**. The nociception pain process describes how pain is transformed from stimuli the body receives into the actual pain sensation. The nociception pain process is responsible for the transmission and perception of pain through the following four processes.

1. **Transduction**. Transduction describes how pain is received by the body. In transduction, the nociceptors in the peripheral body (skin, subcutaneous tissue, or organs) distinguish between noxious (harmful or injurious) and innocuous (innocent or nonharmful) stimuli. If the noxious stimuli is sufficient to cause tissue damage and/or trauma, the body releases substances that allow the pain impulses to reach the spinal cord. Transduction changes noxious stimuli in sensory nerve endings into impulses.

2. **Transmission**. Transmission is the movement of impulses from transduction sites to the brain. Here the impulses ascend to the brain stem, thalamus, and different parts of the brain. The thalamus is a "relay station," sending pain impulses to the brain, where pain can be processed. This "relay station" is sometimes referred to as "the gate," where the

tendency is to allow all noxious stimuli to ascend to the brain and result in pain. It would be difficult to live with all the pain, so the gate control theory comes into play whereby the body "closes the gate" to pain input and prevents some pain transmissions.

3. **Perception of Pain.** At this stage, pain comes into consciousness and is perceived by the person. The body tries to respond to the pain; however, because of the subjectivity of pain, it is not well understood why and how the brain "perceives" pain and/or how it perceives it so differently among individuals.

4. **Modulation.** Modulation is the process by which the brain changes or inhibits the pain impulses. Here the body releases substances that inhibit the transmission of noxious stimuli and produces analgesia.

These four basic processes of the nociception pain process describe how pain becomes a conscious feeling or thought. Basically, a person experiences a pain in the peripheral nervous system outside the central nervous system (brain and spinal cord). The pain is the stimulus that is transferred to the spinal cord as an impulse and is passed through the "relay station." The impulse reaches the brain, which then defines and responds to the pain impulse. The brain releases inhibitory substances to the body depending on the level of pain. For a higher level of pain, the brain produces more inhibitory substances that descend to the body. The lower the pain, the fewer inhibitory substances are produced by the brain.

In summary, both the gate control theory and the nociception pain process provide descriptions that are useful to health-care professionals in the treatment and management of pain.

ASSESSMENT OF PAIN

Pain gives the body warning and usually is accompanied by anxiety or the urge to relieve the pain. Pain is both sensation and emotion. Health-care professionals may find the following mnemonic tool useful for assessing a client in pain:

P = place (client points with one finger to the location of the pain)

A = amount (client rates pain on a scale from 0 [no pain] to 10 [worst pain possible])

I = interactions (client describes what makes the pain worse)

N = neutralizers (client describes what makes the pain less)

The scale of 1 to 10 as described in the mnemonic is a very useful method of assessing pain. Further pain assessment skills include observing the client's appearance and activity. Monitoring the client's vital signs may be of value in assessing acute pain but not necessarily chronic pain.

To assess for children's pain, a "smiley face" model may prove beneficial (Fig. 3.2). The child is told that the first smiley face shows a happy child with no pain or hurt, whereas the last face shows pain that "hurts worst." Ask the child to point to the face that describes his or her smile. Note the faces are on a numeric scale.

ACUTE, CHRONIC, AND CANCER-RELATED PAIN

Acute and chronic pain need to be differentiated before beginning treatment. A third type of pain, cancer-related pain, is discussed separately. *Acute* pain is recent in onset and has been experienced over a period of less than 6 months. Such pain may be manifested as an increase in heart rate, blood pressure, and muscle tension and a decrease in salivary flow and gut motility. Such pain is the result of damage, injury, or surgical pain from traumatized skin, muscle, or visceral organs. Acute pain frequently serves as a warning sign of a disturbance in some physiologic process and usually is accompanied by anxiety.

Chronic pain may be either continuous or intermittent, occurring over a period of longer than 6 months. Chronic pain often cannot be attributed to a specific injury or cause, and when it lasts a long time, it becomes a problem in its own right. It serves no useful purpose. Unlike the acute form, chronic pain may not serve as a warning of physiologic disturbance. It is frequently debilitating, exhausting an individual's physical and emotional resources.

Chronic pain is often difficult to manage. Some diseases have perpetuating factors such as sensory nerve damage that linger long after treatment is initiated. Also, the client may experience psychological effects that cause pain or exacerbate it. Often, the client is depressed and preoccupied with self. Chronic pain may be associated with a decrease in

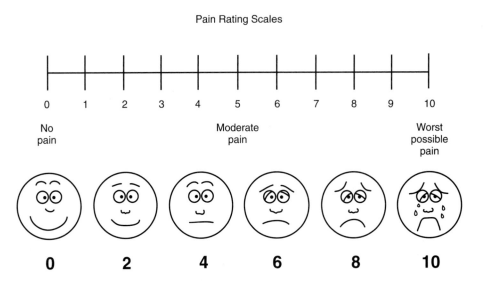

Pain Rating Scales

Figure 3.2 Pain assessment scales for adults and children. (Reprinted from McCaffery M and Pasero C: Pain: Clinical Manual, 2 ed, copyright 1999, p 67, with permission from Elsevier.)

sleep, libido, and appetite. Because the parasympathetic nervous system tends to adapt to a state of chronic pain, there may be few, if any, outward physiologic signs or behavioral changes noted in individuals experiencing such pain.

Although health-care professionals may be familiar with cancer, or malignancy, pain, clients who are terminally ill with diseases other than cancer may also experience pain. Like those with chronic or acute pain, the terminally ill client should be offered analgesia for palliative treatment. The needs of the client's family and caregivers should also be addressed. The assessment of a client with terminal pain is similar to that of any client who is experiencing pain, although the difference with a dying client is that he or she also often deals with emotions of anxiety, fear, anger, and depression, common to people whose condition is terminal. The dying client is facing death in addition to pain.

Cancer-related pain can be either acute or chronic, but it is the type of pain that occurs when the client has a cancer-related condition. Clients with this type of pain may fear the pain as much as the cancer. Cancer-related pain may result directly from the cancer (tumor, abnormal growth), from the treatment of the cancer (surgery, radiation), or from extenuating circumstances relating to the cancer (trauma). Complicated factors for the client with cancer-related pain include increased anxiety, fear, and depression that accompany anyone facing potential death.

TREATMENT OF PAIN

The objective of pain treatment is to remove the cause or to lessen the severity of the pain; however, there may be a lag in time between identifying the cause of the pain and providing relief. The treatment of pain is diverse and can be difficult. A multidisciplinary approach to chronic and cancer-related pain management is being used with success. This team approach involves both medical and nonmedical personnel and may include any of a number of approaches.

Medications

Medications tend to be the treatment of choice for many clients experiencing pain. Analgesics, anesthetics, and anti-inflammatory agents may be prescribed to decrease or eliminate pain, although they do not eliminate the cause of pain. Analgesics can be **opioid** (formerly referred to as narcotic) or **nonopioid** (formerly referred to as non-narcotic), prescription or over-the-counter, and of varying strengths. Opioid analgesics may include morphine-like drugs, whereas nonopioid drugs include acetaminophen and nonsteroidal anti-inflammatory drugs. A third category of drugs called **adjuvant analgesics** include those whose primary purpose is not generally used or prescribed for pain. For example, drugs used for depression may be prescribed to effectively treat pain. Other adjuvant medications include those used for seizure control and corticosteroids. Medication may be administered orally, intravenously, nasally, injection, or skin patch. Additionally, medications may be used alone or in conjunction with other treatment modalities.

In the United States, there is a paradigm shift in the treatment of pain with medication. The old paradigm teaches that the use of pain medicine in the treatment of pain is unsafe, especially when used continually. Further, it teaches that opioid use is addictive and can cause long-term damage to the body. Some believe that clients who ask for more opioids are exhibiting addictive behavior and that when physicians continue to prescribe opioids to clients in pain, they are no different than illicit drug dealers. A new paradigm, supported by years of pain research, has shown that opioid treatment is safe and effective if monitored by physicians.

When clients ask for more pain medication, it means they are experiencing more pain, and if they are given more pain medication, the pain will subside. If clients are treated with adequate pain medication, they no longer have pain and they can lead a productive normal life. Their family and friends will note that their quality of life has improved. Last, the new paradigm shows there is a significant difference between the physician who prescribes pharmaceutical drugs for legitimate pain in a medically controlled environment and the illicit drug dealer who provides drugs in a nonmedical, uncontrolled environment. It is hoped that the new terms do not carry the negative connotations of narcotics and nonnarcotics.

A common treatment of some pain is the patient-controlled analgesia (PCA) pump (Fig. 3.3). The pump allows the client to administer his or her own pain medication, offering the client some sense of control of their pain, which is an important psychologic benefit. In PCA, the amount of drug dispensed by the pump is determined by the physician. The device is designed to not release more than the prescribed amount within a set period of time, thus guarding against overmedication. Clients who should not use a PCA are those with hypersensitivity to the medication used, those with physical impairments

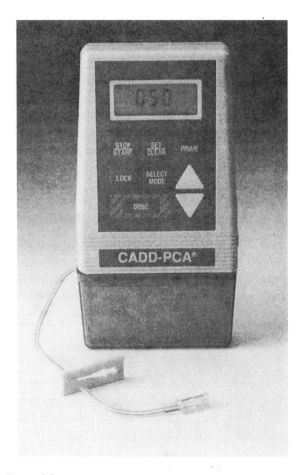

Figure 3.3 Portable infusion pump for patient-controlled analgesia (PCA). (Courtesy of Pharmacia Deltec, Inc., St. Paul, Minnesota; from Phillips, LD: Manual of IV Therapeutics, ed. 2. FA Davis, Philadelphia, 1997, p 211, with permission.)

that make it difficult to activate the pump, and those with any emotional or cognitive disability.

Research indicates that health-care professionals and family members tend to undermedicate for pain because of incorrect assumptions, prevailing attitudes, the complexity of pain assessment, and unfounded fears, mainly those of addiction (psychological dependence). However, no medical research testifies to such an addiction. In fact, the use of opioids is indicated in many cases of pain management, and evidence is overwhelming that the fears of health-care professionals are greatly exaggerated. Untreated pain adversely affects pulmonary, gastrointestinal, and circulatory systems and can cause insomnia, depression, and irritability, if the pain becomes chronic.

An interesting phenomenon is the use of placebos in pain management. A *placebo* is defined as a medication that produces an effect in a client because of its intent rather than because of its specific physical or chemical properties. In the placebo effect, the person is given a medication or treatment because the person believes it to be effective. When such placebos are used, studies show that 20% to 40% of those with objective stimuli report pain relief, at least for a short time. This is a powerful example of the mind-body connection.

The placebo effect results from the natural production of endorphins and enkephalins in the descending control system. The more cues the client received about the placebo's effectiveness, the more likely it will be effective in relieving pain. Obviously, placebos should be used wisely and not as a way to test a client's truthfulness about pain or as first-line treatment. Placebos should not be used to treat cancer pain.

Surgery

Surgery may be necessary to block the transmission of pain or to remove the cause of pain. Surgery for relief of pain may include such procedures as dissection or division of a nerve, or **neurotomy;** surgical division of one or more of the lateral nerve pathways emerging from the spinal cord, or **cordotomy;** and removal of the pituitary gland, or **hypophysectomy**, as well as the removal of any causative factor. Surgery may be helpful to relieve the pain of pancreatic cancer, the severe intractable pain from other malignancies, or intractable abdominal pain.

ALTERNATIVE THERAPIES

The following pain treatments may be used both in traditional medicine and in integrative medicine. These treatments have proved effective in the treatment and management of pain and illustrate the blending of traditional and integrative medicine.

Biofeedback

Biofeedback is aimed at helping an individual gain voluntary control over normally involuntary physiologic functions. Various forms of electronic feedback produced by monitoring physiologic events may promote blood flow and reduce muscle tension, which in turn may reduce the concentration of neurotransmitters at the site of pain. The client has sensors attached to the skin with a device to measure the temperature of the skin site that registers the tension in sore muscles. As the client relaxes, the blood flow increases with the temperature rise. After 10 to 12 sessions, the biofeedback procedure becomes so ingrained that the client is able to call on it whenever pain relief is needed. Currently, biofeedback of four different types is being used to control chronic pain.

1. Electroencephalographic (EEG) feedback
2. Skin temperature feedback
3. Cephalic blood volume–pulse feedback
4. Electromyographic feedback

The Association for Applied Psychophysiology and Biofeedback (www.aapb.org) recommends the use of biofeedback for controlling pain for migraine headaches, tension headaches, certain types of chronic pain, disorders of the digestive system, and Raynaud's disease (refer to Chapter 15).

Relaxation

Relaxation therapy can be used to modify muscle tension that is believed to cause or exacerbate pain. The individual is taught a series of techniques for relaxation to be used any time pain occurs. Audiotapes are used in beginning practice sessions; then the person learns to relax without any assistance. Relaxation therapy is especially successful when used in conjunction with biofeedback and imagery. Almost all people experiencing pain benefit from some form of relaxation. It helps combat fatigue and muscle tension.

Imagery

Imagery is therapy used by a person experiencing pain to produce relaxation and increase the production of endorphins and enkephalins. It may consist of slow, rhythmic breathing with a mental image of comfort and relaxation. The person imagines and concentrates on a pleasant scene or experience and is taught to relax. To be effective, imagery necessitates a positive relationship to the image scene; otherwise, the imagery may only exacerbate the pain. To be effective, the guided imagery should be done for at least 5 minutes three times a day.

Hypnosis

Hypnosis is a state that resembles sleep but is induced by a hypnotist, who makes readily accepted suggestions to the client. Autohypnosis, or self-induced hypnosis, is most effective when a person is motivated—and pain is a strong motivating force. Autohypnosis can be learned in a few hours. The mechanism whereby hypnosis works is thought to be mediated by the endorphin system. It is especially useful in clients with burns. The period of pain relief from hypnosis is from 4 to 6 hours, and the time of relief is extended with repeated hypnotic reinforcement.

Transcutaneous Electrical Nerve Stimulation

Transcutaneous electrical nerve stimulation (TENS) is a therapeutic procedure in which an electrical impulse is induced in the large nerve fibers that carry nonpain information, to block or reduce the transmission of painful impulses. The electrodes are connected by lead wires to a stimulator called a TENS unit, and the frequency and intensity of the electric current can be varied. The current produces a tingling, vibrating, or buzzing sensation in the area of pain. It is used in both acute and chronic pain. For example, it may be used on a surgical client to stimulate the nonpain or noxious receptors. This is consistent with the gate control theory and explains the effectiveness of cutaneous stimulation when applied to the same area as the injury.

Massage

Massage consists of manipulation, methodical pressure, friction, and kneading of the body. A number of oils or creams may be used to increase stimulation. Massage may be performed over or around an area of pain or at trigger points. This type of treatment stimulates blood flow, induces relaxation, and increases the production of endorphins and enkephalins. Massage also promotes comfort because it promotes muscle relaxation.

Humor, Laughter, and Play

Norman Cousins, former editor of the *Saturday Review*, popularized the concept of making laughter and humor an antidote for pain. While quite ill in the hospital, he discovered he could go much longer without his pain medication when he had been doing a great deal of laughing. He watched comedy films and read humor books. Humor and laughter control pain in four ways: (1) by distracting attention, (2) by reducing tension, (3) by changing expectations, and (4) by increasing production of endorphins and enkephalins—the body's natural pain-killers.

Play is another activity that is helpful in reducing pain, even for the severely debilitated person. Play can be childlike or quite adult. Consider the following: Two toddlers, riding tricycles, approach the charge nurse on the floor of the burn unit in a major city hospital. The burns of both are obvious, but their "race" through the corridors has become part of their treatment. One child is quite concerned over the loss of his baseball hat—a gift to all the children from a major league team. The reason for the concern? All the children were leaving shortly to play ball with one of the therapists. Who can play ball without a cap? The tricycle race and the game afterwards focus the child's attention on play—not on pain.

Music

Physicians and dentists have discovered that music helps to alleviate pain. Dentists know that some clients are receptive enough to music to have their teeth extracted without anesthesia. Some hospitals allow music to be piped into their surgical rooms because it puts both clients and practitioners in a more relaxed state.

John Diamond, MD, practices preventive medicine and psychiatry in Valley Cottage, New York, and spent more than 25 years researching music and its therapeutic value and life-enhancing quality. His books, *The Life Energy in Music*, Volumes 1, 2 and 3, would be particularly interesting to any person seeking more knowledge about music therapy and its healing powers.

Acupuncture

Acupuncture, which originated in China more than 5000 years ago, began to receive attention in Western culture in the 1970s and was approved by the U.S. Food and Drug Administration (FDA) in 1997. Acupuncture is a technique for treating certain painful conditions and for producing regional anesthesia via the passage of long, thin needles through the skin to specific points. The free ends of the needles are twirled or, in some cases, used to conduct a weak electric current. Most acupuncturists use only 10 to 12 needles per treatment, and the person feels only a slight pricking sensation when the sterile, disposable needles are inserted. The treatment is painless and can take anywhere from a few seconds to 45 minutes.

Acupuncture appears to stimulate release of the body's natural painkillers, endorphins and enkephalins. It has been suggested that acupuncture influences the production and distribution of neurotransmitters and neuromodulators, which in turn modifies the person's perception of pain. Acupuncture, used as treatment for pain, is most effective in the treatment of postoperative pain, dental pain following surgery, neck pain, myofascial pain syndrome, muscle tension headaches, and migraines.

Aromatherapy

Aromatherapy is the use of essential oils found in plants and herbs to relieve pain. This therapy is used extensively in Europe. Some believe the effects of the oils come from their pharmacologic properties and their small molecular size, making them easier to penetrate the body tissues. Health-care professionals may use essential oils in massage to relieve pain and induce sleep. Oil baths, hot and cold compresses, or a simple topical application can also help alleviate pain.

Therapeutic Touch

Therapeutic touch is a technique that has been taught to thousands of practitioners. The practitioner begins the therapeutic touch session with a client assessment wherein the practitioner places his or her hands 2 to 6 inches above the client's body and makes slow, rhythmic hand motions so that the client's blockages in the energy field can be found. The practitioner's hand motions then replenish the client's energy field.

The session lasts about 20 to 25 minutes. In therapeutic touch, there usually is no physical touching of the client. Sometimes, however, touching may be necessary, especially in pain associated with fractures or physical trauma. Proper use of therapeutic touch has been shown to reduce pain and ease problems associated with the autonomic nervous system.

Yoga Therapy

Yoga, which means "union," is a system of beliefs and practices, the goal of which is to teach mind and body unity. In the Western world, yoga generally is associated with physical postures, relaxation, and regulation of breathing. These are yoga exercises, rather than yoga in the spiritual sense. Yoga is often used in the treatment of pain to promote relaxation, aid circulation, reduce fatigue, lower blood pressure, regulate heart rate, stimulate particular body areas, strengthen muscles, and develop flexibility. For the best results, the regimen has to be practiced regularly.

Summary

Despite its multitude of forms and sometimes highly subjective qualities, pain is real. Pain should be understood and accepted in the terms of the person experiencing it. Each person experiences pain differently. Pain should be managed as aggressively as is its cause. The health professional and the person in pain should be willing to investigate many forms of pain management and seek the one or ones that best suit the individual's needs.

Finally, a useful attitude toward pain management is captured in the following statement by David Black in *The Laughter Prescription*: "Pain is an energy monster, we give it the power to hurt us. And we take that power away—depending on how we choose to view ourselves. All pain is real, but you can change your reality."

CASE STUDIES

■ Case Study 1

Brenda, a 56-year-old carpenter, injured her back years ago, had major surgery, and felt "normal" within 6 months. She returned to work and for 3 years was accident free. Then she reinjured her back four times within a 3-year period. Physical therapy and analgesia were unsatisfactory. Her physician referred her to a multidisciplinary pain clinic. Brenda decided to go to the pain clinic when she began missing too much work and could not pay her bills. At the pain clinic she saw a medical doctor, a psychologist, a social worker, an occupational therapist, and a pharmacist. Her husband was involved in the pain assessment as well and was interviewed separately by team members. At the end of the day-long session, Brenda and her husband met with the team, when they discussed their findings and detailed their treatment plan.

Case Study Questions

1. What do you think the team advised Brenda to do?
2. Why do you think the team involved her husband?
3. What else would you advise?

■ Case Study 2

John, a 35-year-old stockbroker, is near death. His 1-year treatment for pancreatic cancer has been discontinued. He rates his pain as a 9 on a scale of 1 to 10. He is not receiving the maximum dosage of opioids that he could receive. When you as a health professional talk with him, John says, "My wife says I'm strong enough to take it." John's wife is his main caregiver.

Case Study Questions

1. Discuss the assessment of John's pain. Can further pain assessments be done?
2. What strategies would you use working with John? And his wife?

■ Case Study 3

Ten-year-old Madison was riding the brand-new scooter she received from her parents as a birthday gift. Going down a rather steep hill, Madison could not maneuver the scooter around the curve at the base of the hill and side-swiped a tree. Her parents rushed her to the emergency department, where she was treated and sent home with instructions for her care, including a medication for pain. Her parents gave her the acetaminophen every 3 to 4 hours, but it was not adequately addressing her pain. The physician from the emergency department did not want the parents to administer any other medication because it could mask further symptoms.

Case Study Question

1. What other alternative therapies could be used to relieve Madison's pain?

REVIEW QUESTIONS

True/False

Circle the correct answer:

T **F** 1. A person's past pain experiences influence his or her current pain experiences.

T **F** 2. Culture influences how a person perceives pain.

T **F** 3. The longer the duration of pain, the greater is the occurrence of depression.

T **F** 4. Males experience more pain-related symptoms than do females.

T **F** 5. Elderly clients generally require lower doses of pain medication due to their greater ratio of body fat to muscle mass.

Matching

Match the following by placing the correct letter in the column:

_____ 1. Place hands 2 to 6 inches above client, make rhythmic movements

_____ 2. System of beliefs, teaching mind-body unity

_____ 3. Use slow rhythmic breathing with mental image of comfort

_____ 4. Slow rhythmic breathing exercises to decrease muscle tension

_____ 5. State that resembles sleep with suggestions to clients

a. Relaxation

b. Therapeutic touch

c. Hypnosis

d. Imagery

e. Yoga therapy

Short Answer

1. The 1 to 10 scale is a tool for _____.

2. List three major barriers to effective pain management according to the AHRQ:

   a.

   b.

   c.

3. _____ are morphine-like drugs used to control pain.

4. _____ is a type of pain describing clients who have cancer.

5. _____ describes how pain is transformed from stimuli the body receives into actual pain sensation.

Multiple Choice

Place a checkmark next to the correct answer:

1. Which of the following is/are alternative therapy/therapies for the management of pain?

    a. TENS

    b. Hypnosis

    c. Acupuncture

    d. b and c

    e. a, b, and c

2. Biofeedback is an alternative therapy in the treatment of pain for:

    a. Epilepsy

    b. Low blood sugar

    c. Migraine headaches

    d. a and c

    e. a, b, and c

3. Which of the following is/are a variable(s) to be considered when managing a client's pain?

    a. Cultural background

    b. Anxiety and depression

    c. Early pain experiences

    d. a and c

    e. a, b, and c

4. The process(es) of nociception pain process includes which of the following?

    a. Transmission

    b. Modulation

    c. Perceptive pain

    d. a and c

    e. a, b, and c

5. Which of the following statements is true of acute pain?

    a. It usually lasts less than 1 year.

    b. It usually is a result of surgical pain.

    c. It usually is continuous and intermittent.

    d. It serves no useful purpose.

Discussion Questions/Personal Reflection

1. Identify the two definitions of pain given in the text. Define what pain means to you.

2. Of the pain therapies outlined in the text, which have you tried? What works best for you? Which would you like to try the next time you have acute pain? Chronic pain? Which therapy would you never try and why?

Notes

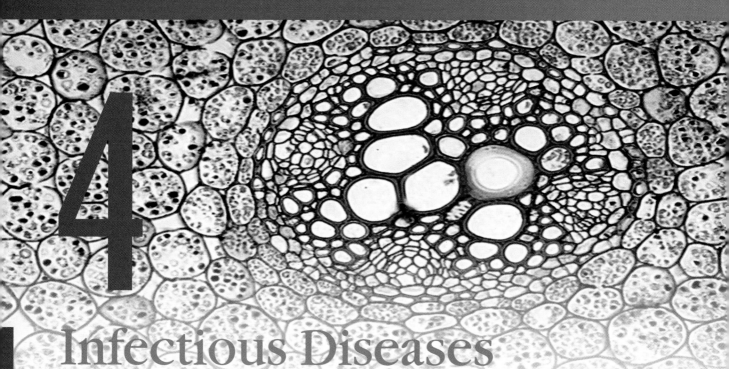

4

Infectious Diseases

CHAPTER OUTLINE

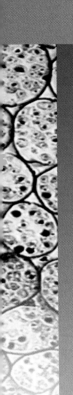

KEY WORDS

Anorexia (ăn•ō•rěk´sē•ă)
Antipruritic (ăntĭ•proo•rĭt´ĭk)
Antipyretic (ăn•tĭ•pī•rět´ĭk)
Arthralgia (ăr•thrăl´jē•ă)
Exanthems (ěg´zăn•thěm)
Leukopenia (loo•kō •pē´nē •ă)
Macule (măk´ūl)
Maculopapular (măk•ū•lō•păp´ū•lăr)
Myalgia (mī•ăl´jē•ă)
Nonvirulent (nŏn•vĭr´ū•lěnt)
Orchitis (ŏr•kī´tĭs)
Papule (păp´ūl)
Pulse oximetry (pŭls ok•sěm´ĭ•trē
Retrovirus (rět´rō•vi•rŭs)
Rhinitis (rī•nī´tĭs)
Scotomata (skă´tō•mă•tă)
Spirochete (spī´rō-kēt)
Vesicle (věs´ĭ•kl)

> *What is to give light must endure burning.*
>
> —VIKTOR E. FRANKL

LEARNING OBJECTIVES

Upon successful completion of this chapter, you will be able to:

- Name and define four emerging infectious diseases.
- Recall the etiology of malaria.
- Restate the preventative methods for West Nile virus.
- Describe variola smallpox.
- Identify the transmission of monkeypox.
- Discuss the etiology of hantavirus pulmonary syndrome
- Identify the etiology and three stages of Lyme disease.
- Discuss the foodborne infection caused by *Escherichia coli* O157:H7.
- Discuss the spread of multidrug-resistant organisms.
- Discuss alternative therapies for the treatment of colds.
- Describe the treatment of influenza.
- Discuss the infectious characteristics of severe acute respiratory syndrome (SARS).
- Define *chronic fatigue syndrome.*
- Restate at least six signs or symptoms of chronic fatigue syndrome.
- Discuss the etiology of human immunodeficiency virus (HIV)/acquired immunodeficiency syndrome (AIDS).
- Recall the incidence of HIV/AIDS in the United States and the world.
- List the most common communicable diseases of childhood and adolescence.
- Recall the etiology of infectious diarrheal diseases.
- Recall the signs and symptoms of measles.
- Distinguish rubeola measles and rubella.
- Describe the infectious period of erythema infectiosum (Fifth disease).
- Define the classic symptoms of mumps.
- Describe the treatment of varicella.
- Explain measures to prevent diphtheria.
- Discuss the two stages of pertussis.
- Describe the signs and symptoms of tetanus.

As we learned in Chapter 1, infection is a major cause of disease. An infectious disease occurs whenever a pathogenic microorganism finds a suitable environment for growth in an appropriate host. A *communicable* (or *contagious*) *disease* is an infectious disease that is readily transmitted from one individual to another, either directly or indirectly. Table 4.1 lists several communicable diseases and their methods of transmission. The authors have used the Centers for Disease Control and Prevention Website (CDC) (www.cdc.gov/) to provide the most up-to-date information on emerging and communicable diseases.

Modern sanitation methods, immunizations, and potent antibiotics have not eradicated infectious diseases. Persons can refuse immunizations, and some infections are resistant to antibiotics; hence, infections flourish. Every hour, 1,500 people worldwide die of an old or a new infectious disease, and more than half of those are children younger than 5 years. According to a report from the Institute of Medicine, a research arm of the U.S. government, there are 13 factors for the surge in new infectious diseases within the past 30 years. These 13 factors are as follows:

- Microbial adaptation and change
- Human susceptibility to infection
- Climate and weather
- Changing ecosystems
- Human demographics and behavior
- Economic development and land use
- International travel and commerce
- Technology and industry
- Breakdown of public health measures
- Poverty and social inequality
- War and famine
- Lack of political will and clout
- Biological warfare

Regardless of the precautions we take, microbes continue to be virulent, appear in unsuspecting places, and cause infection to be a serious illness.

Communicable diseases demand an extra measure of caution. It is helpful to know the infectious period for the disease, so that anyone who has been exposed can be alerted. Isolation may be necessary to prevent further exposure. Table 4.2 shows the incubation period, the onset and duration, and the suggested isolation period for several contagious infections.

Table 4.1

METHODS OF TRANSMISSION OF SOME COMMON COMMUNICABLE DISEASES

DISEASE	HOW AGENT LEAVES THE BODY	HOW ORGANISMS MAY BE TRANSMITTED	METHOD OF ENTRY INTO THE BODY
Acquired immunodeficiency syndrome (AIDS)	Blood, semen, or other body fluids, including breast milk	Sexual contact Contact with blood or mucous membranes or by way of contaminated syringes Placental transmission	Reproductive tract Contact with blood Placental transmission Breastfeeding
Cholera	Feces	Water or food contaminated with feces	Mouth to intestine
Diphtheria	Sputum and discharges from nose and throat Skin lesions (rare)	Droplet infection from patient coughing	Through mouth or nose to throat
Gonococcal disease	Discharges from infected mucous membranes	Sexual activity	Reproductive tract or any mucous membrane

(Continued on following page)

Disease	How Agent Leaves the Body	How Organisms May Be Transmitted	Method of Entry Into the Body
Hepatitis A, viral	Feces	Food or water contaminated with feces	Mouth to intestine
Hepatitis B, viral and delta hepatitis	Blood and serum-derived fluids, including semen and vaginal fluids	Contact with blood and body fluids	Exposure to body fluids including during sexual activity Contact with blood
Hepatitis C	Blood and other body fluids	Parenteral drug use Laboratory exposures to blood Health-care workers exposed to blood (e.g., dentists and their assistants and clinical and laboratory staff)	Infected blood Contaminated needles Cuts; mucosal exposures
Hookworm	Feces	Cutaneous contact with soil polluted with feces Eggs in feces hatch in sandy soil.	Larvae enter through skin (especially of feet), migrate through the body, and settle in small intestine.
Influenza	As for pneumonia	Respiratory droplets or objects contaminated with discharges	As for pneumonia
Leprosy	Cutaneous or mucosal lesions that contain bacilli Respiratory droplets	Cutaneous contact or nasal discharges of untreated patients	Nose or broken skin
Measles (rubeola)	As for streptococcal pharyngitis	As for streptococcal pharyngitis	As for streptococcal pharyngitis
Meningitis, meningococcal	Discharges from nose and throat	Respiratory droplets	Mouth and nose
Mumps	Discharges from infected glands and mouth	Respiratory droplets and saliva	Mouth and nose
Ophthalmia neonatorum (gonococcal infection of eyes of newborn)	Vaginal secretions of infected mother	Contact with infected areas of vagina of infected mother during birth	Directly on conjunctiva
Pertussis	Discharges from respiratory tract	Respiratory droplets	Mouth to nose
Pneumonia	Sputum and discharges from nose and throat	Respiratory droplets	Through mouth and nose to lungs
Poliomyelitis	Discharges from nose and throat, and via feces	Respiratory droplets Contaminated water	Through mouth and nose
Rubella	As for streptococcal pharyngitis	As for streptococcal pharyngitis	As for streptococcal pharyngitis
Streptococcal pharyngitis	Discharges from nose and throat	Respiratory droplets	Through mouth and nose

(Continued on following page)

Table 4.1 (Continued)

METHODS OF TRANSMISSION OF SOME COMMON COMMUNICABLE DISEASES

DISEASE	HOW AGENT LEAVES THE BODY	HOW ORGANISMS MAY BE TRANSMITTED	METHOD OF ENTRY INTO THE BODY
Syphilis	Lesions	Sexual intercourse; contact with skin or mucous membrane lesions	Directly into blood and tissues through breaks in skin or membrane
	Blood	Contaminated needles and syringes	Contaminated needles and syringes
	Transfer through placenta to fetus		
Trachoma	Discharges from infected eyes	Cutaneous contact Hands, towels, handkerchiefs	Directly on conjunctiva
Tuberculosis, bovine		Milk from infected cow	Mouth to intestine
Tuberculosis, human	Sputum	Droplet infection from person coughing with mouth uncovered	Through nose to lungs and intestines
Typhoid fever	Feces and urine	Food or water contaminated with feces, or urine from patients	Through mouth via infected food or water and thence to intestinal tract

Source: Thomas, CL (ed): Taber's Cyclopedic Medical Dictionary, ed 19. FA Davis, Philadelphia, 2001, pp 586–587, with permission.

Medical personnel and hospital staff members are required to notify county and state health departments of confirmed cases of certain communicable diseases. Such reporting helps to monitor epidemics and alerts the medical community to special problems.

EMERGING AND REEMERGING INFECTIOUS DISEASES

The CDC identifies diseases as "emerging and reemerging infectious diseases" when the incidence in humans has increased within the past two decades or threatens to increase in the near future. Many factors may be responsible for this emergence and are similar to those from the Institute of Medicine discussed earlier:

- Global trauma
- Globalization of food supply
- Population growth and increased urban crowding
- War, famine, and natural disaster
- Antimicrobial resistance
- Breakdown in public health measures

Some diseases are increasingly seen in this country because of world travel; some diseases are of concern because of the threat of biological warfare.

Little information is available on alternative therapies for any of the emerging infectious diseases and disorders. It is essential for the individual person to seek immediate medical attention from a primary care physician, who will provide care and treatment for a specific causative agent. Alternative therapies, integrative medicine, or both are likely to encourage client comfort with proper nutrition, fluid balance, and symptomatic treatment.

Table 4.2

INCUBATION AND ISOLATION PERIODS FOR COMMON INFECTIONS*

INFECTION	INCUBATION PERIOD	ISOLATION OF PATIENT†
AIDS	Unclear; antibodies appear within 1–3 months of infection	Protective isolation if T-cell count is very low; enteric precautions with severe diarrhea; private room only necessary with severe diarrhea, bleeding, copious blood tinged sputum if patient has poor personal hygiene habits
Bloodstream (bacteremia fungemia)	Variable; usually 2–5 days	
Brucellosis	Highly variable; usually 5–21 days; may be months	None
Chickenpox	2–3 weeks	1 week after vesicles appear or until vesicles become dry
Cholera	A few hours to 5 days	Enteric precautions
Common cold	12 hours–5 days	None
Dysentery, amebic	From a few days to several months, commonly 2–4 weeks	None
Dysentery, bacillary (e.g., shigellosis)	12–96 hours	As long as stools remain positive
Encephalitis, mosquito-borne	5–15 days	None
Giardiasis	3–25 days or longer; median 7–10 days	Enteric precautions
Gonorrhea	2–7 days; may be longer	No sexual contact until cured
Hepatitis A	15–50 days	Enteric (gloves with infected material; gowns as needed to protect clothing)
Hepatitis B	45–180 days	Blood and body fluid precautions (gloves and plastic gowns for contact with infective materials; mask if risk of coughing or sneezing exists)
Hepatitis C	14–180 days	As for hepatitis B
Hepatitis D	2–8 weeks	As for hepatitis B
Hepatitis E	15–64 days	Enteric precautions
Influenza	1–3 days	As practical
Legionella	2–10 days	None
Lyme disease	3–32 days after tick bite	None
Malaria	7–10 days for *Plasmodium falciparum*; 8–14 days for *P. vivax, P. ovale*; 7–30 days for *P. malariae*	Protection from mosquitoes
Measles (rubeola)	8–13 days from exposure to onset of fever; 14 days until rash appears	From diagnosis to 7 days after appearance of rash; strict isolation from children under 3 yr

(Continued on following page)

Table 4.2 (Continued)

INCUBATION AND ISOLATION PERIODS FOR COMMON INFECTIONS*

INFECTION	INCUBATION PERIOD	ISOLATION OF PATIENT†
Meningitis, meningococcal	2–10 days	Until 24 hours after start of chemotherapy
Mononucleosis, infectious	4–6 weeks	None; disinfection of articles soiled with nose and throat discharges
Mumps	12–25 days	Until the glands recede
Paratyphoid fevers	3 days–3 months; usually 1–3 weeks; 1–10 days for gastroenteritis	Until three stool samples are negative
Plague	2–8 days	Strict; danger of airborne spread (pneumoniae plague)
Pneumonia, pneumococcal	Believed to be 1–3 days	Enteric precautions in hospital Respiratory isolation may be required.
Puerperal fever, streptococcal	1–3 days	Transfer from maternity ward
Rabies	Usually 2–8 weeks; rarely as short as 9 days or as long as 7 years	Strict for duration of illness; danger to attendants
Rubella (German measles)	16–18 days with range of 14–23 days	None; no contact with nonimmune pregnant women
Salmonellosis	6–72 hours, usually 12–36 hours	Until stool cultures are salmonella free on two consecutive specimens collected in 24-hour period
Scabies	2–6 weeks before onset of itching in patients without previous infections; 1–4 days after reexposure	Patient is excused from school or work until day after treatment.
Trachoma	5–12 days	Until lesions disappear, but usually not practical
Tuberculosis	4–12 weeks to demonstrable primary lesion or significant tuberculin reactions	Variable, depending on conversion of sputum to negative after specific therapy and on ability of patient to understand and carry out personal hygiene methods

*Universal precautions and handwashing are assumed.
Source: Thomas, CL (ed): Taber's Cyclopedic Medical Dictionary, ed 19. FA Davis, Philadelphia, 2001, pp 1037–1038, with permission.

The emerging infectious diseases to be considered in this text are malaria, West Nile virus (WNV), smallpox, monkeypox, anthrax, and hantavirus.

Malaria

■ **DESCRIPTION** Malaria is a great masquerader and must be differentiated from other febrile illnesses.

The World Health Organization (WHO) estimates there are 300 to 500 million cases of malaria in the world and that 1 million people die from the infection. There are about 1200 cases diagnosed in the United States each year, most coming from immigrants and travelers entering the country from malaria-risk areas, such as Africa, Central and South America, Haiti, Dominican Republic, India, Southeast Asia, and the Middle East.

■ **ETIOLOGY** Malaria is transmitted from infected mosquitoes to humans. It is a protozoan disease. Once a person is bitten by an infected mosquito, parasites travel to the liver; in the cells of the liver, the parasites multiply and change into another form of parasite (merozoites). Merozoites are released from the liver and enter the red blood cells (RBCs), where they again grow and multiply, causing the RBCs to burst, which frees the parasites and their toxins to attack other RBCs.

■ **SIGNS AND SYMPTOMS** Symptoms are fever and flu-like illness, including shaking chills, headache, muscle aches, and malaise. Nausea, vomiting, and diarrhea may also occur. Malaria can cause anemia and jaundice because of the destruction of RBCs.

■ **DIAGNOSTIC PROCEDURES** The presence of the parasites in the RBCs on peripheral blood smears confirms the diagnosis. An erythrocyte sedimentation rate (ESR) and platelet count are also beneficial.

■ **TREATMENT** The medications that are effective against malaria depend on the strain of malaria diagnosed, the age of the person infected, and the severity of the illness. Antimalaria prescription medications can cure the disease. The medication also depends on resistance of the parasite to the drug, because so many strains of malaria are becoming increasingly resistant to treatment.

ALTERNATIVE THERAPY: *Herbal, Ayurvedic, and traditional Chinese medicine may help but should always be used under the guidance of a practitioner.*

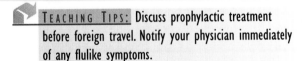

TEACHING TIPS: Discuss prophylactic treatment before foreign travel. Notify your physician immediately of any flulike symptoms.

■ **PROGNOSIS** If the person is treated promptly and correctly, the prognosis is good. However, in many developing countries, malaria is the leading cause of death. Diet and nutrition should be emphasized.

■ **PREVENTION** The best way to prevent malaria is to eliminate the malaria parasite; however, educating people about the spread of malaria is more realistic. In developing countries where mos-

quito control is ineffective, approximately 2 million deaths occur annually, with half occurring in children younger than 5 years. Hence, prompt diagnosis and early treatment are essential. Anyone who is planning to travel to countries with a malaria risk should see his or her health provider 4 to 6 weeks before travel. An antimalarial drug may be prescribed. The use of insect repellent products that contain DEET* (*N,N*-diethyl-*m*-toluamide [www.deetonline.org]) and wearing long pants and long-sleeved shirts are essential to protect against mosquito bites.

West Nile Virus

■ **DESCRIPTION** West Nile virus (WNV) or West Nile encephalitis is an infectious disease that occurs when the virus multiplies in a person's blood, crossing the blood-brain barrier and causing inflammation of the brain. WNV emerged in North America in 1999 with encephalitis reported in humans and horses. Its spread to the United States was rapid. There were 62 disease cases in humans in 1999 and 4,156 cases in 2002.

■ **ETIOLOGY** Much like malaria, WNV is transmitted to humans via the bite of an infected mosquito. Scientists believe that mosquitoes feeding on birds infected with WNV carried the disease to New York, New Jersey, and Connecticut; then it quickly spread to other states. The incubation period from infection to disease symptoms is 3 to 14 days.

■ **SIGNS AND SYMPTOMS** Symptom severity ranges from mild to severe. A mild infection includes fever, headache, body ache, skin rash, and swollen lymph glands. Severe infections include all of the mild symptoms plus stupor, disorientation, tremors, convulsions, coma, paralysis, and, rarely, death.

■ **DIAGNOSTIC PROCEDURES** The West Nile Virus IgM enzyme-linked immunosorbent assay (ELISA) is the test of choice, using a single serum sample that can give a diagnosis within a few hours. This new blood test detects antibodies to the virus that are detectable within the first few days of the onset of the infection.

---

*DEET can be used safely for several weeks. Adults may use repellents that contain 30% to 35% DEET, children should use a maximum of 10%, and infants and pregnant women should not use DEET at all.

■ **TREATMENT** There is no known therapy for West Nile encephalitis and no known cure. Treatment is aimed at alleviating the symptoms.

ALTERNATIVE THERAPY: *Alternative treatment goals are similar to treatment above. Additionally, they are designed to help individuals feel better while dealing with their symptoms.*

 TEACHING TIPS: The best prevention requires the following actions:

• Use an insect repellant that contains DEET when going out at dawn or dusk.
• Wear light, long-sleeved shirts and long pants for protection from mosquito bites.
• Empty any standing water that can become a breeding ground for mosquitoes.
• Install window and door screens.

■ **PROGNOSIS** Mild symptoms last a few days; severe symptoms can last several weeks. The neurologic effect may be permanent. Fortunately, only about 2 of every 10 individuals who are infected experience any illness. Persons over the age of 50 are particularly susceptible to the severe form of the illness.

65 ■ **PREVENTION** See Teaching Tips.

Smallpox (Variola)

■ **DESCRIPTION** Smallpox is a serious, contagious, and sometimes fatal disease caused by the variola poxvirus. Smallpox typically causes systemic disease with rash. The last naturally occurring case of smallpox occurred in Somalia in 1977; the last case in the United States was in 1949. The reason for inclusion here is because of the threat of biological warfare.

■ **ETIOLOGY** Smallpox is spread directly via infected respiratory droplets or dried scales of virus-containing lesions or indirectly through contact with contaminated linens and other objects. Classic smallpox is contagious from onset until the last scab is shed. It affects people of all ages.

■ **SIGNS AND SYMPTOMS** Signs and symptoms are easily confused with those of other diseases and include fever, abrupt onset of chills (10 to 14 days after exposure), headache, backache, severe malaise,

vomiting, and skin lesions that progress from macular to papular, vesicular, and pustular. The pustules rupture, eventually dry, and form scabs that leave permanently disfiguring scars. Two days from onset, symptoms become more severe; then, a day later, the person begins to improve. Sore throat with cough ensues. Generally, after 14 days, the symptoms subside.

■ **DIAGNOSTIC PROCEDURES** A culture of the **vesicles** and pustules confirms the presence of the variola virus. A history of known contact is helpful, as is a physical examination.

■ **TREATMENT** Treatment goals are to reduce contagion, prevent bacterial complications, and introduce symptomatic and supportive measures for the lesions. **Antipyretics** (drugs that reduce fever) and pain medications may be given during the pustular stage.

ALTERNATIVE THERAPY: *No significant alternative therapy is indicated.*

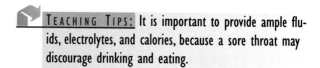 **TEACHING TIPS:** It is important to provide ample fluids, electrolytes, and calories, because a sore throat may discourage drinking and eating.

■ **PROGNOSIS** According to the CDC, in the past, 7 of every 10 smallpox clients survived.

■ **PREVENTION** On December 13, 2002, President George W. Bush, announced a smallpox vaccination program to better protect Americans against the threat of smallpox attack by hostile groups or governments. This program directs state and local health officials on responding to a smallpox emergency. In the event of an outbreak, volunteer Smallpox Response Teams (who are already vaccinated) are to provide critical services to others.

Vaccination of the general public is not recommended at this time. However, the United States currently has sufficient quantities of the vaccine for every person in an emergency.

Monkeypox

■ **DESCRIPTION** Monkeypox is a rare disease caused by the monkeypox virus, a member of the same group of viruses as smallpox virus. In July 2003, the CDC alerted the public to a never-before reported outbreak of monkeypox. Monkeypox is usually found in remote villages of central and western Africa and is thought to have been imported to the United States in a shipment of African rodents.

■ **ETIOLOGY** Monkeypox virus can spread from animals to humans when humans come into close contact with infected animals. In June 2003, monkeypox was reported among individuals who became sick after contact with prairie dogs purchased from an Illinois exotic pet dealer. Other animals that may carry the virus are tree squirrels, rope squirrels, dormice, Gambian rats, brush-tailed porcupines, and striped mice.

Monkeypox also can spread from human to human through large respiratory droplets during prolonged face-to-face contact, by touching body fluids of a sick person or animal, and by touching contaminated bedding or clothing.

■ **SIGNS AND SYMPTOMS** Clinical manifestations may be confused with those of smallpox and include a fever that develops within 1 to 3 days, followed by a rash. The rash spreads and exhibits as raised bumps that fill with fluid and then become crusty, scab over, and fall off. A fever, headache, malaise, backache, and swollen lymph nodes follow.

■ **DIAGNOSTIC PROCEDURES** According to the CDC, the laboratory tests performed for diagnosis are isolation of monkeypox virus in culture, demonstration of monkeypox virus with DNA-based assays, and demonstration of the virus with an electron microscope.

■ **TREATMENT** Treatment is largely symptomatic. Antipyretics and analgesics may be given.

ALTERNATIVE THERAPY: *No significant alternative therapy is indicated.*

> **TEACHING TIPS:** If there is exposure to monkeypox, a discussion with the primary care physician about the use of the smallpox vaccine is warranted. Educate your clients regarding good hygiene and handwashing.

■ **PROGNOSIS** If diagnosed and treated early, the prognosis is good; however, monkeypox can cause death.

■ **PREVENTION** The CDC reports that the smallpox vaccine administered after exposure to monkey-pox may help prevent the disease or make it less severe. Also, the smallpox vaccine is effective in protecting people against monkeypox if administered before they are exposed. Not all persons should receive the smallpox vaccination, especially those with weakened immune systems or those allergic to the ingredients in the vaccine.

Anthrax

■ **DESCRIPTION** Anthrax is an infection that can occur in three forms: cutaneous or skin, inhalation, and gastrointestinal. Farmers and ranchers have been keenly aware of anthrax for many years because of possible exposure to infected cattle and sheep; the cutaneous form of the disease is most common in animals.

■ **ETIOLOGY** Humans develop anthrax after exposure to infected animals or tissue from infected animals and by direct exposure to *Bacillus antracis.* Contact with infected tissue likely occurs during postmortem examination, slaughter, or handling of infected meat or hides. The first cutaneous anthrax in the United States was reported in 1992. Inhalation anthrax is rare but received high publicity in 2001, when it was found in mail that had been distributed to members of the U.S. Senate and to national news media personnel. Gastrointestinal anthrax is the result of consumption of contaminated meat, but there have been no confirmed cases in the United States.

■ **SIGNS AND SYMPTOMS** Cutaneous anthrax infection occurs when the bacterium enters a cut on the skin, causing a raised itchy bump that resembles an insect bite but quickly develops into a vesicle; a painless ulcer usually develops within 1 to 2 days. Symptoms of inhalation anthrax usually resemble those of a cold, with sore throat, mild fever, muscle aches, and malaise. Severe breathing problems and shock can occur. Gastrointestinal anthrax is characterized by acute inflammation of the intestinal tract.

■ **DIAGNOSTIC PROCEDURES** Laboratory diagnosis consists of isolation and confirmation of *B. antracis* from a clinical specimen collected from an affected tissue site. Other laboratory tests include evidence of the *B. antracis* DNA by polymerase chain reaction (PCR) and immunohistochemical staining. A chest x-ray can be used to diagnose inhalation anthrax. Nasal swabs of potentially exposed persons may help determine the extent of exposure.

■ **TREATMENT** Cutaneous anthrax is treated with antibiotic therapy of penicillin or doxycycline. Broad-spectrum antimicrobial agents are beneficial in inhalation anthrax. All treatment should be under the strict supervision of a physician, especially because prolonged treatment is necessary.

ALTERNATIVE THERAPY: *No significant alternative therapy is indicated other than supportive measures to keep individuals comfortable.*

TEACHING TIPS: The fear that a client senses when exposed to inhalation anthrax is real and must be considered in treatment. Help educate the client and family that taking the full course of antibiotics is essential and that treatment may last for some time.

■ **PROGNOSIS** Early treatment of cutaneous anthrax is usually curative; the fatality rate without antibiotics is about 20%. Even with appropriate antimicrobial agents to treat inhalation anthrax, the mortality rate can be as high as 75%.

■ **PREVENTION** The only prevention is postexposure prophylaxis, which includes the use of broad-spectrum antimicrobial agents given under the strict supervision of a physician.

Hantavirus Pulmonary Syndrome

■ **DESCRIPTION** Hantavirus pulmonary syndrome (HPS) is a viral infection that presents with flu-like symptoms.

■ **ETIOLOGY** HPS is caused by hantavirus, which was first isolated in 1977 and first occurred in disease form in the southwestern United States in 1993. The hantavirus strain that causes disease in Europe and Asia is distinctly different than the strain in the United States. HPS is transmitted by rodents, which shed the virus in their urine, droppings, and saliva. People then breathe in contaminated air with the virus when the fresh rodent urine, droppings or nesting materials are stirred up. The tiny droplets become airborne through a process called aerosolization. Rarely does a rodent infect a human through biting and the virus is not transmitted from person to person.

■ **SIGNS AND SYMPTOMS** In general, the signs and symptoms develop within 1 and 5 weeks after exposure to potentially infected rodents and their droppings. Early symptoms include headache, dizziness, chills, and abdominal problems such as nausea, vomiting, diarrhea, and abdominal pain. Deep muscle pain occurs in most cases. Four to 10 days later, symptoms include coughing and shortness of breath. Persons may describe a sensation of a "tight band around the chest and a pillow over their face" due to the lungs filling with fluid. Respiratory distress occurs, and respiratory failure can result.

■ **DIAGNOSTIC PROCEDURES** The CDC uses an ELISA to detect IgM antibodies to specific viral antigens (SNVs) and to diagnose acute infections with other hantaviruses. This test plus a compatible history of exposure to hantavirus is considered diagnostic for HPS.

■ **TREATMENT** There is no specific treatment or cure for hantavirus infection. In all cases, symptomatic treatment includes immediate hospitalization so that the respiratory symptoms can be handled by intubation and oxygen therapy as soon as possible.

ALTERNATIVE THERAPY: *No significant alternative therapy is indicated.*

TEACHING TIPS: Because the symptoms are so similar to those of many other illnesses, it can be helpful to question your clients about their workplace, recent travel, or possible exposure to rodent droppings.

■ **PROGNOSIS** HPS has a high mortality due to respiratory failure.

■ **PREVENTION** The best prevention is to make the environment free of rodents or to minimize contact with them. For example, if camping, keep food and nesting-type material in sealed containers. If a place becomes infected with rodents, disinfect immediately.

Lyme Disease

■ **DESCRIPTION** Lyme disease is caused by *Borrelia burgdorferi,* a tick-transmitted **spirochete**, or bacterium, that has a slender, spiral shape. The disease occurs in stages. Each stage has different clinical manifestations, and between stages there may be remissions and exacerbations. Lyme disease was named for Lyme, Connecticut, a town in which it was

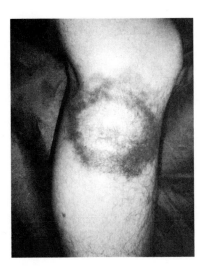

Figure 4.1 Lyme disease rash. (From Thomas, CL [ed]: Taber's Cyclopedic Medical Dictionary, ed 19. FA Davis, Philadelphia, 2001, p 1214, with permission.)

first recognized in 1975. The incidence has increased, and although the disease has spread west, most cases have occurred in the northeastern United States.

■ **ETIOLOGY** *B. burgdorferi* is carried by pinhead-sized ticks found on the white-tailed deer, the white-footed mouse, and even raccoons, rabbits, dogs, horses, cattle, migrating birds, mosquitoes, and flies. The tick injects its saliva into the host's bloodstream, or it deposits fecal material on the skin (Fig. 4.1).

■ **SIGNS AND SYMPTOMS** Stage I signs include a rash called erythema chronicum migrans (ECM), which appears at the site of the bite. ECM is very distinct, with a dark-red rim and faded center. ECM does not occur in all cases. Other signs of stage I include flulike symptoms such as fatigue, headache, fever, chills, stiff neck, and joint and muscle pain, which can last from several weeks to several months. Stage II symptoms affect the central nervous system, causing such diverse problems as meningitis, nerve damage, and facial palsy. Stage III symptoms include chronic arthritis and continuing neurologic problems. Stage I usually lasts for several weeks; stage II occurs during the following several months; and stage III occurs months to years after the onset of the initial infection. Except for fatigue and lethargy, which are often constant, the early signs of the disease are typically intermittent and changing.

■ **DIAGNOSTIC PROCEDURES** Blood tests are used to assist in diagnosis; however, it can take more than 6 weeks for the antibodies to appear in the blood, making diagnosis by this method alone inconclusive. The most common laboratory abnormalities are a high ESR, an elevated total serum IgM level, or an increased aspartate aminotransferase level.

■ **TREATMENT** The treatment of choice in all three stages is the use of antibiotics, such as penicillin, or erythromycin for those allergic to penicillin.

ALTERNATIVE THERAPY: *Along with the anitbiotic therapy, alternative medicine practitioners suggest avoidance of alcohol and sugar, because the bacteria feed on them. Proper nutrition can help bolster immune function. Practice stress reduction techniques and use herbal supplements under the guidance of a trained specialist.*

TEACHING TIPS: Because the disease occurs in stages and may have exacerbations and remissions, your client needs different support systems during the course of the disease. Encourage your client to follow the treatment plan, especially taking the medication as directed. Eating a balanced diet and drinking lots of fluids are recommended. Be sure to educate the client about exacerbations and remissions.

■ **PROGNOSIS** Although minor recurrences of headaches, musculoskeletal pain, or lethargy are consistent with the disease, eventually, complete recovery occurs with proper treatment.

■ **PREVENTION** The best prevention is to cover as much of the body as possible when in the woods. Look for tiny pinpoint specks on your body and clothing. Use an insect repellent on clothes and exposed areas of arms and hands as directed. Make certain pets who go outside have protection against fleas and ticks and inspect them after outings.

Escherichia coli O157:H7

■ **DESCRIPTION** *Escherichia coli* O157:H7 is only one of hundreds of strains of the bacterium *E. coli*. Most strains are harmless and live in the intestinal tract of healthy humans and animals, but the O157:H7 strain produces a powerful toxin and can cause serious illness. *E. coli* O157:H7 is an emerging cause of foodborne illness, with an estimated 73,000 cases of infection and 61 deaths in the United States each year. The infection, associated with eating undercooked, contaminated ground beef, consuming sprouts, lettuce, and salami, or drinking unpasteurized milk and fruit juices, often leads to bloody diarrhea.

■ **ETIOLOGY** The organism, which can be found on some cattle ranches, lives in the intestines of healthy cattle. Meat may become contaminated during slaughter. Organisms can be thoroughly mixed into beef when it is ground. Bacteria present on the cow's udders or on equipment may get into raw milk. Swimming in sewage-contaminated water also can cause infection. Bacteria in the diarrheal stools of infected persons can be passed from one person to another if handwashing and personal hygiene is inadequate.

■ **SIGNS AND SYMPTOMS** The infection causes severe bloody diarrhea and abdominal cramps, although in some cases, the person is asymptomatic. Usually no fever is present and the illness will resolve in 5 to 10 days. In elderly persons and children, the infection can cause a complication called *hemolytic uremic syndrome*. This syndrome is the leading cause of acute kidney failure in children in the United States. The syndrome is associated with death and long-term complications in a small percentage of individuals. Complications include end-stage renal disease, hypertension, or seizures, blindness, and paralysis.

■ **DIAGNOSTIC PROCEDURES** The infection from *E. coli* O157:H7 is diagnosed by detecting the bacteria in the stool. Some laboratories in the United States do not routinely test for this bacteria, and it is not considered a reportable disease in some states. Therefore, it may be necessary to request that the stool specimen be tested specifically for the organism in all individuals who suddenly have bloody diarrhea.

■ **TREATMENT** Persons with only diarrhea usually recover without specific treatment in 5 to 10 days. However, hospitalization may be necessary in severe cases, such as those with hemolytic uremic syndrome, which is life-threatening and treated aggressively. Blood transfusions and kidney dialysis are usually required.

ALTERNATIVE THERAPY: *Alternative therapy is supportive only and designed to make the client more comfortable.*

▶ **TEACHING TIPS:** The disease process may be acute or can linger with complications; hence, it is wise to educate your client to specifically follow the treatment plan. Rest, eating a balanced diet, and drinking ample fluids is recommended.

■ **PROGNOSIS** Persons with only diarrhea usually recover completely. The prognosis is good with bloody diarrhea symptoms only; it is guarded if hemolytic uremic syndrome develops. About one third of people with the syndrome either develop abnormal kidney function or require long-term dialysis.

■ **PREVENTION** Consumers can prevent the illness by cooking all ground beef thoroughly to an internal temperature of at least 160° F, by consuming only pasteurized milk and fruit juices, and by making certain that all persons, especially children, wash their hands carefully with soap and water. Washing counters, utensils, and surfaces where raw meat has been may help prevent cross-contamination. Washing fruit and vegetables thoroughly is important as well. Meat processing plants are more regulated as a result of *E. coli* O157:H7.

MULTIDRUG-RESISTANT ORGANISMS

The CDC has made drug resistance one of its target areas in their plan *Preventing Emerging Infectious Diseases: A Strategy for the 21st Century*. In their report, they recommend physicians educate parents

In 1942, *a woman was hospitalized for a month with a life-threatening streptococcal infection. One night she was delirious, and her temperature soared to almost 107 degrees F. Various treatments had been tried; none worked to break the fever. As a last resort, her physicians administered a tiny amount of penicillin, an obscure experimental drug at the time. Her hospital records showed that she had a sharp drop in temperature the following morning. This woman was the first person to receive penicillin. She lived until 1999, dying at the age of 90.*

why antibiotics should not be given for most colds, coughs, sore throats, and runny noses. The CDC is encouraging physicians to "write a prescription" for treating viral illnesses for which antibiotics would be inappropriate.

Unfortunately, the public has demanded antibiotics and physicians have continued to prescribe them, oftentimes when the specific microorganism has not yet been isolated and identified. Now, bacteria and other microorganisms have developed resistance to antimicrobial drugs both inside and outside of the hospital settings. Antibiotics are no longer the "miracle drugs" they once were. In fact, antimicrobial resistance already affects virtually all pathogens previously considered to be easily treatable.

According to the CDC, the most common organisms to develop resistance are methicillin/oxacillin-resistant *Staphylococcus aureus* (MRSA); vancomycin-resistant enterococci (VRE); extended-spectrum beta-lactamase (which is resistant to cephalosporins and monobactams; ESBL); and penicillin-resistant *Streptococcus pneumoniae* (PRSP). MRSA and VRE are more common in nonhospital health-care settings such as hemodialysis centers, long-term care facilities, and in-home care. Staphylococci are one of the most common causes of skin infections in the United States; over the years, staphylococci have become resistant to various antibiotics. PRSP is more common in physician offices and clinics, especially in pediatric settings. *Streptococcus pneumoniae* is the leading microorganism in most cases of pneumonia, otitis media and meningitis. These specific diseases are detailed in Chapter 11, "Respiratory Diseases and Disorders" (pneumonia), Chapter 13, "Nervous System Diseases and Disorders" (meningitis), and Chapter 17, "Eye and Ear Diseases and Disorders" (otitis media). MRSA tends to be more common, and is discussed here.

■ **ORIGINS OF MRSA:** An individual may have *staphylococci* present in or on the body and not cause illness. This is known as colonization. The CDC reports that approximately 25% to 30% of the population are colonized in the nose with *staphylococci* at a given time. Infection occurs when the *staphylococci* causes disease. Spread of MRSA among clients in outpatient departments generally occurs through close or direct contact with infected individuals. MRSA is not spread through the air. Indirect contact by touching contaminated objects may occur when infected towels,

wound dressings, clothes, or sports equipment are involved. Infections can result from sharing contaminated items, having recurrent skin diseases, and living in crowded areas; in addition, players in close-contact sports and persons in intimate relationships can spread infection. Sometimes it is unknown how the person contacted the infection.

Risk factors include severity of the MRSA infection, previous exposure to antimicrobial agents, invasive procedures including dialysis, repeated contact with the health-care system, any underlying diseases or conditions, children, and those who are advanced in age.

■ **SIGNS AND SYMPTOMS** Signs and symptoms depend on where the infection causes disease. For example, if the infection occurs in a wound, the wound will be painful, reddened, swollen, and warm to the touch. If the skin infection spreads to the lung causing pneumonia or to the blood stream, then the symptoms will be more systemic. Also, any antibiotic therapy prescribed may have little or no affect upon the particular illness.

■ **DIAGNOSTIC PROCEDURES** Culture and sensitivity is the best diagnostic tool strictly following The National Committee for Clinical Laboratory Standards (NCCLS) at www.nccls.org. However, it can be difficult to detect the exact organism and its sensitivity.

■ **TREATMENT** Sometimes draining a skin sore may be all the treatment that is necessary. However, in most cases, the treatment of choice is still antibiotic therapy, with doctors and pharmacists working together to determine the best antibiotic to use. Vancomycin often is the drug of choice for treatment for MRSA; however, it is not effective against VRE.

ALTERNATIVE THERAPY: *No significant alternative therapy is indicated.*

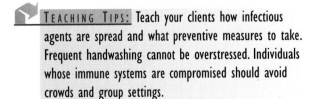

TEACHING TIPS: Teach your clients how infectious agents are spread and what preventive measures to take. Frequent handwashing cannot be overstressed. Individuals whose immune systems are compromised should avoid crowds and group settings.

■ **PROGNOSIS** MRSA can be difficult to treat and can progress to life-threatening blood or bone infections, lung infections, or skin/tissue infections.

The prognosis may also depend on how quickly or aggressively the client is treated and on the client's general health.

■ **PREVENTION** It is essential to use Universal Precautions at all times in physicians' offices, outpatient departments, group homes, schools, group activities, and other settings. Handwashing is paramount. Some urgent care facilities and outpatient departments require staff and infected clients to wear masks while in the facility. Healthy people generally are at low risk of becoming infected through casual contact. Infants and elderly people are at increased risk.

COMMUNICABLE DISEASES

Common Cold

■ **DESCRIPTION** The *common cold (acute coryza)* is an acute infection that causes inflammation of the upper respiratory tract. Colds occur more frequently in children and are the leading cause of time lost from work or school. The highest incidence of colds is during the winter months.

■ **ETIOLOGY** Colds are caused by hundreds of different viruses. These microorganisms are transmitted by airborne respiratory droplets. Some colds, however, result from infection by a group of microorganisms called *Mycoplasma*.

■ **SIGNS AND SYMPTOMS** The onset of symptoms is gradual and may include nasal congestion, pharyngitis, headache, malaise, burning and watery eyes, and low-grade fever (in children). A productive or nonproductive cough may be present. The symptoms commonly last from 2 to 4 days, but nasal congestion may persist for an indefinite period. Reinfection is common, but complications are rare. The cold is contagious for 2 to 3 days after onset.

■ **DIAGNOSTIC PROCEDURES** There is no specific diagnostic test for the common cold. Diagnosis should rule out disorders that produce similar symptoms.

■ **TREATMENT** Treatment of the cold is symptomatic and includes mild analgesics, ample fluid intake, and rest. Decongestants, nasal sprays, throat lozenges, and steam may be helpful. In a child with fever, acetaminophen is the drug of choice. If secondary bacterial infections are suspected, antibiotics

may be prescribed, but they are not a cure for the common cold.

ALTERNATIVE THERAPY: *A person with a cold will find it helpful to get extra sleep and drink large amounts of water and herbal teas, vegetable juices, and broths. Stress can increase susceptibility to disease. Saline nasal sprays will keep nasal passages moist. Baths with eucalyptus, lavender, lemon, or peppermint can be soothing to someone with a cold. The additional fluids help rehydrate the body and increase immune function. Taking additional vitamin C may prove helpful. Some find taking the herb echinacea, in tablet form or as an herbal tea, helpful during a cold. Large doses of any vitamin or herb supplement should be taken only under the supervsion of an alternative medicine practitioner or a medical doctor.*

> **TEACHING TIPS:** If clients are infectious, teach them how to minimize the transmission of their cold. Handwashing and proper care and disposal of tissues and utensils are important. Encourage the person to drink plenty of fluids and to eat a balanced diet throughout the course of the cold.

■ **PROGNOSIS** The disease is self-limiting, but it can lead to secondary bacterial infection.

■ **PREVENTION** There is no known prevention. Frequent handwashing and avoiding crowds may lessen the likelihood of contracting a cold.

Influenza

■ **DESCRIPTION** Influenza (flu) is an acute, contagious respiratory disease characterized by fever, chills, headache, and muscle pain or tenderness (**myalgia**). The disease may affect anyone, but school-age children and elderly persons are especially susceptible. Flu often occurs in epidemic outbreaks, particularly in the winter and spring.

■ **ETIOLOGY** Flu is caused by viruses that are members of the Orthomyxoviridae family. For diagnostic and treatment purposes, the viruses are classified as either type A, B, or C based on their antigenic properties. Influenza viruses frequently mutate, creating new strains that easily infect populations that had acquired immunity to previous strains of the virus.

Transmission generally occurs via cough, sneeze, hand-to-hand contact, and other personal contact.

■ **SIGNS AND SYMPTOMS** The onset generally is abrupt, with fever, chills, croup in children, malaise, muscle aches, headache, nasal congestion, laryngitis, and a cough.

■ **DIAGNOSTIC PROCEDURES** Because the signs and symptoms of flu resemble those of so many other illnesses, it is frequently difficult to diagnose solely on the basis of symptomatology, unless there is an ongoing epidemic. A throat culture may be performed to isolate the virus or to rule out bacteria, or various immunofluorescence techniques may be performed to detect viral antigens.

■ **TREATMENT** Treatment consists of bed rest, adequate fluid intake, and analgesics and antipyretics. *Note:* Aspirin should not be used to treat fever and muscle pain in children and adolescents with flu, because of its association with an increased incidence of Reye's syndrome (see Chapter 12, Cardiovascular System Diseases and Disorders, Reye's Syndrome). Acetaminophen may be given to children.

ALTERNATIVE THERAPY: *Alternative therapies noted for colds are appropriate for the treatment of influenza. The use of antibiotics is not indicated, and therefore they are to be avoided. Warm baths may relieve myalgia.*

TEACHING TIPS: Instruct the client, especially if elderly, to rest, drink ample fluids, and eat a balanced diet. It is important to handle all tissue, utensils, and bedding with the usual precautions to prevent the spread of the disease. Encourage the elderly client to continue as many of the activities of daily living as possible to avoid the need for later rehabilitation from physical inactivity.

■ **PROGNOSIS** The prognosis is good with proper care. Complications include sinusitis, otitis media, bronchitis, and pneumonia.

■ **PREVENTION** Influenza vaccines prepared from the most recent strains of A- and B-type viruses are useful in preventing these particular strains of influenza. The vaccines may produce reactions in some, especially people who are allergic to egg products or other components of the vaccine. The CDC recommends influenza vaccine for children and adults, especially those with certain risk factors, such as diabetes, cardiac disease, and asthma. Proper disposal of contaminated tissues and frequent handwashing is important.

Severe Acute Respiratory Syndrome (SARS)

■ **DESCRIPTION** Severe acute respiratory syndrome (SARS) is a respiratory illness that may present in varying degrees of severity. SARS has been reported in Asia, North America, and Europe. Physicians indicated that tourists, business travelers, and physicians carried the virus from Hong Kong to Hanoi, Singapore, and Toronto. SARS set a record for speed of continent-to-continent transmission.

■ **ETIOLOGY** The CDC has detected a previously unrecognized coronavirus in patients with SARS, and the leading hypothesis is that this virus is the infective agent. SARS is spread via close person-to-person contact, especially through respiratory secretions. Studies showed the virus survived for at least 24 hours on a plastic surface at room temperature and that the microbe remained viable for as long as 4 days in human waste. Consequently, potential ways to contact SARS include touching the skin of other people or objects that are contaminated with infectious droplets and then touching your eye(s), mouth, or nose. Most people have been infected when caring for or living with a person with SARS. Most cases of SARS in the United States have occurred among travelers returning to the country from other parts of the world where SARS has been diagnosed. Infection has also been spread as a result of close contact with family members and health-care workers.

■ **SIGNS AND SYMPTOMS** Individuals with SARS may be asymptomatic or experience a mild respiratory illness. The more moderate and severe form of SARS may begin with a temperature of greater than 100.4° F. Other symptoms include headache, an overall feeling of discomfort, and body aches. With the moderate or severe forms of SARS, people develop a dry cough, have trouble breathing, and may show evidence of pneumonia or respiratory distress syndrome (severe impairment of respiratory function). The onset of symptoms in the moderate and severe forms is generally 2 to 7 days after exposure.

■ **DIAGNOSTIC PROCEDURES** Testing should include chest radiography, **pulse oximetry**, blood and sputum cultures, and testing for viral respiratory pathogens. Any available clinical specimens should be saved for additional testing until a specific diagnosis is made. The CDC has asked medical personnel to conduct extensive laboratory testing of clinical specimens from suspected SARS clients to identify the cause of the disease. Medical personnel should contact health authorities for the most recent SARS information and for reporting purposes.

■ **TREATMENT** The CDC recommends that therapy include treatment for both typical and atypical organisms. Treatment choices generally are symptomatic and may be influenced by the severity of the illness. For example, oxygen therapy may be required as well as bed rest. It is imperative to practice frequent handwashing and to wear gloves when working with persons with SARS. The CDC has recommended, but not required, isolation of individuals with SARS. It has not required quarantine of those who have been exposed.

ALTERNATIVE THERAPY: *Alternative therapy includes additional fluids, proper nutrition with some additional supplements, and supportive measures to keep clients comfortable.*

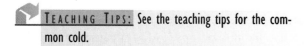 **TEACHING TIPS:** See the teaching tips for the common cold.

■ **PROGNOSIS** Thus far, in the United States, 80% to 90% of SARS clients have improved without intervention. Of the 10% to 20% who have needed inpatient intensive care, 7% to 15% have died.

■ **PREVENTION** Prevention includes good hygiene, especially in situations where someone in the family has SARS or is suspected to have SARS. Limit interactions with those suspected of having SARS. Disposable gloves and eye protection should be worn. Careful washing of shared eating utensils, towels, and bedding is good prevention as well.

IMMUNOSUPPRESSANT SYNDROMES

Chronic Fatigue Syndrome

■ **DESCRIPTION** Chronic fatigue syndrome (CFS), although not fully understood, is aptly named.

Individuals suffer from debilitating chronic fatigue, and the illness presents a host of symptoms. Another name for the illness is myalgic encephalomyelitis. The symptoms are many and varied, and individuals may suffer for weeks or even years from CFS. It is twice as prevalent in women as it is in men, and generally it affects persons 25 to 45 years of age.

■ **ETIOLOGY** There is no current agreement on the cause of CFS. It is most likely multifactorial. It was once thought to be attributed to the Epstein-Barr virus, but that hypothesis has been set aside. Viruses currently suspected include human herpesvirus 6, enteroviruses, or **retroviruses.** Other predisposing factors that may be partly responsible include the state of a person's immune system, genetic makeup, age, hormonal balance, sex, environment, and previous illness.

■ **SIGNS AND SYMPTOMS** Two major criteria must be met for CFS to be diagnosed: persistent/relapsing fatigue for at least 6 months that does not resolve with bed rest and is severe enough to reduce daily activity by at least 50%. In addition, at least 4 of the 8 following minor criteria must be present:

- Fever or chills
- Sore throat; nonexudative pharyngitis
- Painful cervical or axillary lymph nodes
- Unexplained generalized muscle weakness
- Muscle discomfort and myalgia
- Migratory **arthralgia** or joint pain without joint swelling or redness
- Neuropsychological symptoms including photophobia, forgetfulness, transient visual **scotomata** or an island-like blind spot on the visual field of the eye, irritability, confusion, depression, inability to concentrate, difficulty thinking
- Sleep disturbance
- Individual describes initial onset as acute or subacute

■ **DIAGNOSTIC PROCEDURES** A complete history and physical examination are essential for diagnosis. Laboratory testing including complete blood cell count (CBC), ESR, electrolytes, thyroid-stimulating hormone (TSH), and a urinalysis is used to rule out other possible causes. The challenge in diagnosis is that CFS remains a syndrome of symptoms and a diagnosis that comes from exclusion.

■ **TREATMENT** Treatment is supportive. The physician will want to reassess the disease process frequently so that new symptoms can be treated. Nonsteroidal anti-inflammatory drugs (NSAIDs) may be beneficial in the treatment of headache, pain, and fever. Medications to improve energy and emotional state may be used. At times, a psychiatric evaluation may be necessary if the person becomes depressed. Lifestyle changes may be needed in the areas of sleeping and exercise. A holistic approach is essential.

ALTERNATIVE THERAPY: *There are numerous recommendations for CFS. Diet is crucial to reinforcing the immune system. Clients should concentrate on high-nutrition, high-protein, complex carbohydrate foods. A basic multivitamin/ multimineral supplement with adequate amounts of trace minerals is beneficial. Herbal medications, acupuncture, and Chinese medicine have shown promise.*

TEACHING TIPS: Assure your client that although the disease may be chronic in nature, it is possible to make some lifestyle changes and live with the disease. Joining a support group may prove helpful. Encourage your client to eat a balanced diet and drink ample fluids.

■ **PROGNOSIS** The disease is debilitating and may last for months or years. Some individuals respond to a variety of treatment protocols based on symptoms. Research is under way to determine effective treatment.

■ **PREVENTION** No prevention is known.

Human Immunodeficiency Virus Infection/Acquired Immunodeficiency Syndrome

■ **DESCRIPTION** Acquired immunodeficiency syndrome (AIDS) is a severe illness associated with human immunodeficiency virus (HIV) infection. Sexual contact is the major mode of transmission of HIV, but it can also be transmitted via blood, blood products, and shared needles. In addition, infants born to HIV-infected woman may become infected before or during birth via transplacental, partuition, or postpartum transmission. The virus also can be transmitted via breast milk.

■ **ETIOLOGY** AIDS, which was first diagnosed in the United States in 1981, is caused by HIV. HIV is a member of the class of retroviruses. These very simple viruses carry their genetic material in the form of ribonucleic acid (RNA) rather than DNA. HIV predominantly infects cells called T4 lymphocytes (T4-helper cells), which are critical to the operation of the body's immune system. HIV replicates by taking over the genetic machinery of the T cell it invades. The replication process continues until the host cell is destroyed. The newly produced HIV-infected cells can then infect other T4 lymphocytes. This progressive and inevitable destruction of T4 cells leaves the body open to opportunistic infections.

In the United States, the majority of individuals with AIDS are male homosexuals and bisexuals; the next largest group consists of intravenous drug users. Other individuals with AIDS include children born to mothers infected with HIV, sexual partners of those infected with HIV, and persons who have received blood products and transfusions infected with HIV (before screening of blood and blood products was possible).

■ **SIGNS AND SYMPTOMS** After exposure to HIV, the majority of individuals experience no recognizable symptoms. Some persons, however, may develop a mononucleosis-like syndrome characterized by fever and flulike symptoms. The syndrome resolves spontaneously, with seroconversion usually occurring 8 to 10 weeks later. When symptoms of HIV occur later, the most common are generalized persistent lymphadenopathy, weight loss, fever, fatigue, neurologic symptoms such as opportunistic infections, and malignancy.

The pulmonary, gastrointestinal, and neurologic systems may be involved, and several forms of malignancy and chronic illnesses may result.

Pulmonary symptoms include shortness of breath, dyspnea, coughing, chest pain, and fever; usually caused by a variety of opportunistic infections. The most common pulmonary infection is *Pneumocystis jiroveci* (formerly *Pneumocystis carinii*) pneumonia, which has a high mortality rate. There is an increased incidence of tuberculosis.

Gastrointestinal symptoms of AIDS may include loss of appetite, nausea, vomiting, oral and esophageal candidiasis, and chronic diarrhea or gastroenteritis. Diarrhea occurs in more than half of all clients with AIDS.

Neurological symptoms may include memory loss, headache, depression, fever, confusion, and visual disturbances. Dementia and depression may also be seen.

Malignancies commonly associated with AIDS include Kaposi's sarcoma, a neoplasm evidenced by multiple vascular nodules in the skin and other organs. This malignant neoplasm is especially prevalent in the lymph nodes, the gastrointestinal tract, and the lungs. The purple lesions characterizing Kaposi's sarcoma may appear on the skin and grow rapidly until wounds are produced, which increase the client's susceptibility to infections. Studies show that women infected with HIV experience a higher incidence of cervical cancer.

Chronic illness results because AIDS sufferers are often severely immunocompromised. Nearly all infected persons will eventually develop one or more chronic opportunistic infections during the course of the disease. Such illnesses may complicate treatment and produce debilitating symptoms.

■ **DIAGNOSTIC PROCEDURES** The most widely used screening test is the ELISA, followed by the Western blot test for confirmation. These tests can take several days for results. Additional tests to help evaluate the severity of immunosuppression may be performed. In November 2002, the U.S. Food and Drug Administration approved a test for HIV that can return results in 20 minutes, known as OraQuick Rapid HIV-1 Antibody Test (Abbott Laboratories). This blood test uses a plastic stick that stains red-purple in the presence of HIV. A positive HIV test does not mean that a person has AIDS.

It is necessary to obtain a complete client history (including risk factors) and to perform a physical examination. Laboratory studies are essential to determine the extent of immune system impairment, the presence of any opportunistic infections, and the presence of HIV antibodies.

According to the CDC, the disease progression of HIV infection can be measured even before symptoms occur. A diagnosis of AIDS is made by a physician using certain clinical and laboratory criteria. When HIV establishes itself in the body, the number of CD4 lymphocytes begins to decline. If the number falls below 300, individuals are at heightened risk for one or more opportunistic infections. If the CD4 cell number drops below 200, an individual is said to have AIDS.

■ **TREATMENT** There is no cure for AIDS. Currently there is no effective treatment to stop the HIV infection and the immunodeficiency it causes. Through research, zidovudine (AZT), didanosine (DDI), and other antiretroviral drugs were developed, which impair the ability of HIV to insert itself into a host cell. Protease inhibitors, another class of antiretroviral agents, have greatly increased life expectancy for persons with AIDS. HIV resistance to some antivirial agents prompts the need for combination of alternating therapies with multiple aniretroviral agents. It is important to manage the opportunistic infections and malignancies as aggressively as possible, using antimicrobial agents for infections and radiation therapy or chemotherapy for the malignancies. Chronic illnesses may require symptomatic treatment for malnutrition, weakness, immobility, diarrhea, skin lesions, and altered mental state.

ALTERNATIVE THERAPY: *Treatment focuses on the prevention of opportunistic infections, and alternative therapies focus on enhancing overall health. Vitamin supplementation with herbal medicines may be tried. Acupuncture has shown success in reducing fatigue, night sweats, and diarrhea. Mind-body therapies have shown promise, because there is such an important relationship between an individual's emotional state and his or her immune system. Massage can improve circulation as well as reduce emotional and mental stress.*

TEACHING TIPS: Encourage your client to join an HIV/AIDS support group in the local area; this will provide education, support, and resource information that could prove invaluable. Although the medication regimen can be daunting, teach your client the importance of following the regimen as closely as possible. Eating a balanced diet is important, as is an exercise program to fit the individual's needs. Because financial resources may be limited due to the cost of treatment, a referral to a social worker may be helpful.

■ **PROGNOSIS** Recurrent bouts of opportunistic infections, with or without malignancies, usually cause the death of individuals with AIDS. In the United States, the number of deaths attributed to HIV infection fell 42% from 1996 to 1997. The decline has since leveled off, with 15,000 dying of AIDS in the United States in 2001. Worldwide statistics are dismal; everyday, 14,000 people worldwide are infected with HIV, which is a total of 15 million people who are infected per year. Approximately 50% of the 42 million people infected in the world are women. There has been growing evidence of a "superinfection" with more than one strain of HIV. Such a superinfection makes the development of a vaccine a serious challenge.

■ **PREVENTION** After years of research, there is still no effective vaccine against the infection. Education is the first defense against this epidemic. To avoid exposure to HIV, a person should practice safe sex. The use of latex condoms for any form of sexual intercourse is essential. Body fluids and items such as used hypodermic needles should be considered potentially infective. Health-care workers must practice Universal Precautions when handling blood and body fluids. Eliminating risk factors for HIV-infected people can be as beneficial as treating the HIV infection. Eliminating malnutrition and needle sharing among drug users is extremely important, and purifying blood-clotting factors for hemophiliacs has been very beneficial.

COMMUNICABLE DISEASES OF CHILDHOOD AND ADOLESCENCE

 Infectious Diarrheal Diseases

■ **DESCRIPTION** Infectious diarrheal disease usually affects children under 5 years of age. The disease can be highly contagious and occurs frequently in day care centers. It is estimated that more than 20 million episodes of infectious diarrheal diseases occur in children younger than 5 years and that 400 deaths per year occur as a result.

■ **ETIOLOGY** Diarrheal infections generally are transmitted via the oral-fecal route and possibly respiratory. Individuals have natural defenses to combat pathogens taken in while eating, including normal flora, gastric acid, intestinal motility, and cellular immunity. However, when an individual ingests more than the host can combat, infection occurs. The incubation period from ingestion to infection generally is 48 hours. The most common causative agents are rotaviruses and bacteria; the latter include *E. coli* O157:H7, *Salmonella, Shigella, Campylobacter,* and *Yersinia* spp. Parasitic infections can also cause infectious diarrheal disease, generally from contaminated food and drink ingested by people who travel to high-risk areas in other countries of the world. Parasitic organisms include *Giardia* and *Cryptosporidium* spp.

■ **SIGNS AND SYMPTOMS** The most common symptom, diarrhea, may be bloody and may be preceded or accompanied by vomiting, nausea, and abdominal cramping. A low-grade fever may be present. In severe cases, dehydration, electrolyte imbalance, acidosis, and kidney failure may occur.

■ **DIAGNOSTIC PROCEDURES** History and physical examination with clinical presentation is important. Stool is examined for parasites, bacteria, and/or white blood cells. Repeat stool specimens may be required to confirm the infecting organism. Special laboratory tests may be needed, especially for *E. coli* O157:H7. A careful review of the person's diet for the previous 3 or 4 days may be helpful in determining the cause. The level of dehydration needs to be assessed.

■ **TREATMENT** Rehydration is most important and must start immediately. If vomiting continues, it is better to rehydrate by offering small amounts of liquid frequently. If the infectious disease is caused by a virus, no medication generally is given; however, if the causative agent is bacterial, antibiotics may be administered. In parasitic infectious diarrheal disease, the drug of treatment is determined by the specific parasite involved. Intake and output of fluids should be continually measured, as well as noting the frequency of the stool. The infected person needs to maintain a high caloric intake and avoid foods high in sugar; however, food may have to be offered slowly and in small amounts at first. The importance of good hygiene cannot be overstressed, especially good handwashing when changing diapers or feeding children.

ALTERNATIVE THERAPY: *Alternative therapy recommends dietary limitations and appropriate nutritional therapy to replace fluid and electrolytes.*

TEACHING TIPS: Because the disease is highly contagious, it is paramount to teach all caregivers the proper care of the client during the contagious stage. Handwashing is essential, as is the proper handling of diapers and bedding. Encourage a balanced diet and ample fluids.

■ **PROGNOSIS** The prognosis is good if detected early, hydration is started immediately, and antimicrobial treatment is begun. Unfortunately, if the infection is severe, a child can die within hours. Some children, especially those younger than 2 years, may die of complications such as dehydration, shock, and bacteremia.

■ **PREVENTION** In the case of *E. coli,* thoroughly cook all meat. Avoid swimming in ponds, lakes, or any stagnant bodies of water. Good hygiene cannot be overemphasized.

Rubeola (Measles)

■ **DESCRIPTION** Measles is a highly communicable disease whose diagnostic signs are fever and the appearance of a characteristic rash. The disease is most common in school-age children, with outbreaks occurring in the winter and spring. Recently, though, the disease has occurred with increasing frequency among high school and college students who were not vaccinated as children or those who were vaccinated between 1957 and 1980 with an ineffective vaccine.

■ **ETIOLOGY** Measles is caused by the morbillivirus rubeola virus through direct contact with infectious droplets and occasionally through the air. The virus has an incubation period of 10 to 20 days.

■ **SIGNS AND SYMPTOMS** The onset of symptoms is usually gradual. Initial symptoms may include inflammation of the nasal mucosa (**rhinitis**), cough, cold or coryza, drowsiness, loss of appetite (**anorexia**), and a slow but progressive rise in temperature to 101° or 103° F by the second day. Small red spots with bluish white centers or Koplik's spots appear on the oral mucosa by the second or third day. Photophobia and cough soon follow. By about the fourth day, the fever usually reaches its maximum (as high as 104° to 106° F) and the characteristic rash appears. The rash first appears on the face as tiny

maculopapular lesions that contain both discolored spots of skin called **macules** and red, raised areas of skin called **papules**. These rapidly enlarge and spread to other areas of the body. The lesions may be so densely clustered in certain areas that the skin surface appears generally swollen and red.

■ **DIAGNOSTIC PROCEDURES** The clinical picture of symptoms is usually a sufficient basis for a diagnosis of measles. Blood testing may reveal an abnormal decrease in the number of circulating white blood cells, or **leukopenia**, and antibody titers are used to detect the presence of measles antibody in both the acute and convalescent phases.

■ **TREATMENT** Treatment for measles is essentially symptomatic. Bed rest is indicated, usually in a darkened room to alleviate the discomfort of photophobia. Antipyretics and liquids may be recommended. Avoid the use of aspirin as its use has been linked to Reye's syndrome (see Chapter 12, Cardiovascular System Diseases and Disorders, Reye's Syndrome). The affected individual should be kept isolated until the rash disappears.

ALTERNATIVE THERAPY: *No significant alternative therapy is indicated.*

TEACHING TIPS: Educate any caregivers about the incubation period, the spread of infection, and how to handle bedding, discarded tissues, and dishes. It is important to have your client rest, drink ample fluids, and eat a balanced diet.

■ **PROGNOSIS** Measles is usually a benign disease, running its course in about 5 days after the rash appears. An attack of measles usually confers permanent immunity. Complications may arise, including croup, conjunctivitis, myocarditis, hepatitis, and opportunistic respiratory tract infections from staphylococci, streptococci, or *Haemophilus influenzae.*

■ **PREVENTION** Measles can be prevented within 5 days of exposure by administration of gamma globulin, a protein formed in blood that functions as an antibody to provide rapid, temporary immunity to the disease. Active immunization can be produced by administration of measles vaccine, preferably containing the live attenuated virus. Handwashing and discarding tissues contaminated with respiratory secretions may help prevent the spread of measles within a family.

Rubella (German Measles)

■ **DESCRIPTION** Rubella is an acute infectious disease characterized by fever and rash. It closely resembles measles, but it differs in its short course, mild fever, and relative freedom from complications. Rubella is not as contagious as measles, and it occurs most frequently among teenagers and young adults.

■ **ETIOLOGY** The disease is caused by the rubella virus. This virus has an incubation period of 14 to 21 days.

■ **SIGNS AND SYMPTOMS** The onset of the disease is sometimes characterized by malaise, headache, slight fever, and sore throat. From 25% to 50% of cases are asymptomatic, especially among children. The rash typically appears the first or second day after onset. It may be composed of pale red, slightly elevated, discrete papules, or the rash may be highly diffuse and bright red. The rash begins on the face, spreads rapidly to other portions of the body, and usually fades so rapidly that the face may clear before the extremities are affected. Rash-covered portions of skin may itch or peel.

■ **DIAGNOSTIC PROCEDURES** Because rubella can be easily confused with other diseases, a definitive diagnosis can be reached with cultures of the throat, blood, and urine or with antibody titers. The latter is generally done in the acute and convalescent phases.

■ **TREATMENT** Treatment is nonspecific and symptomatic. Bed rest is indicated. Topical **antipruritics** or warm water baths may be recommended to relieve itching. Antipyretics may be prescribed.

ALTERNATIVE THERAPY: *No significant alternative therapy is indicated.*

> TEACHING TIPS: Because many clients are asymptomtic, teaching opportunities may be limited; however, it is a good idea to encourage your client to eat a balanced diet and drink ample fluids. Measures to reduce itching may be helpful.

■ **PROGNOSIS** The prognosis for an individual with rubella is usually good. The disease is benign, seldom produces complications, and runs its course in 3 days. Rubella is dangerous, however, when it occurs in pregnant women, especially during the first trimester of pregnancy; the virus is capable of producing severe fetal malformation.

■ **PREVENTION** Lasting immunization can be conferred through use of a live rubella vaccine. This vaccine must not be administered to pregnant women or to those who may become pregnant within 3 months after immunization. Administration of gamma globulin shortly after exposure may prevent development of the disease, but it still may not prevent transfer of the virus to the fetus if exposure occurs during pregnancy. Prevention includes good handwashing and disposing of contaminated tissues with respiratory secretions.

Erythema Infectiosum (Fifth Disease)

■ **DESCRIPTION** Erythema infectiosum is a common infection occurring predominantly in children with flulike symptoms and diffuse redness of the skin or erythema. It is called fifth disease because it was classified in the late nineteenth century as the fifth in a series of six childhood **exanthems**, rashes that occur on the skin as opposed to those rashes that occur on the mucous membranes (**enanthems**). It is a mild illness that exhibits a rash that develops quickly.

■ **ETIOLOGY** Fifth disease is caused by the human parvovirus B19 and is transmitted through respiratory secretions or direct contact. Parvovirus B19 can be transmitted during therapy with clotting factor concentrate. Its incubation period is generally 4 to 14 days but can be as long as 20 days. Unfortunately, the person is contagious before the onset of the symptoms. It is most prevalent in elementary and junior high school children during winter and spring.

■ **SIGNS AND SYMPTOMS** The child has an occasional fever and a red facial rash that looks like a "slapped cheek." There is a circumoral pallor and symmetric lacy rash on the trunk and limbs. The rash can recur for weeks with exposure to the sun, heat, stress, or exercise. Between 20% and 60% of the children in outbreaks are symptomatic, and many are asymptomatically infected.

■ **DIAGNOSTIC PROCEDURES** B19 can be detected in throat swabbings, respiratory tract secretions, and serum. The B19 specific antibodies can be detected with commercially available immunoassay kits.

■ **TREATMENT** Generally, no treatment is needed; however, it is important to manage any fever. Children can attend school after the appearance of the rash because they are not contagious once the rash appears.

ALTERNATIVE THERAPY: *No significant alternative therapy is indicated.*

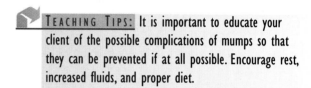 **TEACHING TIPS:** Inform the caregivers that your client is not contagious after the onset of a rash so he or she can continue to attend school or work. Although the exact route of transmission is unknown, it is important to discard any used tissues appropriately and to encourage your clients to drink ample fluids and practice good handwashing.

■ **PROGNOSIS** Complications include arthralgia and arthritis.

■ **PREVENTION** Good hygiene and proper disposal of tissues with contaminated respiratory secretions are necessary.

Mumps

■ **DESCRIPTION** Mumps is an acute contagious disease characterized by fever and inflammation of the parotid salivary glands. The disease is most common among children and young adults in late winter and spring.

■ **ETIOLOGY** The disease is caused by the mumps paramyxovirus, which has an incubation period of 18 days. The disease is transmitted via little droplets of saliva or the airborne route.

■ **SIGNS AND SYMPTOMS** The classic symptoms of mumps are unilateral or bilateral swollen parotid glands. Headache, malaise, fever, and earache may occur, and other salivary glands may become swollen.

■ **DIAGNOSTIC PROCEDURES** The clinical picture of mumps and a history of recent exposure usually are sufficient for diagnosis. A nasopharyngeal culture is done. A complement-fixation test may be ordered.

■ **TREATMENT** Analgesics, antipyretics, and adequate fluid intake are recommended. Isolation of the affected individual is important during the contagious period.

ALTERNATIVE THERAPY: *No significant alternative therapy is indicated.*

TEACHING TIPS: It is important to educate your client of the possible complications of mumps so that they can be prevented if at all possible. Encourage rest, increased fluids, and proper diet.

■ **PROGNOSIS** The prognosis for an individual with mumps is good. Complications can occur, however, and include **orchitis**, pancreatitis, and various central nervous system manifestations. Orchitis, which causes swelling of the testes in adult men, is extremely uncomfortable but rarely causes sterility, as is often feared.

■ **PREVENTION** The best prevention is to receive the mumps vaccine and to avoid exposure to the disease during its period of communicability. Good handwashing and proper disposal of contaminated tissues is essential for prevention.

Varicella (Chickenpox)

■ **DESCRIPTION** Varicella (chickenpox) is a highly contagious disease characterized by the appearance of a distinctive rash that passes through stages of macules, papules, small fluid-filled blisters or vesicles, and crusts. The disease occurs most commonly among children and may occur in epidemic outbreaks.

■ **ETIOLOGY** The disease is caused by the varicella-zoster virus (VZV), a herpesvirus. Its incubation period is 2 to 3 weeks, usually between 13 and 17 days, and is spread via respiratory secretion and direct contact.

■ **SIGNS AND SYMPTOMS** The sign of chickenpox is a pruritic rash, which begins as erythematous macules that produce papules and then clear vesicles. The rash usually contains a combination of papules, vesicles, and scabs in all stages. Anorexia, malaise, and fever may accompany the rash (Fig. 4.2).

■ **DIAGNOSTIC PROCEDURES** The clinical signs are usually sufficient for the diagnosis. A history that indicates recent exposure helps confirm the diagnosis.

■ **TREATMENT** Isolation is important during the infectious period—usually until all the scabs disappear. The only treatment necessary is to reduce the itching. Antihistamines may be given. Calamine lotion, cool bicarbonate of soda, or oatmeal baths can be very helpful. It is best not to scratch the lesions.

ALTERNATIVE THERAPY: *No significant alternative therapy is indicated.*

 TEACHING TIPS: Chickenpox requires strict adherence to proper handwashing, disposal of tissues, and proper cleaning of bedding and clothing. Teach your client or caregivers how to apply any lotions or medications to alleviate itching. Encourage bedrest and push fluids. Caregivers should be reminded not to give children aspirin-containing products because of its linkage to Reye's syndrome.

■ **PROGNOSIS** The prognosis for an individual with varicella is good. The disease runs its course in about 2 to 3 weeks. Complications may include secondary bacterial infections of the skin as a result of scratching open lesions, thrombocytopenia, arthritis, hepatitis, and Reye's syndrome.

■ **PREVENTION** In certain situations, varicella-zoster immune globulin (VZIG) may be administered within 72 hours of exposure to stop the development of the disease. Good hygiene, including proper disposal of tissues contaminated with respiratory secretions, is important.

Diphtheria

■ **DESCRIPTION** *Diphtheria* is an acute, life-threatening infectious disease. It is characterized by a membranelike coating that forms over mucous membrane surfaces, particularly along the respiratory tract, and by a toxic reaction primarily affecting the heart and peripheral nerves. The disease may occasionally involve the skin. Most cases occur in children younger than age 10, but older children and adults also may be affected.

■ **ETIOLOGY** Diphtheria is caused by *Cornebacterium diphtheriae*. The bacterium has an incubation period of 2 to 5 days. Most strains of *C. diphtheriae*

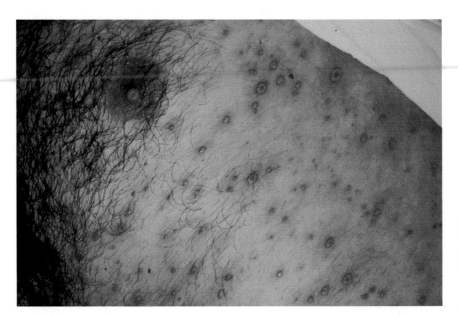

Figure 4.2 Chickenpox (varicella). (From Goldsmith, LA, Lazarus, GS, and Tharp, MD: Adult and Pediatric Dermatology: A Color Guide to Diagnosis and Treatment. FA Davis, Philadelphia, 1997, p 312, with permission.)

also release a highly potent toxin capable of damaging the heart, kidneys, and peripheral nerves. Transmission is through intimate contact with discharges from the nose, throat, eye, and skin lesions.

■ **SIGNS AND SYMPTOMS** The specific symptoms vary with the site of infection. In typical cases, a slight headache, malaise, and a mild fever (100° to 101° F) occur. There may be a strong, foul odor to the breath. Some individuals infected with *C. diphtheriae* remain asymptomatic but become carriers of the disease.

■ **DIAGNOSTIC PROCEDURES** The appearance of the characteristic membrane may be sufficient to establish a diagnosis of diphtheria. A definitive diagnosis can be made only by identifying the bacterium in nose and throat cultures.

■ **TREATMENT** The only specific treatment is administration of sufficient quantities of diphtheria antitoxin as early in the course of the disease as possible. The affected individual must be isolated, and bed rest is required. A soft or liquid diet is recommended. Emergency measures may be required to maintain an airway or to control cardiac complications. Carriers of diphtheria are usually treated with antibiotics.

ALTERNATIVE THERAPY: *No significant alternative therapy is indicated.*

> **TEACHING TIPS:** Educate family members about diphtheria. Any nonimmunized members should receive diphtheria toxoid appropriate to age. Hospitalization of the infected child is often necessary for proper treatment and observation for complications.

■ **PROGNOSIS** The prognosis for an individual with diphtheria varies according to the severity of the disease. Mild cases of diphtheria resolve in 3 to 4 days, or a week in moderate cases. Complications include thrombocytopenia, myocarditis, and vocal cord paralysis. Even with antitoxin therapy, death may result.

■ **PREVENTION** Diphtheria is highly preventable. Innoculation with diphtheria toxoid at the age of 3 months is normally routine. Booster doses should be administered at appropriate intervals during early childhood (see Table 4.3). Diphtheria toxoid is usually administered along with the vaccine for pertussis and the toxoid for tetanus (the DPT shot), because higher levels of antibodies are produced when all three vaccines are administered simultaneously rather than individually.

Pertussis (Whooping Cough)

■ **DESCRIPTION** Pertussis is an acute, highly infectious respiratory tract disease characterized by a repetitious, paroxysmal cough and a prolonged, harsh or shrill sound during inspiration (the "whoop"). Pertussis affects infants and children more frequently and more severely than it does adults.

■ **ETIOLOGY** Most cases of pertussis are caused by *Bordetella pertussis*. This bacterium has an incubation period of 7 to 10 days. The bacterium induces a mucopurulent secretion and hampers the natural ability of the respiratory tract to clear such secretions. Consequently, mucus accumulates in the airways and obstructs airflow. The bacterium also may produce a mild toxic reaction.

■ **SIGNS AND SYMPTOMS** The signs and symptoms of pertussis can be divided into three stages. The *catarrhal stage* is marked by the gradual onset of coldlike symptoms—mild fever, running nose, dry cough, irritability, and anorexia. This stage lasts from 1 to 2 weeks, during which the disease is highly communicable. The *paroxysmal stage* is marked by the onset of the classic cough, consisting of a series of several short, severe coughs in rapid succession followed by a slow, strained inspiration, during which a "whoop" (stridor) may be heard. The coughing occurs in periodic attacks. This stage, lasting 3 to 4 weeks, may be accompanied by weight loss, dehydration, vomiting, epistaxis, and hypoxia. After several weeks, a period of *decline* begins, marked by the gradual diminishment of coughing.

■ **DIAGNOSTIC PROCEDURES** A history of exposure to another infected individual and the presence of the classic cough may be sufficient to establish the diagnosis. A very high white blood cell count is a further distinguishing feature of pertussis. A definitive diagnosis depends on a nasopharyngeal culture.

■ **TREATMENT** Antibiotics administered during the catarrhal stage may check the development of the disease; if administration is delayed past this stage, antibiotics have little effect. The individual with pertussis requires meticulous care to ensure adequate nutrition, hydration, and clearance of mucous secretions.

ALTERNATIVE THERAPY: *Fluids are encouraged. Light foods can be taken. Avoid all dairy products during the acute stage. Fruits, vegetables, brown rice, clear vegetable soups, potatoes, and whole grain toast may be tried. Aromatherapy with basil, chamomile, eucalyptus, peppermint, and lavender in steam inhalation may be useful. Osteopathic manipulation may be able to reduce the severity of the cough.*

TEACHING TIPS: Remind caregivers that the characteristic cough may sound worse than it is but that they need to be aware that mucus may accumulate and require attention. Encourage proper fluid intake and a balanced diet. Educate your clients about the necessity of following the treatment plan, including taking all of the prescribed medication.

■ **PROGNOSIS** The prognosis for an individual with pertussis varies from case to case. Uncomplicated pertussis may run its course in 12 weeks. Recovery may be considerably extended, however, particularly among infants. Complications and possible death can occur as a result of seizures, encephalopathy, and pneumonia.

■ **PREVENTION** A child can be rendered less susceptible to pertussis by receiving a series of immunizations with pertussis vaccine, starting around the age of 3 months. Good handwashing and proper disposal of contaminated tissue from respiratory secretions are essential.

Tetanus (Lockjaw)

■ **DESCRIPTION** Tetanus is an acute, life-threatening infectious disease characterized by persistent, painful contractions of skeletal muscles. The disease may affect any person at any time, but children are at greater risk because of their tendency to develop skin wounds as a result of play activities.

■ **ETIOLOGY** The disease is caused by *Clostridium tetani*, a bacterium commonly found in soil. The bacillus becomes pathogenic when its spores enter the body through a puncture wound. Burns, surgical incisions, and chronic skin ulcers may also provide opportunities for *C. tetani* spores to enter the body, as may generalized conditions such as otitis media and dental infections. The spores produce a powerful toxin that attacks the central nervous system and that also acts directly on voluntary muscles to produce contraction.

■ **SIGNS AND SYMPTOMS** The onset of symptoms may be either gradual or abrupt. Stiffness of the jaw, esophageal muscles, and some neck muscles is often the first sign of the disease. Later, in the most common manifestation of tetanus, the jaws become rigidly fixed (lockjaw), the voice is altered, and the facial muscles contract, contorting the individual's face into a grimace. Finally, the muscles of the back and the extremities may become rigid or the individual may experience extremely severe convulsive spasms of muscles. This final phase of the disease often is accompanied by high fever, profuse sweating, tachycardia, dysphagia, and intense pain.

■ **DIAGNOSTIC PROCEDURES** Tetanus is diagnosed on the basis of its classic symptomatology.

■ **TREATMENT** The site of the wound or the point of infection must be thoroughly cleaned and debrided. Human tetanus immune globulin (TIG) often will be administered. Muscle relaxants may be prescribed. Meticulous care and support are required to maintain adequate nutrition and hydration and to avoid the development of decubitus ulcers. Tracheostomy is routinely performed in moderate to severe cases of tetanus to prevent choking.

ALTERNATIVE THERAPY: *No significant alternative therapy is indicated.*

TEACHING TIPS: The disease process can be frightening; however, educating the client and caregivers helps alleviate anxiety and fears. It is important to follow your client and watch for any complications during the disease. Special attention should be given to ensure a proper diet and ample fluids.

■ **PROGNOSIS** The mortality rate is high. The disease usually runs its course in about 6 to 7 weeks, seldom producing any lasting disability. However, despite effective treatment measures, tetanus is frequently fatal, especially among unimmunized people. Death may result from asphyxiation, a host of possible complications, and sometimes from sheer exhaustion.

■ **PREVENTION** Surprisingly enough, having tetanus does not confer future immunity to the disease. Immunization with tetanus toxoid should be routinely started at 3 months of age. Boosters are required periodically throughout life. The risk of contracting tetanus also can be minimized by wearing protective clothing and by prompt cleansing and care of wounds and other skin lesions.

IMMUNIZATION

Immunizations are important for protection against certain communicable diseases. Medical personnel maintain accurate records of immunizations, but in the current mobile society and with the ever-present changes in primary care providers due to insurance restrictions within the United States, parents should keep a separate and complete record of their children's and their own immunizations. Additional health immunizations are required for travel to some other countries. County health departments have specific information on recommended or required immunizations for world travel.

Four excellent resources of information on immunizations are:

- Centers for Disease Control and Prevention (www.cdc.gov)
- National Center for Infectious Diseases (www.cdc.gov/ncidod)
- Morbidity and Mortality Weekly Report (www.cdc.gov/mmwr)
- National Center for Health Statistics (www.cdc.gov/nchs)

The incidence of certain communicable diseases in the United States has steadily decreased. Children and adolescents are no longer the routine victims of many diseases, thanks to advances in medical knowledge, general improvements in living conditions, and government-mandated immunization programs. Poliomyelitis, for example, once endemic in the United States, occurs only rarely since the advent of the Salk vaccine.

Caution cannot be thrown to the wind, however. A serious outbreak of rubeola occurred recently on a college campus, where a substantial number of students had not been vaccinated against the disease owing to their religious beliefs. In the inner cities of the United States, limited access to medical care, lack of knowledge, and distrust of government-sponsored health outreach programs have conspired to leave significant numbers of children unprotected by vaccines. In the absence of the effective immunization provided by vaccines, communicable disease can still cause major epidemics.

A *vaccine* is a suspension of infectious agents, components of the agents, or genetically engineered antigens. It is given for the purpose of establishing resistance to an infectious disease. There are two general classes of vaccines:

- Use of live, generally attentuated, infectious agents (e.g., measles virus)
- Use of inactivated agents or products obtained through genetic recombination (acellular pertussis vaccines)

Both approaches are used in many diseases (poliomyelitis and influenza).

Whatever its makeup, a vaccine stimulates the development of specific defense mechanisms that should result in permanent protection from the disease. Table 4.3 is an immunization schedule that lists the vaccines commonly administered during childhood and adolescence.

The immunization schedules are generally based on the consensus of the Advisory Committee on Immunization Practices (ACIP) of the CDC, the American Academy of Pediatrics (AAP), and the American Academy of Family Physicians (AAFP). The current schedule is updated annually (see www.cispimmunize.org/ill/ill_main.html for annual reports).

ALTERNATIVE THERAPY: *One of the areas where alternative medicine practitioners and traditional physicians disagree is on the use of vaccinations to prevent communicable diseases. The majority of alternative practitioners believe that it is better to allow the communicable disease to run its course and provide subsequent immunity rather than risking the side effects of vaccinations. Alternative therapy practitioners recommend making the child comfortable, while providing proper hydration and nutrition.*

Table 4.3

RECOMMENDED CHILDHOOD AND ADOLESCENT IMMUNIZATION SCHEDULE UNITED STATES - JULY–DECEMBER 2004

Vaccine ▼ / Age ▶	Birth	1 mo	2 mo	4 mo	6 mo	12 mo	15 mo	18 mo	24 mo	4-6 y	11-12 y	13-18 y
			Range of Recommended Ages							Catch-up Immunization	Preadolescent Assessment	
Hepatitis B[1]	HepB #1	only if mother HBsAg (-)	HepB #2			HepB #3					HepB series	
Diphtheria, Tetanus, Pertussis[2]			DTaP	DTaP	DTaP		DTaP			DTaP	Td	Td
Haemophilus influenzae Type b[3]			Hib	Hib	Hib	Hib						
Inactivated Poliovirus			IPV	IPV		IPV				IPV		
Measles, Mumps, Rubella[4]						MMR #1				MMR #2	MMR #2	
Varicella[5]						Varicella				Varicella		
Pneumococcal[6]			PCV	PCV	PCV	PCV			PCV	PPV		
Influenza[7]					Influenza (Yearly)					Influenza (Yearly)		
Hepatitis A[8]										Hepatitis A Series		

Vaccines below red line are for selected populations

This schedule indicates the recommended ages for routine administration of currently licensed childhood vaccines, as of April 1, 2004, for children through age 18 years. Any dose not given at the recommended age should be given at any subsequent visit when indicated and feasible. ▨ Indicates age groups that warrant special effort to administer those vaccines not previously given. Additional vaccines may be licensed and recommended during the year. Licensed combination vaccines may be used whenever any components of the combination are indicated and the vaccine's other components are not contraindicated. Providers should consult the manufacturers' package inserts for detailed recommendations. Clinically significant adverse events that follow immunization should be reported to the Vaccine Adverse Event Reporting System (VAERS). Guidance about how to obtain and complete a VAERS form can be found on the Internet: www.vaers.org or by calling 800-822-7967.

1. Hepatitis B (HepB) vaccine. All infants should receive the first dose of hepatitis B vaccine soon after birth and before hospital discharge; the first dose may also be given by age 2 months if the infant's mother is hepatitis B surface antigen (HBsAg) negative. Only monovalent HepB can be used for the birth dose. Monovalent or combination vaccine containing HepB may be used to complete the series. Four doses of vaccine may be administered when a birth dose is given. The second dose should be given at least 4 weeks after the first dose, except for combination vaccines which cannot be administered before age 6 weeks. The third dose should be given at least 16 weeks after the first dose and at least 8 weeks after the second dose. The last dose in the vaccination series (third or fourth dose) should not be administered before age 24 weeks.

Infants born to HBsAg-positive mothers should receive HepB and 0.5 mL of Hepatitis B Immune Globulin (HBIG) within 12 hours of birth at separate sites. The second dose is recommended at age 1–2 months. The last dose in the immunization series should be administered before age 24 weeks. These infants should be tested for HBsAg and antibody to HBsAg (anti-HBs) at age 9–15 months.

Infants born to mothers whose HBsAg status is unknown should receive the first dose of the HepB series within 12 hours of birth. Maternal blood should be drawn as soon as possible to determine the mother's HBsAg status; if the HBsAg test is positive, the infant should receive HBIG as soon as possible (no later than age 1 week). The second dose is recommended at age 1–2 months. The last dose in the immunization series should not be administered before age 24 weeks.

2. Diphtheria and tetanus toxoids and acellular pertussis (DTaP) vaccine. The fourth dose of DTaP may be administered as early as age 12 months, provided 6 months have elapsed since the third dose and the child is unlikely to return at age 15–18 months. The final dose in the series should be given at age ≥4 years. **Tetanus and diphtheria toxoids (Td)** is recommended at age 11–12 years if at least 5 years have elapsed since the last dose of tetanus and diphtheria toxoid-containing vaccine. Subsequent routine Td boosters are recommended every 10 years.

3. Haemophilus influenzae type b (Hib) conjugate vaccine. Three Hib conjugate vaccines are licensed for infant use. If PRP-OMP (PedvaxHIB or ComVax [Merck]) is administered at ages 2 and 4 months, a dose at age 6 months is not required. DTaP/Hib combination products should not be used for primary immunization in infants at ages 2, 4 or 6 months but can be used as boosters following any Hib vaccine. The final dose in the series should be given at age ≥12 months.

4. Measles, mumps, and rubella vaccine (MMR). The second dose of MMR is recommended routinely at age 4–6 years but may be administered during any visit, provided at least 4 weeks have elapsed since the first dose and both doses are administered beginning at or after age 12 months. Those who have not previously received the second dose should complete the schedule by the visit at age 11–12 years.

5. Varicella vaccine. Varicella vaccine is recommended at any visit at or after age 12 months for susceptible children (i.e., those who lack a reliable history of chickenpox). Susceptible persons age ≥13 years should receive 2 doses, given at least 4 weeks apart.

6. Pneumococcal vaccine. The heptavalent **pneumococcal conjugate vaccine (PCV)** is recommended for all children age 2–23 months. It is also recommended for certain children age 24–59 months. The final dose in the series should be given at age ≥12 months. **Pneumococcal polysaccharide vaccine (PPV)** is recommended in addition to PCV for certain high-risk groups. See MMWR 2000;49(RR-9):1-35.

7. Influenza vaccine. Influenza vaccine is recommended annually for children aged ≥6 months with certain risk factors (including but not limited to asthma, cardiac disease, sickle cell disease, HIV, and diabetes), healthcare workers, and other persons (including household members) in close contact with persons in groups at high risk (see MMWR 2004;53;[RR-6]:1-40) and can be administered to all others wishing to obtain immunity. In addition, healthy children aged 6–23 months and close contacts of healthy children aged 0–23 months are recommended to receive influenza vaccine, because children in this age group are at substantially increased risk for influenza-related hospitalizations. For healthy persons aged 5–49 years, the intranasally administered live, attenuated influenza vaccine (LAIV) is an acceptable alternative to the intramuscular trivalent inactivated influenza vaccine (TIV). See MMWR 2004;53;[RR-6]:1-40. Children receiving TIV should be administered a dosage appropriate for their age (0.25 mL if 6–35 months or 0.5 mL if ≥3 years). Children aged <8 years who are receiving influenza vaccine for the first time should receive 2 doses (separated by at least 4 weeks for TIV and at least 6 weeks for LAIV).

8. Hepatitis A vaccine. Hepatitis A vaccine is recommended for children and adolescents in selected states and regions and for certain high-risk groups; consult your local public health authority. Children and adolescents in these states, regions, and high-risk groups who have not been immunized against hepatitis A can begin the hepatitis A immunization series during any visit. The 2 doses in the series should be administered at least 6 months apart. See MMWR 1999;48(RR-12):1-37.

For additional information about vaccines, including precautions and contraindications for immunization and vaccine shortages, please visit the National Immunization Program Web site at www.cdc.gov/nip/ or call the National Immunization Information Hotline at 800-232-2522 (English) or 800-232-0233 (Spanish).

Approved by the Advisory Committee on Immunization Practices (www.cdc.gov/nip/acip), the American Academy of Pediatrics (www.aap.org), and the American Academy of Family Physicians (www.aafp.org).

TEACHING TIPS: It is important that all individuals be given information related to the particular vaccine and any side effects that might occur. Respect must be given to those who refuse vaccinations, however, it can be helpful to make certain they are properly informed of the dangers of communicable diseases.

Summary

Infectious diseases emerge and reemerge in our lives. One disease is eradicated, only to have another surface. Smallpox, once completely eradicated from the world, is again a threat. Infectious diseases that once responded to antibiotics are now resistant. SARS has made us look at a prevention method not practiced for many years—isolation and quarantine.

CASE STUDIES

■ **Case Study 1**

Austin is a 40-year-old architect who has been fighting AIDS for 13 years. With the consent of his primary care physician, he removes himself from all medications. He improves. His appetite improves, and his stamina increases. He thinks about returning to work. Six months later, he returns to his physician weaker and sicker than before. At this point, Austin and his physician decide to seek alternative therapies.

Case Study Questions

1. What alternative therapies might be considered?
2. How will the integration of alternative therapies and the primary care physician's therapies be carried out?

■ **Case Study 2**

In the United States, the CDC lists a shortage of five vaccines, including DPT.

Case Study Questions

1. Why do we have childhood immunizations?
2. What happens when there is a shortage?
3. What economic and political factors are considered here?

REVIEW QUESTIONS

True/False

Circle the correct answer:

T   F   1. Another name for the common cold is acute coryza.

T   F   2. Influenza is most apt to occur in summer and fall.

T   F   3. Aspirin is the analgesic of choice for children.

T   F   4. Diphtheria, pertussis, and tetanus are preventable through inoculation.

T   F   5. Exposure to German measles during pregnancy can cause fetal complications.

Matching

Match the following by placing the correct letter in the column:

_____   1. Acupuncture, massage, mind-body therapies

_____   2. Avoid alcohol and sugars; proper nutritional supplements

_____   3. Herbal teas, vegetable juices, and broths

_____   4. Soothing baths, vitamin C, lots of fluids

_____   5. High-protein diet with complex carbohydrates, vitamin/
mineral supplements

a. Measles, chickenpox

b. HIV/AIDS

c. Colds and influenza

d. CFS

e. Lyme disease

Short Answer

1. Koplik's spots are characteristic of what childhood disease? _____.

2. Another name for German measles is _____.

3. Another name for tetanus is _____.

4. The _____ virus causes mumps.

5. Another name for chickenpox is _____. It is caused by
_____.

6. DPT stands for _____, _____ , and
_____.

Multiple Choice

Place a checkmark next to the correct answer:

1. Which of the following statements is true about CFS?

   a. CFS is easily diagnosed with laboratory testing.

b. CFS occurs more frequently in young adults.

c. CFS is a debilitating illness characterized by at least 6 months of unresolved fatigue.

d. CFS is treatable and curable.

2. Lyme disease

a. Is caused by tick-transmitted spirocete.

b. Progresses in two stages.

c. Is treated by strict bed rest and a low-salt diet.

d. Has no preventative measures.

3. SARS

a. Can present as asymptomatic, as a moderate respiratory infection, or as a severe infection.

b. Has a specific viral cause.

c. Is transmitted only via respiratory secretions.

d. Occurs only in China and Europe.

4. HIV infection/AIDS

a. Are curable.

b. Have leveled off in the United States due to a new vaccine.

c. Are showing evidence of a "superinfection."

d. Are caused by a virulent bacterium that depresses the immune system.

5. *E. coli* O157:H7

a. Is a viral infection of the gastrointestinal tract.

b. Is highly contagious from human to human.

c. Is found in undercooked beef.

d. Rarely is fatal.

Discussion Questions/Personal Reflection

1. Contact your county health department to ascertain which communicable diseases must be reported in your geographic location.

2. Contact a grade school or day care center, and compare their recommendations with those of your local health deparment for immunizations to have when starting school.

3. The United States is seeing a leveling off of HIV infection/AIDS; however, the rest of the world is experiencing an epidemic. Discuss this. Consider economics, politics, and availability of health-care resources.

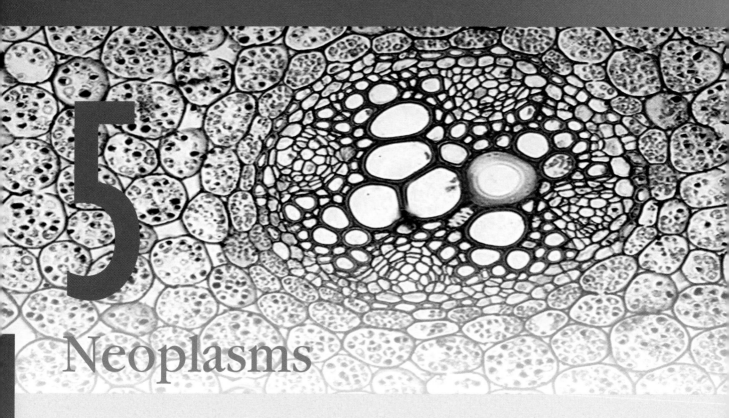

5

Neoplasms

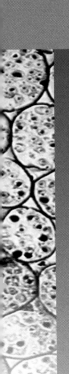

Anaplasia (ăn•ă•plā′zē•ă)
Carcinogen (kăr•sĭn′ō•jĭn)
Carcinoma in situ (kăr•sĭn•ō•mă ĕn si•tū′)
Choriocarcinoma (kō•rē•ō•kăr•sĭ•nō′mă)
Dysplasia (dĭs•plā′zē•ă)
En bloc (ĕn blŏk′)
Epithelial (ĕp•ĭ•thē′lē•ăl)
Erythema (ĕr•ĭ•thē′mă)
Exfoliative cytology (ĕks•fō′lē•ă•tĭv sī•tŏl′ō•jē)
Hyperplasia (hī•pĕr•plā′zē•ă)
Leukocyte (loo′kō•sit)
Leukopenia (loo•kō•pē′nē•ă)
Metastasis (mĕ•tăs′tă•sĭs)
Palliative (păl′ē•ă•tĭv)
Papanicolaou test (pă•pē′nē•kĕ•laŭ tĕst)
Radioisotope (rā•dē•ō•ī′sō•tōp)
Reed-Sternberg cell (rēd stĕrn′ bĕrg sĕl)

> *In the hour of adversity be not without hope, for crystal rain falls from black clouds.*
>
> —PERSIAN POEM

LEARNING OBJECTIVES

Upon successful completion of this chapter, you will be able to:

• Define *neoplasm.*
• Compare benign and malignant tumors.
• Recall death statistics on cancer.
• Identify at least eight suggestions for cancer prevention.
• List the seven warning signals of cancer.
• Describe the three main classifications for cancer.
• Identify the grading and staging of neoplasms and their use.
• List at least four possible causes of cancer.
• Discuss four major forms of cancer treatment and their advantages and disadvantages.
• Describe circumstances in which a physician and client may choose a combination of the five major cancer treatments.

S ome new growth in our bodies is necessary and advantageous; repair of bone and skin is an example. Other new growth (neoplasm) can be frightening, perplexing, and life-threatening. *Neoplasm* is a new formation or new growth that serves no useful purpose. In fact, the growth is uncontrollable and progressive, and it may be detrimental to other parts of the body. The term *tumor*, a swelling or an enlargement, may be used interchangeably with *neoplasm.*

A tumor may be benign or malignant depending on its growth pattern, cell characteristics, potential for the cells to move from one part of the body to another (**metastasis**), tendency to recur, and capacity to cause death. A *benign* tumor is one that grows slowly and has cells that closely resemble normal cells of the tissue from which the tumor originated. The tumor usually is encapsulated and does not infiltrate surrounding tissue; it does not tend to recur when removed. A favorable recovery is likely.

A *malignant* tumor, by comparison, is one that is invasive, grows rather rapidly, is sometimes **anaplastic** (has lost its cell definition and function), and has the capability of metastasizing through the blood or lymph. These tumor cells are not normal. If untreated, a malignancy generally progresses, and death may result. We commonly refer to malignant tumors as cancer. Henceforth in this chapter, the two terms are used interchangeably (Table 5.1).

Cancer is a focus of attention in American society because of its toll in lives, the suffering it causes, and the economic losses it produces. Cancer strikes people of all ages, both men and women, and is the second-leading cause of death in the United States, preceded only by heart disease. About 77% of all cancers are diagnosed at age 55 or older. According to the American Cancer Society, the lifetime risk for men developing cancer is a little less than 1 in 2. For women, the risk is a little greater than 1 in 3. Figure 5.1 illustrates the estimated incidence of new cancer cases and deaths by site and sex.

In the United States, more than 1.3 million new cases of cancer are diagnosed each year. Cancer is the cause of death for more than 556,500 people in this country every year, more than 1500 deaths per day. Almost half of all deaths from cancer are from the four most frequently diagnosed kinds: lung and bronchus, prostate, breast, and colorectal cancer. For males, prostate cancer is the most frequently diagnosed kind of cancer; for women, breast cancer is the most frequently diagnosed. Lung and bronchus cancers remain the leading cause of cancer death for both men and women. Colorectal cancer occurs at about the same frequency in men and women.

One way to measure the overall success of cancer treatment is to see how many patients remain alive at specific time intervals (e.g., 5, 10, and 15 years) after they are diagnosed. The 5-year survival rate is a widely used marker. In treating cancer, much depends on the stage of the cancer at the time it is diagnosed. A *localized* cancer is one in which the cancer cells have not yet spread from the site of the original tumor. In the *regional* stage, the cancer has spread to sites within the same region of the body. The cancer is said to be in the *distant* stage when cancerous cells have entered the bloodstream and been

Table 5.1

BENIGN AND MALIGNANT TUMORS

	GROWTH PATTERN	APPEARANCE	TISSUE DESTRUCTION	RECURRENCE
Benign	Grows slowly Remains localized (no metastasis) Expands	Cells closely resemble mature, normal cells. Cells are well differentiated. In many cases, the tumor is encapsulated	Usually slight unless location interferes with blood flow	Rare when surgically removed
Malignant	Grows rapidly	Cells are not well differentiated.	Extensive infiltration and metastic lesions	May recur after surgery due to surrounding tissue infiltration
Carcinoma	Infiltrates surrounding tissues	Tumor is seldom encapsulated.		
Sarcoma	Spreads via blood and lymph			
Leukemias	Establishes secondary tumors			

ESTIMATED NEW CANCER CASES AND DEATHS BY SEX FOR ALL SITES, US, 2004*

	Estimated New Cases			Estimated Deaths		
	BOTH SEXES	MALE	FEMALE	BOTH SEXES	MALE	FEMALE
All sites	1,368,030	699,560	668,470	563,700	290,890	272,810
Oral cavity & pharynx	28,260	18,550	9,710	7,230	4,830	2,400
Tongue	7,320	4,860	2,460	1,700	1,100	600
Mouth	10,080	5,410	4,670	1,890	1,070	820
Pharynx	8,250	6,330	1,920	2,070	1,460	610
Other oral cavity	2,610	1,950	660	1,570	1,200	370
Digestive system	255,640	135,410	120,230	134,840	73,240	61,600
Esophagus	14,250	10,860	3,390	13,300	10,250	3,050
Stomach	22,710	13,640	9,070	11,780	6,900	4,880
Small intestine	5,260	2,750	2,510	1,130	610	520
Colon†	106,370	50,400	55,970	56,730	28,320	28,410
Rectum	40,570	23,220	17,350			
Anus, anal canal, & anorectum	4,010	1,890	2,120	580	210	370
Liver & intrahepatic bile duct	18,920	12,580	6,340	14,270	9,450	4,820
Gallbladder & other biliary	6,950	2,960	3,990	3,540	1,290	2,250
Pancreas	31,860	15,740	16,120	31,270	15,440	15,830
Other digestive organs	4,740	1,370	3,370	2,240	770	1,470
Respiratory system	186,550	102,730	83,820	165,130	95,460	69,670
Larynx	10,270	8,060	2,210	3,830	3,010	820
Lung & bronchus	173,770	93,110	80,660	160,440	91,930	68,510
Other respiratory organs	2,510	1,560	950	860	520	340
Bones & joints	2,440	1,230	1,210	1,300	720	580
Soft tissue (including heart)	8,680	4,760	3,920	3,660	2,020	1,640
Skin (excluding basal & squamous)	59,350	31,640	27,710	10,250	6,590	3,660
Melanoma-skin	55,100	29,900	25,200	7,910	5,050	2,860
Other nonepithelial skin	4,910	2,400	2,510	2,340	1,540	800
Breast	217,440	1,450	215,990	40,580	470	40,110
Genital system	323,210	240,660	82,550	59,250	30,530	28,720
Uterine cervix	10,520		10,520	3,900		3,900
Uterine corpus	40,320		40,320	7,090		7,090
Ovary	25,580		25,580	16,090		16,090
Vulva	3,970		3,970	850		850
Vagina & other genital, female	2,160		2,160	790		790
Prostate	230,110	230,110		29,900	29,900	

(Continued on the following page)

(Continued)

ESTIMATED NEW CANCER CASES AND DEATHS BY SEX FOR ALL SITES, US, 2004*

	Estimated New Cases			Estimated Deaths		
	BOTH SEXES	MALE	FEMALE	BOTH SEXES	MALE	FEMALE
Testis	8,980	8,980		360	360	
Penis & other genital, male	1,570	1,570		270	270	
Urinary system	98,400	68,290	30,110	25,880	17,060	8,820
Urinary bladder	60,240	44,640	15,600	12,710	8,780	3,930
Kidney & renal pelvis	35,710	22,080	13,630	12,480	7,870	4,610
Ureter & other urinary organs	2,450	1,570	880	690	410	280
Eye & orbit	2,090	1,130	960	180	110	70
Brain & other nervous system	18,400	10,540	7,860	12,690	7,200	5,490
Endocrine system	25,520	6,950	18,570	2,440	1,140	1,300
Thyroid	23,600	5,960	17,640	1,460	620	840
Other endocrine	1,920	990	930	980	520	460
Lymphoma	62,250	33,180	29,070	20,730	11,090	9,640
Hodgkin disease	7,880	4,330	3,550	1,320	700	620
Non-Hodgkin lymphoma	54,370	28,850	25,520	19,410	10,390	9,020
Multiple myeloma	15,270	8,090	7,180	11,070	5,430	5,640
Leukemia	33,440	19,020	14,420	23,300	12,990	10,310
Acute lymphocytic leukemia	3,830	2,110	1,720	1,450	820	630
Chronic lymphocytic leukemia	8,190	5,050	3,140	4,800	2,730	2,070
Acute myeloid leukemia	11,920	6,280	5,640	8,870	4,810	4,060
Chronic myeloid leukemia	4,600	2,700	1,900	1,570	940	630
Other leukemia‡	4,900	2,880	2,020	6,610	3,690	2,920
Other & unspecified primary sites‡	31,090	15,930	15,160	45,170	22,010	23,160

*Rounded to the nearest 10; excludes basal and squamous cell skin cancers and in situ carcinomas except urinary bladder. Carcinoma in situ of the breast accounts for about 59,390 new cases annually, and in situ melanoma accounts for about 40,780 new cases annually. †Estimated deaths for colon and rectum cancers are combined. ‡More deaths than cases suggests lack of specificity in recording underlying causes of death on death certificates.

Source: Estimates of new cases are based on incidence rates from 1979 to 2000, National Cancer Institute Surveillance, Epidemiology, and End Results program. Estimates of deaths are based on data from US Mortality Public Use Data Tapes, 1969 to 2001, National Center for Health Statistics, Centers for Disease Control and Prevention, 2003.

©2004, American Cancer Society, Inc., Surveillance Research

carried to other sites in the body (metastasis). Successful treatment is more likely with localized tumors and least likely in the distant stage.

Medical researchers continue to develop improved treatment procedures for various forms of cancer. For all cancers combined, the 5-year survival rate is 62%. Current information on cancer incidence, survival rates, and deaths are easily accessed through the American Cancer Society Website. (www.cancer.org). From their home page, click on "facts and figures" or "statistics" for the latest data. Another useful Website is the National Cancer Institute (www.nci.nih.gov), which also lists statistics and facts and figures.

CANCER RISK FACTORS AND PREVENTIVE MEASURES

There is no single cause of cancer. Research indicates that all cancers arise because of alterations in DNA resulting from unrestrained cellular proliferation. These cell mutations are most often caused by substances or agents to which humans are exposed that increase the risk of the development of cancer. Such an element is termed a **carcinogen**. Carcinogens include many kinds of chemicals and certain kinds of high-frequency radiation such as ultraviolet and ionizing radiation that damages the DNA.

The use of tobacco is a significant factor in the cause of respiratory cancers. All cancers caused by cigarette smoking and heavy use of alcohol could be prevented completely. A high incidence of colon cancer may be linked to a high-fat, low-fiber diet, which is very popular in American households. About 1 million skin cancers diagnosed could be prevented by protection from the sun's rays.

The American Cancer Society recommends the following preventive measures:

1. Do not smoke. The risk of developing lung cancer increases 15 to 25 times for the smoker and poses risks to those near smokers. If a pregnant woman smokes, she passes on the smoke and risk to her baby. Smoking and drinking alcohol are even riskier.

2. Limit alcoholic intake to one or two drinks per day. Heavy drinking increases the risk of cancer of the esophagus, mouth, throat, larynx, and liver.

3. Protect the skin from UV rays. Limit excessive sun exposure, especially between 10 A.M. and 4 P.M. Wear protective covering and/or apply sun screen with SPF 15 or higher. Do not use sun lamps or tanning salons.

4. Refuse needless x-rays. Special precautions must be taken to protect the unborn child if x-rays are necessary.

5. Limit exposure to chemicals such as asbestos, aniline dyes, arsenic, chromium, nickel compounds, vinyl chloride, benzene, and certain products of coal, lignite, oil shale, and petroleum. Wear protective clothing and follow directions exactly if working with harmful chemicals or fibers.

6. Take hormone therapy to relieve menopausal symptoms only if and as long as necessary. However, the use of progesterone with estrogen helps decrease the cancer risk.

7. Avoid heavily polluted air and long exposure to household solvent cleaners, paint thinners, and similar products. Follow label instructions carefully when using pesticides, fungicides, and other home, garden, and lawn chemicals.

8. Monitor caloric intake, and exercise properly. Eat less fatty foods and more high-fiber foods such as bran, whole grains, and fibrous vegetables and fruits.

9. Regular screening and self-examinations can detect cancers of the breast, tongue, mouth, colon, rectum, cervix, prostate, testes, and skin.

10. Limit how much meat you eat, and limit consumption of salt-cured, smoked, and nitrite-cured foods. Trim the skin off of turkey and chicken.

Have regular checkups by physicians. The American Cancer Society, the National Cancer Institute, and the U.S. Department of Health and Human Services recommend a mammogram every 1 to 2 years for woman older than age of 40. A sonogram is recommended if suspicious or abnormal results are found. Also, the **Papanicolaou test** (also known as the *Pap smear* or *Pap test* [discussed later]) should be performed at regular intervals. Men should be regularly checked for prostate cancer. This check includes a yearly digital examination for men older than 40, a yearly blood test to detect prostate-specific antigen (PSA) in men older than 50, and ultrasonography if abnormal results are found. A rectal examination should be part of every medical checkup for men and women, and stool samples should be examined for blood, which may be an indication of colon cancer.

CLASSIFICATION OF NEOPLASMS

Neoplasms are classified for diagnostic, treatment, and research purposes, as well as to aid in reporting cancer statistics. One commonly accepted system classifies neoplasms according to the type of body tissue in which they appear. Using this method, neoplasms are divided into three categories: carcinomas, sarcomas, and blood and lymph neoplasms.

Carcinomas, the largest group, are solid tumors

of **epithelial** tissue of external and internal body surfaces. Benign tumors of epithelial origin usually are named using the suffix -*oma* added to the type of tissue involved. For example, an *adenoma* is a benign tumor of a gland. Malignant tumors of epithelial origin, however, are named with the term -*carcinoma* added to the type of tissue involved. For example, an *adenocarcinoma* is a malignant tumor of a gland. Such terminology often is confusing for the layperson, who may believe that *all* tumors are cancerous.

Sarcomas, which are less common than carcinomas, arise from supportive and connective tissue such as bone, fat, muscle, and cartilage. Again, benign tumors of connective tissue are named by appending the suffix -*oma* to the type of tissue involved, and malignant tumors of connective tissue are named by adding the term -*sarcoma* to the type of tissue involved. Thus, *osteoma* is a benign tumor of bone, and *osteosarcoma* is a malignant tumor of bone.

Neoplasms of *blood* and *lymph* include leukemias, Hodgkin's disease, and non-hodgkin's lymphoma.

Leukemias are sometimes considered to be sarcomas, but the fact that leukemias do not form solid tumors suggests the need for a separate category. Leukemias rise from the body's blood-forming tissues within the bone marrow. The abnormal tissue proliferates, crowding out normal blood-forming cells, and releases large quantities of abnormal white blood cells called **leukocytes** into the circulating blood.

Leukemias are further subdivided into chronic and acute forms (see Chapter 12). The chronic leukemias include chronic myelocytic leukemia and chronic lymphocytic leukemia. The acute leukemias include acute myeloblastic leukemia. The pathologic course of leukemia is characterized by the infiltration of leukemic cells into numerous organs, which subsequently become enlarged, soft, and pale. The lymph nodes, spleen, and bone marrow are particularly susceptible, but no organ is exempt from this infiltration.

Hodgkin's disease is a lymphoma characterized by an unusual giant cell, the **Reed-Sternberg cell**. The disease is characterized by painless enlargement of lymph nodes beginning in the cervical region and moving to all lymphoid structures.

Non-Hodgkin's lymphomas, also known as malignant lymphomas, are more common than Hodgkin's disease and are increasing in incidence, especially in clients with autoimmune disorders. These are characterized by painless lymph node swelling. The difference between Hodgkin's disease and non-Hodgkin's lymphoma, other than the Reed-Sternberg cell, is that non-Hodgkin's lymphoma may involve lymphoid tissue other than lymph nodes, such as the gut and skin.

ETIOLOGY OF NEOPLASMS

As discussed in Chapter 1, the actual cause of neoplasms is not known, but some alteration in the cell chromosomes does occur, allowing independent and uncontrollable cell growth. Such a mutated cell is abnormal in that it is not subject to normal control mechanisms. It is suspected that mutations occur fairly frequently but that the body's immune response is able to destroy the abnormal cells as soon as they occur. Therefore, a malignancy may represent a failure of the body's immune system.

With the alteration in the cell chromosome, it is known that genetics play an etiologic role in neoplasms, but most neoplasms are not inherited. There are, however, a few examples deserving of discussion. Cancer of the breast generally is more common in female relatives of affected women than in the general population. The uncommon condition polyposis coli* is inherited through an autosomal dominant gene and eventually leads to carcinoma of the colon. Another rare cancer, retinoblastoma,† is inherited as a Mendelian dominant trait and usually is present at birth.

There is some evidence that viruses may cause some kinds of cancers, and this is an area of active research. It has been shown that viruses can cause tumors in animals, but the situation is not so clear in humans. A herpeslike virus, the Epstein-Barr virus, often associated with infectious mononucleosis, is thought to be a causative factor in Burkitt's lymphoma.‡ The herpes simplex virus appears to be more common in individuals with cervical cancer.

Carcinogens were mentioned briefly earlier in this chapter. They can be either physical or chemical

---

*A highly malignant condition marked by multiple adenomatous polyps lining the intestinal mucosa, beginning about puberty.

†A tumor arising from retinal germ cells, a common malignancy of the eye in childhood.

‡A malignant neoplasm composed of undifferentiated lymphoreticular cells that form a large osteolytic lesion in the jaw or an abdominal mass. It is seen chiefly in Africa.

agents, and hundreds have been identified. Physical agents include excessive exposure to ultraviolet rays of sun and repeated exposure to diagnostic x-ray procedures or radiation therapy. Chemical agents include smoking or exposure to tobacco smoke, chewing tobacco, or repeated exposure to pesticides, formaldehydes, asbestos, and nickel and zinc ores. *Carcinogenesis* is the process by which compounds act directly on cells to cause cancer.

The process may take many years to occur in humans; it may stop at any point and occasionally is reversible. Generally, there is a progressive evolution of cancer cells through different states—**hyperplasia** (excessive growth of cells), **dysplasia** (abnormal growth of cells), **carcinoma in situ** (a cancerous growth that remains in place), to carcinomas that **metastasize** (spread through the circulatory system).

Disturbances in hormonal balance may influence tumor growth either through the body's own changes or from the administration of exogenous hormones. Additionally, increased pregnancies are associated with a decrease in ovarian, breast, and endometrial cancers.

Chronic irritation is not usually considered to be a cause of cancer, but it is thought to be a precursor in some instances. A chronic irritation that is not eliminated can cause abnormal cell changes that may become cancerous. For example, chronic skin ulcers sometimes are complicated by the development of squamous cell carcinomas.

DIAGNOSIS OF NEOPLASMS

Responsibility for early detection lies partly with the individual. Because any delay in the diagnosis and treatment of cancer can significantly alter the disease course, the American Cancer Society recommends the following:

- A cancer-related checkup by a physician every 3 years for persons aged 20 to 39 and annually for those aged 40 and over.
- Persons at greater risk for certain cancers may require more frequent testing.
- Checkups should include health counseling on topics such as cessation of smoking, use of sun blocks, and so on.
- Checkups should include examinations for cancer of the breast, uterus, cervix, ovaries, prostate, testes, colon, rectum, mouth, skin, thyroid, and lymph nodes.

Any suspicion of a neoplasm or cancer should include a thorough medical history and a physical examination. Specific tests for early detection have been quite helpful and include ultrasonography, radiography, endoscopy, isotope scanning, computed tomography (CT) scanning, and magnetic resonance imaging (MRI). The single most helpful tool is probably the biopsy. Tissue samples can be taken for biopsy through curettage, fluid aspiration, fine-needle aspiration biopsy, dermal punch, endoscopy, and surgical excision.

Another tumor marker, carcinoembryonic antigen (CEA), can alert physicians to malignancies of the colon, stomach, pancreas, lungs, and breasts. CEA can also serve as a baseline during chemotherapy to determine tumor spread, to regulate drug dosage, to detect cancer recurrence, and to prognosticate after surgery or radiation. The PSA, mentioned earlier in this chaspter, is used to detect and monitor prostatic cancer.

To help in the diagnosis of the disease, a Pap test and a biopsy may be performed. The Pap test was developed by Dr. George N. Papanicolaou (1883–1962) to detect cancer, commonly of the uterus and cervix. It is a simple test using an **exfoliative cytology** staining procedure, and it can be performed on any body excretion, such as urine and feces; secretion, such as sputum, prostatic fluid, and vaginal fluid; or tissue scrapings, such as from the uterus or the stomach. The specimen sample is placed on a slide, stained, and studied under the microscope for abnormal cells. For a person at average risk who has had two negative Pap tests 1 year apart, the American Cancer Society recommends subsequent Pap tests every 3 years. The Pap test is highly effective in detecting early cancer of the cervix or the uterus.

GRADING AND STAGING OF NEOPLASMS

Part of the diagnosis is the grading and staging of neoplasms. Pathologists grade neoplasms by studying the microscopic appearance of suspected tumor cells to determine their degree of **anaplasia**. The grading helps in the diagnosis and in treatment planning. Usually four grades are used, as follows:

- Grade I: Tumor cells are well differentiated, closely resembling normal parent tissue.

- Grades II and III: Tumor cells are intermediate in appearance, moderately or poorly differentiated.
- Grade IV: Tumor cells are so anaplastic that recognition of the tumor's tissue origin is difficult.

Persons with grade I tumors typically have a high survival rate, whereas persons with grade IV tumors have a much poorer likelihood of survival. Grading also is used when evaluating cells from body fluids in preventive screening tests, such as Pap smears of the uterine cervix.

Staging neoplasms involves estimating the extent to which a tumor has spread. As with grading, staging is important in determining a proper course of treatment. A TNM system is commonly used and is summarized here. This system stages tumors according to three basic criteria: T refers to the size and extent of the primary *tumor*, N refers to the number of area lymph *nodes* involved, and M refers to any *metastasis* of the primary tumor. The grading and staging system will be specific and more greatly detailed according to the site of the disease.

TREATMENT OF NEOPLASMS

Treatment of cancer is continually changing as new technology develops. The treatment may offer symptomatic relief to the client, be used in conjunction with some primary course of treatment, and, perhaps, cure the cancer. The five major types of treatment against cancer are surgery, radiation therapy, chemotherapy, immunotherapy or biotherapy, and hormonal therapy. The physician may recommend one or any combination of these treatment procedures to combat a particular form of cancer. Following the presentation of the more traditional types of cancer treatment, the integration of alternative thereapies will be discussed.

Surgery

Surgery now is more precise because of improved diagnostic equipment and operating procedures and advances in preoperative and postoperative care. Surgery for cancer may be specific, **palliative**, or preventive.

Specific surgery is done to remove all of the cancerous tissue and, it is hoped, to cure the person. The types of cancers that respond well to this type of surgery are those of the lung, skin, stomach, large intestine, breast, and endometrium.

Palliative surgery is done to sustain the individual with cancer or to alleviate the pain that directly or indirectly results from the cancer. Examples include treating complications of cancer such as abscesses, intestinal perforation and bleeding, or intestinal obstructions. Reconstructive surgery may also be used, especially in the breasts, skin, head, and neck cancers. In advanced cancers, palliative surgery may be done to sever nerves to alleviate pain.

Preventive surgery may be done to prevent the development of cancer. For example, polyps of the colon may be removed because they are thought to be precancerous.

Types of surgery include excisional, or **en bloc**, which is removal of the primary tumor, lymph nodes, adjacent involved structure, and surrounding tissues. En bloc procedure is done during a radical mastectomy, colectomy, or gastrectomy. *Electrocautery* is the burning of cancer tissue with electric current. This is the preferred method of treating cancers of the rectum.

Radiation Therapy

Radiation may be used alone or in combination with other forms of cancer treatment. More than half of all persons with cancer receive some type of radiation therapy. Radiation may be used to cure, to control the disease, or to prevent malignant leukemias from infiltrating the brain or spinal cord. There are two types of radiation: (1) electromagnetic rays and (2) particles. In the former, radiation consists of x-rays and gamma rays, and in the latter, the particles are electrons, protons, neutrons, and alpha particles. The radiation may be applied externally or internally. In the external mode, an x-ray machine or a radioactive form of an element called a **radioisotope** may be used. In the internal mode, a radioisotope is placed into catheters, beads, seeds, ribbons, or needles and implanted inside the body.

The goal of radiation therapy is to destroy as much of the tumor as possible without affecting surrounding healthy tissue. Unfortunately, some cancers are situated where radiation would cause serious harm to surrounding tissues. Moreover, some cancers are *radioresistant*, meaning they are not affected by radiation within the safe dosage range.

The effects of radiation on the body include cell death, because ionizing radiation disrupts DNA and interferes with cell replication and growth. Recovery from radiation damage to normal tissue does occur between doses, but the degree varies, depending on the radiosensitivity of the normal tissue. The radiation dose is determined by the size, type, and location of the tumor.

The adverse effects of radiation generally occur in the skin, mucous membranes, and bone marrow. Hair may begin to fall out, **erythema** or redness of the skin may develop, and eating may be difficult because of the nausea, vomiting, and mucosal damage to the mouth and stomach. These distressing side effects generally subside, either between radiation treatments or after the therapy is complete. Late effects of radiation therapy may be more severe and chronic, especially when combined with other treatment modalities. New developments in cancer radiology are continually appearing for both curative and palliative purposes.

Chemotherapy

Chemotherapy may be used alone or in combination with other cancer treatments. It is especially effective against cancers that spread, such as leukemias and some solid cancers, including **choriocarcinoma** (an extremely rare but highly malignant neoplasm, usually of the uterus) and Hodgkin's disease. The goals of chemotherapy are to cure, to control, or to use as a palliative agent. As with radiation, chemotherapeutic drugs affect normal cellular growth and replication, especially of rapidly proliferating cells. The chemotherapeutic agents are used alone or in combination for the treatment of malignancy. Many of the chemotherapeutic drugs are experimental and can be used only by oncologists. Chemotherapeutic drugs of similar action generally are grouped together.

Most of these drugs are toxic and have adverse effects on the gastrointestinal tract, skin, and bone marrow. The most common side effects of chemotherapeutic drugs include nausea, vomiting, anorexia, anemia, an abnormal decrease in white blood cells (**leukopenia**), and loss of hair. The person receiving chemotherapy will be monitored closely with laboratory testing and physical examination to evaluate the efficacy of the treatment and to detect potentially serious side effects.

Immunotherapy (Biotherapy)

A treatment that is used in combination with radiation and chemotherapy is *immunotherapy* or *biotherapy,* or biological treatment of tumors. Biotherapy stimulates or restores, and strengthens the body's own immune system, allowing it to recognize and attack cancer cells. Thus, biotherapy is used to lessen side effects that may be caused by some cancer treatments. Some tumors overwhelm the body's immune system; radiation and chemotherapy may also suppress the immune system. Thus, treatment to enhance the immune system's response may be indicated. Biotherapy is most effective in the early stages of cancer. The use of interferon, a naturally occurring body protein that is capable of killing cancer cells or stopping their growth in high-risk melanomas, has been useful. Bone marrow transplantation has proved effective in restoring hematologic and immunologic properties in clients with some cancers, such as Hodgkin's disease and multiple myeloma. Other transplantations used include peripheral blood stem cell transplantation and cord blood transplantation.

Hormonal Therapy

Hormonal therapy is treatment that adds, blocks, or removes hormones. It is based on research that shows that certain hormones affect the growth of certain cancers. Surgical removal of glands that produce the hormones may be necessary or administration of synthetic hormones may be tried to block the body's natural hormones. In women, estrogen promotes the growth of about two-thirds of breast cancers, according to the American Cancer Society. Hence, hormonal therapy is aimed at blocking the effects of estrogen or lowering estrogen levels in the treatment of breast cancer. After breast surgery, drugs such as Tamoxifen or Raloxifene may be prescribed for 5 years. In metastatic prostate cancer, hormonal deprivation therapy is the main treatment, especially in men with less advanced prostate cancer. More and more drugs for hormonal therapy are available for physicians to use in the treatment of prostate cancer. Whether or not to consider hormonal therapy requires an assessment of the client's needs including the stage and extent of the client's cancer, the side effects of the treatment, and the cost of the treatment.

Alternative Therapy

Most individuals diagnosed with cancer have considered or participated in some form of alternative medicine therapy. In some circles, the debate rages on with traditional therapies on one side and alternative therapies on another. Refer to Chapter 2 for a more detailed discussion of the use of alternative therapies.

Increased benefit may be achieved if persons with cancer carefully consider both traditional or conventional treatments and alternative treatment therapies. Many will choose to embrace both simultaneously and will want to seek physicians who are willing and able to offer both or to work cooperatively in an integrative way with the client's wishes in mind.

Alternative practitioners recognize the three major forms of conventional cancer treatment and understand the wisdom of each. Most, however, prefer that their clients wait for any chemotherapy or radiation treatment (both of which can be either very toxic to the body or cause inherent health hazards) until after alternative therapies have had a chance at success. However, if chemotherapy and/or radiation is deemed necessary, alternative therapies can, in some cases, reduce many side effects or enhance the effectiveness of chemotherapy and radiation. Proponents of alternative therapies consider that cancer is a manifestation of an unhealthy body whose defenses are so seriously out of balance that they can no longer destroy cells that turn cancerous.

Alternative therapies hold the premise that cancer is a result of the dysfunction of the body as a whole rather than a single disease. The goal of alternative therapy is to strengthen the body's immune system. These therapies may include treatments that rely on biopharmaceutical, immune enhancement, metabolic, nutritional, and herbal nontoxic methods.

Cancer is very complex and can be life threatening. It requires professional medical care. Some alternative remedies may actually make cancer worse if not used properly, just as conventional methods can be so toxic that a person succumbs to the treatment rather than the disease itself. Any alternative methods should become a part of a cancer treatment program that is guided and monitored by a qualified physician experienced in integrative medicine and treatment.

Summary

Cancer is a life-threatening disease that can strike any person at any age. It can strike with or without warning and has been a recognized disease for more than 100 years. Prevention is the best line of defense. Early detection, diagnosis, and prompt treatment form the best course of action. If the spread is not controlled or checked, cancer can result in death; however, many cancers can be cured if detected and treated promptly. Integrative medicine may offer the best solution to enhance cancer treatment.

CASE STUDIES

■ Case Study 1

Kai Simpson has surfed since he was a young teenager through his young adulthood years off the coast of Maui, where he was born and raised. Every time the surf was up and the sun was out, he was on his board. Twenty years later, he is diagnosed with malignant melanoma.

Case Study Questions

1. What protective measures might Kai have taken as a young surfer?
2. Identify possible treatment measures that might be taken.

■ Case Study 2

A 72-year-old man, Keith Wilson, was diagnosed with lung cancer and died less than a year later. In reviewing his history, it was noted that he remembered aspirating peanuts, husks and all, when he was a child; no treatment was available. Keith was a heavy smoker since his teenage years and smoked cigars into his 50s. Keith's wife and son vividly recall taking many family automobile trips to Canada and Mexico, crisscrossing the nation, with Keith smoking in the enclosed automobile.

Case Study Questions

1. What is the effect of secondary smoke to Keith's wife and son?
2. What preventative measures could have Keith taken early in life?
3. Describe how debilitating lung cancer can be.

REVIEW QUESTIONS

True/False

Circle the correct answer:

T   F   1. About 50,000 diagnosed cases of skin cancer could be prevented by protection from the sun's rays.

T   F   2. Leukemias are sometimes considered to be sarcomas.

T   F   3. Non-Hodgkin's lymphomas are also known as malignant lymphomas.

T   F   4. Palliative surgery may be done to alleviate pain.

T   F   5. Chemotherapy drugs are nontoxins and are preferred by alternative medicine practitioners.

Matching

Match each of the following definitions with its correct term:

_____   1. System used to estimate extent to which a tumor spreads

_____   2. Neoplasms of blood-forming tissues

_____   3. Cancers made up of supportive and connective tissue

_____   4. System used to determine cell degree of anaplasia

_____   5. Largest group of cancers; solid tumors of epithelial tissue

a. Carcinomas

b. Sarcomas

c. Leukemia

d. Grading

e. Neoplasms

f. TNM

Short Answer

1. _____ is a new formation that serves no useful purpose; it is uncontrollable and progressive.

2. _____ is a new formation that grows slowly; cells resemble cells of tissue from which the tumor originates.

3. _____ is a new formation that is invasive, grows rather rapidly, is anaplastic, and is capable of metastasis.

4. Cancer of the _____ is the leading cause of cancer death in both men and women.

5. _____ , _____ , and _____ are the three most common cancer sites for females.

Multiple Choice

Place a check next to the correct answers:

1. Which of the following is a definitive diagnostic tool of neoplasms?

    a. Early recognition of cancer warning signals

    b. Breast self-examination

    c. Testicular self-examination

    d. Pap test

    e. Biopsy by needle aspiration, endoscopy, or surgical incision

2. Which of the following is/are treatment(s) for cancer?

    a. Surgery

    b. Radiation

    c. Chemotherapy

    d. Biopsy

    e. Immunotherapy/biotherapy

    f. Hormonal therapy

3. Immunotherapy includes

    a. Hormonal therapy.

    b. Nutritional methods.

    c. Interferon.

    d. Radiation by electromagnetic rays.

4. Which of the following statements is true about the cause of cancer?

    a. Genetic factors are the cause of cancer.

    b. All cancers are inherited.

    c. Specific bacteria can cause cancer.

    d. There is no one single cause of cancer.

5. Surgery for cancer can be

    a. Palliative.

    b. Curative.

    c. Preventative.

    d. a, b, and c

    e. a and c

HARPER COLLEGE LIBRARY
PALATINE, ILLINOIS 60067

Discussion Questions/Personal Reflection

1. Discuss the integrated medicine approach to the treatment of cancer.

2. Consider how you might personally prevent cancer in your life. Consider your family history and lifestyle.

Notes

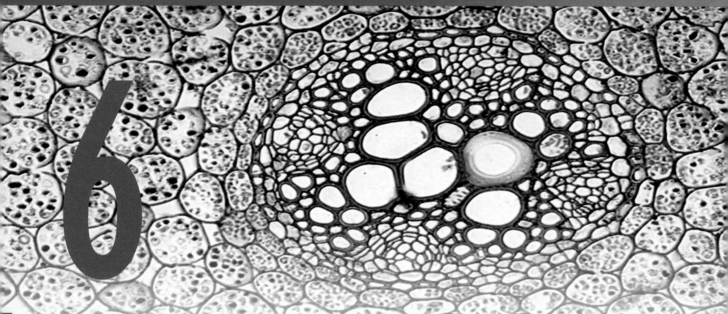

6

Congenital Diseases and Disorders

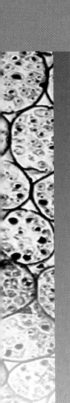

KEY WORDS

Acetabulum (ăs•ĕ•tăb′ ū•lŭm)
Alveoli (ăl•vē′ ō•lī)
Anastomosis (ă•năs•tō•mō′sĭs)
Angiography (ăn•jē •ŏg′ră•fē)
Anoxia (ăn•ŏk′sē•ă)
Atelectasis (ăt•ĕ•lĕk′tă•sĭs)
Auscultation (aws•kŭl•tā′shŭn)
Bronchiole (brong′kē•ŏl)
Cardiomegaly (kăr•dē•ō•mĕg′ă•lē)
Chyme (kīm)
Claudication (klaw•dĭ•kā′shŭn)
Colostomy (kō•lŏs′tō•mē)
Cyanosis (sī•ăn•ō′sĭs)
Ductus arteriosus (dŭk′tŭs ăr•tē•rē•ō•sĭs)
Dystonia (dĭs•tō′nē•ă)
Epigastrium (ĕp•ĭ•găs′trē•ŭm)
Epistaxis (ĕp•ĭ•stăk′sĭs)
Excoriated (ĕk′skŏr•ē•āt•ĕd)
Excretory urography (ĕks′krē•tō-rē ū•rŏg′ ră-fē)
Fontanelle (fŏn•tă•nĕl′)
Ganglion (găng′lē•ŏn)
Hematuria (hē•mă•tū′rē•ă)
Hydronephrosis (hī•drō•nĕf•ro′sĭs)
Hydroureter (hī•drō•ū•rē′tĕr)
Hypertrophy (hī•pĕr′trŏ•fē)
Ileostomy (ĭl•ē•ŏs′tō•mē)
Lumen (lū′mĕn)
Macrocephaly (măk•rō•sĕf′ă•lē)
Meconium (mĭ-kō•nē•ĕm)
Meninges (mĕn•ĕn′jēz)
Nephrectomy (nĕf•rĕk′tō•mē)
Nevus (nē′vŭs)
Nystagmus (nĭs•tăg′mŭs)
Ortolani's sign (ŏr′tĕl•ĕn•ez sĭn)
Parasympathetic (păr•ă•sĭm•pă•thĕt′ĭk)
Peristalsis (pĕr•ĭ•stăl′sĭs)
Pylorus (pī•lŏr′ŭs)
Reflux (rē′flŭks)
Resection (rē•sĕk′shŭn)
Septum (sĕp′tŭm)
Tachypnea (tăk•ĭp•nē′ă)
Teratogen (tĕr-ăt′ō•jĭn)
Thrill (thrĭl)
Toxemia (tŏks•ē′mē•ă)

The last of the human freedoms is to choose one's attitudes.

—VIKTOR E. FRANKL

LEARNING OBJECTIVES

Upon successful completion of this chapter, you will be able to:

• Describe the three types of cerebral palsy.
• Identify the signs and symptoms of spina bifida, meningocele, and myelomeningocele.
• Recall the diagnostic procedures used for hydrocephalus.
• Identify the etiology of pyloric stenosis.
• Discuss Hirschsprung's disease.
• Describe cleft lip and palate.
• Compare and contrast the various congenital defects of the heart.
• Define *cryptorchidism.*
• Compare and contrast the congenital defects of the ureter, bladder, and urethra.
• List the four common forms of clubfoot.
• Recall the etiology of congenital hip dysplasia.
• Describe the signs and symptoms of cystic fibrosis.
• Restate the diagnostic procedures for phenylketonuria (PKU).

In Chapter 1, a basic description of genetic factors relating to the body's disease processes was given. Here, the term *congenital diseases* refers to problems that are present at birth and have genetic causes, nongenetic causes, or a combination of the two. The clinical manifestations of congenital disease may be minor and inconsequential, or they may be life-threatening. Some may be detected at birth; others are not apparent until later in infancy or childhood. All congenital diseases, however, require the attention of physicians and the involvement of the entire family.

NERVOUS SYSTEM DISEASES AND DISORDERS

Cerebral Palsy

■ **DESCRIPTION** *Cerebral palsy* (CP) is bilateral, symmetrical, nonprogressive paralysis resulting from developmental defects of the brain or trauma during or after the birth process.

■ **ETIOLOGY** CP is caused by central nervous system damage that occurs before, during, or after birth. Prenatal causes can include maternal rubella (especially in the first trimester), maternal diabetes, absence of oxygen (**anoxia**), or **toxemia** (a condition of pregnancy-induced hypertension). Causes related to the birth process include trauma during delivery, prematurity, or asphyxia from the umbilical cord becoming wrapped around the infant's neck. Postnatal causes include head trauma, meningitis, or poisoning. The occurrence of CP is highest in premature infants, and it is the most common cause of crippling in children. There are three types: spastic, athetoid, and ataxis.

■ **DIAGNOSTIC PROCEDURES** *Spastic cerebral palsy* affects about 70% of CP children and is characterized by hyperactive reflexes, rapid muscle contraction, muscle weakness, and underdevelopment of limbs. Children with this form of CP typically walk on their toes, crossing one foot in front of the other.

Athetoid cerebral palsy affects 20% of CP children and is characterized by involuntary muscle movements and impaired muscle tone or **dystonia**. The arms are more often affected than the legs, and speech may be difficult. The body movements in athetoid CP are increased during times of stress and are not apparent during sleep.

Roughly 10% of CP persons show signs of ataxic CP. They have difficulty with balance and coordination and show signs of rhythmic, involuntary movement of the eyeball, or **nystagmus**, muscle weakness, and tremor. Sudden movements are almost always impossible.

A few children will exhibit signs of all three types of CP. Mental retardation occurs in about 40% of CP children. Seizure disorders, impaired motor function, and impaired speech or vision often are present. Many may have dental abnormalities, and vision and hearing defects.

■ **DIAGNOSTIC PROCEDURES** Careful neurological assessment, including examination and history, is necessary. The spontaneous movement and behavior of the child are observed for characteristic signs, such as (1) inability to suck or keep food in the mouth, (2) difficulty in voluntary movements, (3) difficulty in separating the legs during diaper changes, and (4) use of only one hand or both hands, but not the legs.

■ **TREATMENT** CP has no cure, and treatment is directed toward helping children overcome any functional or intellectual disability. The treatment process typically involves the entire family. Treatment may include the use of braces and special appliances, range-of-motion exercises, orthopedic surgery, and medications to decrease seizures and spasticity. The family may benefit from a referral to the local chapter of the United Cerebral Palsy Association.

ALTERNATIVE THERAPY: *Alternative practitioners have recommended avoidance of any food allergens that may increase or intensify symptoms of the disease, mostly due to decreased immune functioning because the body is dealing with the allergen. Other therapies include acupuncture, biofeedback training, and traditional Chinese medicine.*

▶ TEACHING TIPS: Parents will need assistance from physicians, social workers, and other health-care professionals for the child's rehabilitation.

■ **PROGNOSIS** The prognosis varies. If impairment is mild, a near-normal life may be possible.

■ **PREVENTION** Early prenatal care and good maternal health are preventive measures.

Neural Tube Defects: Spina Bifida, Meningocele, and Myelomeningocele

■ **DESCRIPTION** The neural tube defects (NTDs), *spina bifida, meningocele,* and *myelomeningocele* (Fig. 6.1), are developmental defects of the first trimester of pregnancy that are characterized by incomplete closure of the bones encasing the spinal cord. *Spina bifida occulta* is the most common but least severe of these defects. It is marked by an

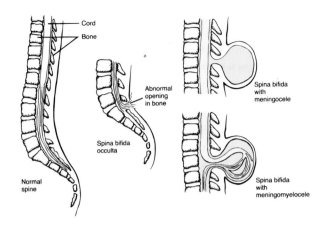

Figure 6.1 Neural tube defects. (Adapted from Rothstein, JM, Roy, SH, and Wolf, SL: The Rehabilitation Specialist's Handbook, ed 2. FA Davis, Philadelphia, 1998, p 704, with permission.)

incomplete closure of one or more vertebrae, with no protrusion of the spinal cord or the membranes covering the brain and spinal cord, called the **meninges**. In *meningocele*, the incomplete closure of the vertebra is accompanied by a protrusion of the spinal fluid and meninges into an external sac. *Myelomeningocele* results when the external sac contains meninges, cerebrospinal fluid, and a portion of the spinal cord or its nerve roots.

■ ETIOLOGY Between 20 and 23 days of gestation, the neural tube should be complete except for the opening at each end. What causes the failure to close or a later reopening is essentially unknown. NTDs may be isolated birth defects, or they may result from exposure to a **teratogen**, anything that adversely affects normal cellular development in the embryo or fetus, such as certain chemicals, some therapeutic and illicit drugs, and radiation. Risk factors associated with these conditions include exposure to radiation and viruses. There may also be genetic factors. Research has identified a lack of folic acid in the pregnant woman's diet. Spina bifida affects about 5% of the population.

■ SIGNS AND SYMPTOMS Spina bifida occulta may show no visible signs or may be manifested by a dimple in the skin, hair tuft, or a port-wine birthmark (**nevus**) along the posterior surface of the body, in the midline above the buttocks. In general, spina

bifida does not cause neurologic dysfunction, although there may be associated foot weakness or bowel or bladder disturbances. With meningocele and myelomeningocele, a saclike structure protrudes from the spinal area. Spina bifida and meningocele may cause little or no neurologic deficit, but myelomeningocele frequently results in permanent neurologic difficulties.

■ DIAGNOSTIC PROCEDURES Prenatal detection of some open NTDs is possible through ultrasonographic examination between the 14th and 16th weeks of gestation or through the use of amniocentesis, which shows high levels of acetylcholinesterase. A fetal karyotype may be done because 5% to 7% of NTDs are associated with chromosomal abnormalities. After birth, meningocele and myelomeningocele are obvious on examination. Spina bifida occulta may show as a dimple, depression, tuft of hair, soft fatty deposits, or a combination of these, or it may not be evident on visual inspection. Accordingly, x-ray, pinprick examination of the legs and trunk, and myelography are other procedures used to diagnose the condition and to show the level of sensory and motor involvement.

■ TREATMENT Spina bifida occulta usually requires no treatment. Meningocele and myelomeningocele require surgical repair of the sac and closure of the bone defect and supportive measures to promote independence and to decrease the possibility of complications.

ALTERNATIVE THERAPY: *Alternative therapy for NTDs includes administering folic acid to pregnant women as a preventative measure.*

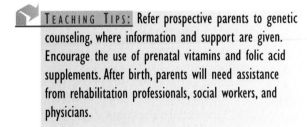

TEACHING TIPS: Refer prospective parents to genetic counseling, where information and support are given. Encourage the use of prenatal vitamins and folic acid supplements. After birth, parents will need assistance from rehabilitation professionals, social workers, and physicians.

■ PROGNOSIS The prognosis is dependent on the extent of neurologic deficit that accompanies the condition. The prognosis is worse for individuals with large open spinal lesions, neurogenic bladder, or leg paralysis and much better for those with only spina bifida occulta. In the latter, many affected individuals may be able to live a normal life. In the most severe cases of spina bifida, waist supports, leg braces, and management of fecal incontinence and neurogenic bladder are necessary.

■ **PREVENTION** Because spinal cord defects occur more often in offspring of women who have previously had a child with a similar defect, genetic counseling may be helpful. Refer parents to the Spina Bifida Association of America.

Hydrocephalus

■ **DESCRIPTION** *Hydrocephalus* is a condition marked by too much cerebrospinal fluid in the *ventricles* of the brain. If hydrocephalus occurs before the cranial sutures have fused, the ventricles expand beyond the point of obstruction, the cranial sutures separate, the head expands, and the **fontanelles**, commonly called "soft spots" of the skull, bulge. The condition is called noncommmunicating hydrocephalus when there is an obstruction in cerebrospinal fluid flow. If the problem is faulty absorption of cerebrospinal fluid, the condition is called communicating hydrocephalus. This condition is more common in newborns but may occur in adults as the result of injury or disease.

■ **ETIOLOGY** Noncommunicating hydrocephalus may result from problems in fetal development, an infection, a tumor, or a blood clot. In communicating hydrocephalus, faulty absorption of the cerebrospinal fluid may be a consequence of surgery to repair myelomeningocele or a meningeal hemorrhage.

■ **SIGNS AND SYMPTOMS** The classic symptom of noncommunicating hydrocephalus is the enlarged head; communicating hydrocephalus produces bulging fontanelles as the only visible sign. The scalp skin may be thin and fragile appearing, with the veins clearly visible. Hydrocephalic infants often have high-pitched cries and abnormal muscle tone in their legs. Projectile vomiting often occurs. Seizures, weakness, and uncoordinated movements are common.

■ **DIAGNOSTIC PROCEDURES** The head circumference is measured; an abnormally large head may indicate the diagnosis. Magnetic resonance imaging (MRI) and computed tomography (CT) scanning confirm the diagnosis. Angiography (x-ray of the blood vessels shown on film) also may be used.

■ **TREATMENT** Surgical correction is the treatment of choice for hydrocephalus. A shunt is usually placed from the affected ventricles of the brain into the peritoneal cavity or into the right atrium of the heart, where the excess fluid makes its way into the venous circulation.

ALTERNATIVE THERAPY: *No significant alternative therapy is indicated.*

> **TEACHING TIPS:** Help parents focus on rehabilitation after surgery, building on the infant's abilities and potential. Parents require information about what to watch for in shunt malfunction. The child may require special education programs.

■ **PROGNOSIS** The prognosis is guarded even with early detection and surgical correction. Mental retardation, vision loss, and impaired motor function often occur. Without surgery, the mortality rate is high.

■ **PREVENTION** There is no known prevention to

DIGESTIVE SYSTEM DISEASES AND DISORDERS

Pyloric Stenosis

■ **DESCRIPTION** *Pyloric* stenosis is narrowing of the **pylorus (pyloric sphincter)**, the lower opening of the stomach leading into the upper part of the intestine, or duodenum. This condition causes obstruction of the flow into the small intestine of **chyme**, the nearly liquid mixture composed of partially digested food and gastric secretions. Pyloric stenosis is much more common in male than in female infants and adolescents.

■ **ETIOLOGY** The cause is unknown, but the disease may be hereditary. It is one of the most common developmental abnormalities of the digestive system.

■ **SIGNS AND SYMPTOMS** The classic symptom is projectile vomiting, beginning about the second to fourth week after birth. The infant may eject vomitus a distance of 3 to 4 feet. Signs of dehydration and starvation may be evident if the pyloric sphincter closes completely. There may be decreased elasticity of the skin, abdominal distention, and a palpable tumor in the **epigastrium**, the region of the abdomen over the pit of the stomach.

■ **DIAGNOSTIC PROCEDURES** The history and physical examination may suggest the condition. Other studies may include upper gastrointestinal x-ray and laboratory tests, with the latter being used to detect dehydration and electrolyte imbalances. Pyloric stenosis must be distinguished from feeding difficulties associated with colic or disturbed mother-child relationships.

■ **TREATMENT** The standard treatment is incision and suture of the pyloric sphincter. The procedure, called pyloromyotomy, is relatively simple, safe, and effective.

ALTERNATIVE THERAPY: *No significant alternative therapy is indicated.*

TEACHING TIPS: This disorder can be particularly unnerving for parents and caregivers. Reassurance is important. Prepare the family for the infant's surgery and necessary follow-up care.

■ **PROGNOSIS** The prognosis is excellent with proper care and surgical correction.

■ **PREVENTION** There is no known prevention.

Hirschsprung's Disease (Congenital Aganglionic Megacolon)

■ **DESCRIPTION** Hirschsprung's disease is the obstruction and dilation of the colon with feces as a result of inadequate intestinal motility. Feces are not moved past the aganglionic segment of the colon. Pressure from accumulating feces then distends the preceding portion of the colon. The amount of intestinal wall affected varies; involvement may be limited to the internal sphincter or may extend to the entire colon. The disease more frequently affects white female infants and adolescents. Often, the disease occurs with other congenital anomalies.

■ **ETIOLOGY** The cause of the disease is unknown, but it appears to be a hereditary, usually familial disease. Hirschsprung's disease may occur with other congenital anomalies, such as trisomy 21. The condition is due to an absence of autonomic **parasympathetic** (involuntary) **ganglion** cells, that are masses of nervelike cell bodies in the colorectal walls, resulting in the absence of the involuntary wavelike contractions (**peristalsis**) in the affected portion.

■ **SIGNS AND SYMPTOMS** Clinical manifestations typically appear during infancy, but they may not appear until adolescence. In infancy, the newborn fails to pass the first feces, or **meconiun,** within 48 hours of birth. Signs and symptoms include severe abdominal distention and feeding difficulties. After the neonatal period, symptoms may include fever, failure to thrive, and explosive watery diarrhea. In adolescence, symptoms may include chronic constipation, abdominal distention, and palpable fecal masses. The child also may be anemic and appear poorly nourished.

■ **DIAGNOSTIC PROCEDURES** Diagnosis is confirmed with a rectal biopsy that reveals the absence of ganglion cells in the colorectal wall. In older infants and adolescence, a barium enema, upright x-ray of the abdomen, or rectal manometry may be ordered.

■ **TREATMENT** Surgical treatment generally involves a two-stage procedure. First, a temporary colostomy is created in the normal bowel. The colostomy allows the infant to evacuate feces, allows the bowel to rest, and allows the infant to gain weight. The second-stage surgery is a pull-through procedure wherein the affected segment of the bowel is resected or removed and the normal bowel is anastomosed to the rectum. During this second state, the colostomy is also closed. More recently, a one-stage procedure has been used with the pull-through as described above only without a temporary colostomy. The benefit with a one-stage surgical procedure is that it is only one operation and there is no colostomy care. Another type of procedure is called a laparascope-assisted pull-through. In this procedure, a laparoscope is put through the anus, allowing the surgeon to pull the affected bowel segment through the opening. In all of these procedures, fluid and electrolyte balance must be maintained. Antibiotics may also be prescribed to reduce intestinal flora.

ALTERNATIVE THERAPY: *No significant alternative therapy is indicated.*

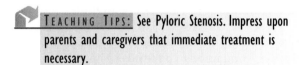

TEACHING TIPS: See Pyloric Stenosis. Impress upon parents and caregivers that immediate treatment is necessary.

■ **PROGNOSIS** With prompt treatment, the prognosis is good. If untreated, death is likely from enterocolitis, severe diarrhea, and shock.

■ **PREVENTION** There is no known prevention.

Cleft Lip and Palate

■ **DESCRIPTION** Cleft lip is a congenital birth defect in which there are one or more clefts in the upper lip. Cleft palate is a birth defect that is characterized by a hole in the middle of the roof of the mouth. The cleft may extend completely through the hard and soft palates into the nasal area. The defects appear singly or together and vary in severity. Major problems are difficulty by the infant in sucking and the infant's facial appearance.

■ **ETIOLOGY** These disorders are thought to represent a multifactorial genetic disorder that results in a failure in the embryonic development of the fetus. The combination of cleft lip and cleft palate occurs in approximately 1 in 1,000 births.

■ **SIGNS AND SYMPTOMS** The described physical symptoms are apparent at birth.

■ **DIAGNOSTIC PROCEDURES** Symptoms confirm the diagnosis and may include seeing formula or the mother's milk come through the nose of the infant.

■ **TREATMENT** Surgery is the treatment of choice and usually is done as soon as possible because sucking can be difficult. Some deformities require that surgery be performed in stages. Special feeding devices and techniques can be tried. A team of practitioners is likely to be required. Specialists such as plastic surgeons, neurosurgeons, orthodontists, otolaryngologists, speech pathologists, and audiologists are likely to be involved into adulthood.

ALTERNATIVE THERAPY: *No significant alternative therapy is indicated.*

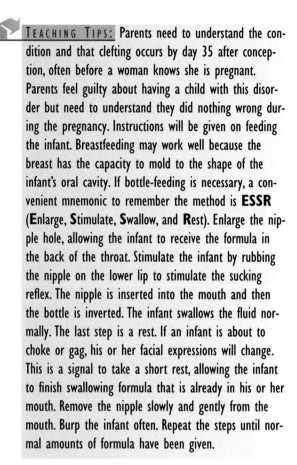

TEACHING TIPS: Parents need to understand the condition and that clefting occurs by day 35 after conception, often before a woman knows she is pregnant. Parents feel guilty about having a child with this disorder but need to understand they did nothing wrong during the pregnancy. Instructions will be given on feeding the infant. Breastfeeding may work well because the breast has the capacity to mold to the shape of the infant's oral cavity. If bottle-feeding is necessary, a convenient mnemonic to remember the method is **ESSR** (**E**nlarge, **S**timulate, **S**wallow, and **R**est). Enlarge the nipple hole, allowing the infant to receive the formula in the back of the throat. Stimulate the infant by rubbing the nipple on the lower lip to stimulate the sucking reflex. The nipple is inserted into the mouth and then the bottle is inverted. The infant swallows the fluid normally. The last step is a rest. If an infant is about to choke or gag, his or her facial expressions will change. This is a signal to take a short rest, allowing the infant to finish swallowing formula that is already in his or her mouth. Remove the nipple slowly and gently from the mouth. Burp the infant often. Repeat the steps until normal amounts of formula have been given.

■ **PROGNOSIS** The prognosis is good with corrective surgery. A child may need speech therapy as he/she begins to talk.

■ **PREVENTION** There is no known prevention.

CARDIOVASCULAR DISEASES AND DISORDERS

Congenital Heart Defects

■ **DESCRIPTION** *Congenital heart defects* can be broadly classified according to whether or not poorly oxygenated blood entering from the veins mixes in the heart with the freshly oxygenated blood reentering the systemic circulation. *Acyanotic defects* are those in which there is no mixing of poorly oxygenated blood with the blood reentering the systemic circulation. *Cyanotic defects* are those in which

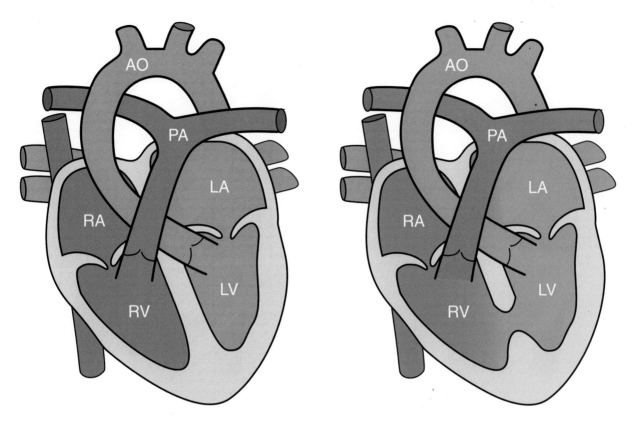

Figure 6.2 Ventricular septal defect. AO, aorta; PA, pulmonary artery; LA, left atrium; LV, left ventricle; RA, right atrium; RV, right ventricle. (From http://www.kumc.edu/instruction/medicine/pedcard/cardiology/pedcardio/vsddiagram.gif, courtesy of The University of Kansas Medical Center © 1996. Accessed October 14, 2003.)

poorly oxygenated blood mixes with the blood reentering the systemic circulation.

Acyanotic defects include the following:

- *Ventricular septal defect* (*VSD*), a congenital heart defect in which there is an abnormal opening between the wall, or **septum**, of the right and left ventricles (Fig. 6.2). The extent of the opening may vary from pin size to complete absence of the ventricular septum, creating one common ventricle. This defect typically accompanies other congenital anomalies, especially Down syndrome, renal defects, or other cardiac defects. VSD is the most commonly occurring congenital heart defect.
- *Atrial septal defect* (*ASD*), an abnormal opening between the right and left atria. The size

and location of the opening determine the severity of the defect.

- *Coarctation of the aorta*, a malformation in a portion of the wall of the aorta that causes narrowing of the aortal opening or **lumen** at the point of the defect (Fig. 6.3). Consequently, blood pressure is increased proximal to the defect and decreased distal to it.
- *Patent ductus arteriosus* (*PDA*), a defect resulting from the failure of the **ductus arteriosus,** a connection between the aorta and the pulmonary artery in the fetus, to close after birth. During the prenatal period, much of the fetal circulation bypasses the lungs through this blood vessel, which connects the pulmonary artery to the aorta. When this fetal structure fails to close after birth, blood

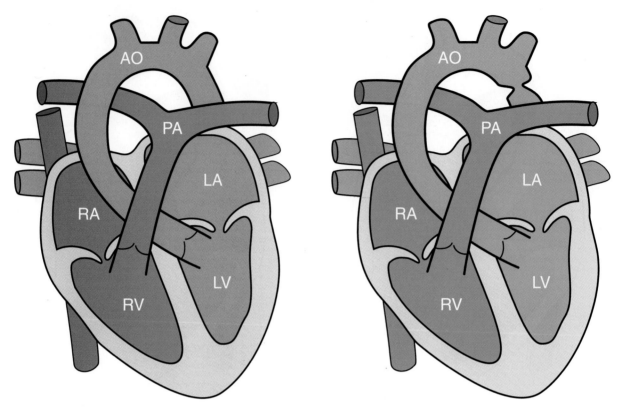

Figure 6.3 Illustration of a normal aorta and coarctation of the aorta. AO, aorta; PA, pulmonary artery; LA, left atrium; LV, left ventricle; RA, right atrium; RV, right ventricle. (From http://www.kumc.edu/instruction/medicine/pedcard/cardiology/pedcardio/coarctationdiagram.gif, courtesy of The University of Kansas Medical Center © 1996. Accessed October 14, 2003.)

from the aorta flows back into the pulmonary artery.

Cyanotic defects include the following:

- *Tetralogy of Fallot*, a combination of four congenital heart defects, including (1) pulmonary stenosis, a narrowing of the opening into the pulmonary artery from the right ventricle; (2) VSD, an abnormal opening in the septum between the left and right ventricles; (3) dextroposition of the aorta, in which the opening of the aorta bridges the ventricular septum, receiving blood from both the left and right ventricles; and (4) right ventricular **hypertrophy**, an increase in size or volume. Tetralogy of Fallot is the most common cyanotic heart defect.

- *Transposition of the great vessels*, a condition in which the two major arteries of the heart are reversed, with the aorta arising from the right ventricle and the pulmonary artery from the left ventricle. The result is two noncommunicating circulatory systems—one circulating blood in a closed loop between the heart and lungs, and the other, between the heart and systemic circulation.

■ **ETIOLOGY** The etiology of congenital heart defects is unknown, but genetic anomalies are strongly suspected. Predisposing factors may include maternal infections, use of certain drugs during gestation, diabetes, alcoholism, and poor maternal nutrition.

Clinical features vary with age and seriousness of the defect.

Signs and Symptoms of Acyanotic Defects

- *VSD:* The classic clinical feature is a loud, early systolic murmur heard during **auscultation,** or the listening to sounds produced by the internal organs. The typical murmur is described as blowing or rumbling.
- *ASD:* The classic clinical feature is a crescendo-decrescendo type of systolic ejection murmur.
- *Coarctation of the aorta:* The clinical features vary with age (Fig. 6.4). A murmur may or may not be present. An infant may exhibit dyspnea, pulmonary edema, an abnormally rapid heartbeat (**tachycardia**), and failure to thrive. Symptoms appearing after adolescence may include dyspnea, lameness (**claudication**), headache, nosebleed (**epistaxis**), and hypertension.
- *PDA:* The clinical feature is a "machinery" murmur usually associated with an abnormal tremor accompanying a cardiac murmur or **thrill** and often accompanied by a widened pulse pressure. Respiratory distress is common.

Signs and Symptoms of Cyanotic Defects

- *Tetralogy of Fallot:* A bluish discoloration of the skin and mucous membranes, or **cyanosis,** is often evident at birth or within several months of birth and is considered the hallmark of the disorder. The child may exhibit other signs of poor oxygenation, such as increasing dyspnea on exertion, diminished exercise tolerance, and delayed physical growth and development.
- *Transposition of the great vessels:* The infant is typically severely cyanotic at birth and has tachypnea. Signs of congestive heart failure and **cardiomegaly,** or an increase in the volume of the heart or the size of the heart muscle tissue, follow.

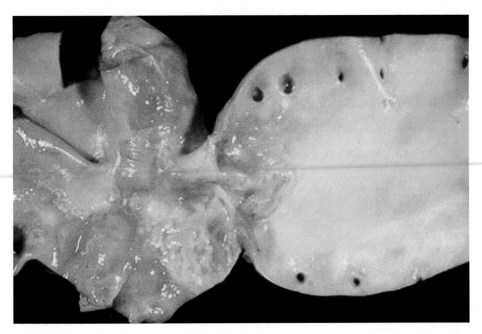

Figure 6.4 The aorta is opened longitudinally to reveal a coarctation. In the region of narrowing, there was increased turbulence that led to increased atherosclerosis. (From The Internet Pathology Laboratory for Medical Education, http://www-medlib.med.utah.edu/WebPath/CVHTML/CV082.html, courtesy of Edward C. Klatt, MD. Accessed October 14, 2003.)

■ **DIAGNOSTIC PROCEDURES** A history and physical examination are essential and may be all that are necessary to diagnose tetralogy of Fallot. Other diagnostic procedures may include x-rays, an electrocardiogram (ECG), an echocardiogram, and heart catheterization. Laboratory studies may be ordered to determine the degree of cyanosis and to detect possible acidosis.

■ **TREATMENT** Some congenital heart defects require no treatment because the infant has spontaneous closure of the defects. When surgery is necessary, it usually is done during the first year of life. When the defect is complex, however, more surgical procedures will be required. Some surgical procedures may be delayed until the child is old enough to withstand the surgery.

ALTERNATIVE THERAPY: *No significant alternative therapy is indicated.*

> **TEACHING TIPS:** Any heart defect is frightening to all involved. Reassurance is important and should include explanations to the parents of surgical procedures to be performed. The March of Dimes has a Website that can be a quick reference for parents who are trying to understand what is happening and why.

■ **PROGNOSIS** The prognosis is dependent on the type of defect, its location, and its severity. If the defect is small and surgery is successful, the prognosis is often good; otherwise, the prognosis is guarded.

■ **PREVENTION** There is no known prevention other than proper prenatal care and minimizing suspected risk factors.

GENITOURINARY DISEASES AND DISORDERS

Undescended Testes (Cryptorchidism)

■ **DESCRIPTION** This congenital condition is the failure of the testes to descend into the scrotal sac from the abdominal cavity. The condition may be unilateral or bilateral; it more commonly affects the right testis. The testes can be either retractable or ectopic. A retractable testis is descended but readily retracts with examination or physical stimulation, whereas an ectopic testis is found outside the normal path of descent. It can be in the groin, perineum, or abdominal wall. A retractable testis does not represent cryptorchidism.

■ **ETIOLOGY** The cause is unknown, but it may be linked to inadequate or improper hormone levels in the fetus. The testes normally descend into the scrotal sac during the eighth month of gestation, so the condition is most often seen in premature births and those with low birth weight.

■ **SIGNS AND SYMPTOMS** When the condition is unilateral, the testis on the affected side is not palpable in the scrotum. In bilateral cryptorchidism, the scrotum will appear to be underdeveloped.

■ **DIAGNOSTIC PROCEDURES** Physical examination reveals cryptorchidism. A serum gonadotropin test will confirm the presence of testes, because it assesses the level of circulating hormone produced by the testes. Ultrasound may be used to determine their location.

■ **TREATMENT** In many cases, the testes descend during the infant's first year. Otherwise, the treatment of choice is surgical correction between the ages of 2 and 4 years. Human chorionic gonadotropin may be tried to stimulate descent.

ALTERNATIVE THERAPY: *No significant alternative therapy is indicated.*

> **TEACHING TIPS:** The goal of teaching is to offer information to caregivers to help alleviate any fear or anxiety about treatment or lack thereof. Answering questions about sexuality or fertility is paramount.

■ **PROGNOSIS** The prognosis is good with proper attention. Corrected cryptorchidism generally does not cause sexual dysfunction later in life. Testes that have not descended by the time of adolescence will atrophy, causing sterility, but testosterone levels remain normal. A child with undescended testes has a 20% to 44% increase in risk for developing a malignant testicular tumor in adulthood.

■ **PREVENTION** Because the cause is essentially unknown, prevention also is unknown.

Congenital Defects of the Ureter, Bladder, and Urethra

The causes of congenital defects of the ureter, bladder, and urethra are unknown. Some of the problems are obvious at birth; others are not apparent until later, when they produce symptoms. The following is a brief discussion of the most common congenital urinary tract anomalies, together with their symptoms and possible treatments. Diagnostic tests include an x-ray of the urinary tract after the introduction of a contrast medium, or **excretory urography**, voiding cystoscopy, cystourethrography, urethroscopy, and ultrasonography.

Duplicated ureter means that each kidney has two ureters rather than one. Sometimes the two ureters join before they enter the urinary bladder. The common symptoms may include frequent urinary infections, urinary frequency and urgency, diminished urine output, and flank pain. Surgery is the treatment of choice to remove the unnecessary ureter.

Retrocaval ureter occurs when the right ureter passes behind the inferior vena cava before entering the urinary bladder. The symptoms may include the swelling of the ureter with urine (**hydroureter**), right flank pain, urinary tract infection, renal calculi, and blood in the urine (**hematuria**). Surgical excision (**resection**) and surgical formation of a connection called **anastomosis** of the ureter constitute the treatment of choice.

Ectopic orifice of the ureter occurs when the ureteral opening inserts into the vagina in females or in the prostate or vas deferens in males. The symptoms may include urinary obstruction, a flowing back of urine (**reflux**), incontinence, flank pain, and urinary urgency. Resection and ureteral reimplantation into the bladder are necessary for correction.

Stricture or stenosis of the ureter means that one of the ureters is tightened or partially closed. The affected ureter may become enlarged, and a swelling of the renal pelvis of the kidney with urine (**hydronephrosis**) may result. Surgical repair is necessary. Removal of the kidney (**nephrectomy**) may be required if severe renal damage has occurred as a result of hydronephrosis.

Ureterocele is the bulging of the ureter into the urinary bladder, sometimes almost filling the bladder. There will be urinary obstruction difficulties and recurrent urinary tract infections. Surgical excision or resection of the ureterocele is necessary.

Exstrophy of the bladder is a congenital malformation in which the lower portion of the abdominal wall and the anterior wall of the bladder are missing. Consequently, the inner surface of the posterior wall of the bladder is everted through the opening in the abdominal wall. In effect, the bladder appears turned inside out. The skin covering the hole in the abdominal wall is easily **excoriated**, or roughened by accumulating urine, and infection typically results. Surgical closure of the defect is necessary. Reconstruction of the bladder and abdominal wall is required, and urinary diversion may be necessary.

Congenital bladder diverticulum is caused by a pouching out (diverticulum) of the bladder wall. Fever, urinary frequency, and pain on urination are common. Surgery is the treatment of choice to correct the herniation and reflux.

Hypospadias is an abnormal opening of the male urethra onto the undersurface of the penis, or of the female urethra into the vagina. *Epispadias* is an abnormal opening of the male urethra onto the upper surface of the penis, or of the female urethra through a fissure in the labia minora and clitoris. In all these instances, normal urination is difficult or impossible. Surgical repair is almost always necessary.

ALTERNATIVE THERAPY: *No significant alternative therapy is indicated.*

 TEACHING TIPS: It is important to support parents during the diagnosis, treatment, and recovering phases of these congenital defects. Providing adequate information and education is essential.

MUSCULOSKELETAL DISEASES AND DISORDERS

Clubfoot (Talipes)

■ **DESCRIPTION** *Clubfoot* is a nontraumatic, frequently occurring congenital deformity in which the foot is permanently bent. The four basic forms are (1) *talipes varus*, an inversion or inward bending of the foot; (2) *talipes valgus*, an eversion or outward bending of the foot; (3) *talipes equinus*, or plantar flexion, in which the toes are lower than the heel; and (4) *talipes calcaneus*, or dorsiflexion, in which the toes are higher than the heel. An individual also may have a combination of these basic forms: for example, talipes equinovarus, in which the toes point downward and the body of the foot bends inward.

■ **ETIOLOGY** The exact cause is unknown, but a combination of genetic and environmental factors in utero has been implicated. It is twice as common in boys as in girls.

■ **DIAGNOSTIC PROCEDURES** The deformity is usually obvious at birth.

■ **SIGNS AND SYMPTOMS** Clubfoot varies greatly in severity; however, in all cases the talus is deformed, the Achilles' bursa is shortened, and the calcaneus is flattened and shortened. It is painless.

■ **TREATMENT** Treatment is aimed at correcting the deformity and maintaining the corrected position. Simple manipulation and casting may be done and repeated several times. Corrective surgery may be required. Maintenance treatment includes special exercises, night splints, and orthopedic shoes. Close follow-up observation is essential.

ALTERNATIVE THERAPY: *No significant alternative therapy is indicated.*

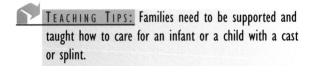 TEACHING TIPS: Parents need to be taught how to care for an infant with casts, splints, or orthopedic shoes. Exercising may be ordered so parents need to be shown and educated to perform the exercises at home.

■ **PROGNOSIS** The prognosis is good with prompt treatment.

■ **PREVENTION** There is no known prevention.

Congenital Hip Dysplasia

■ **DESCRIPTION** Hip dysplasia is an abnormality of the hip joint that may take three forms: (1) unstable hip dysplasia, in which the hip can be dislocated manually; (2) incomplete dislocation, in which the femoral head is on the edge of the **acetabulum**, the rounded cavity on the outer surface of the hip bone that receives the femur; and (3) complete dislocation, in which the femoral head is outside the acetabulum.

■ **ETIOLOGY** The cause is not known; however, two unproved etiologies have been proposed. First, hormones that relax the maternal ligaments during labor also may relax the hip ligaments of the infant. Second, hip dislocation may result if the fetus is not positioned correctly within the uterus before and during birth.

■ **SIGNS AND SYMPTOMS** Physical examination shows asymmetric folds in the thigh of newborns with limited abduction of the affected hip. A shortening of the femur is noted when the knees and hips are flexed at right angles. The signs are typically quite obvious when children attempt to walk, if the condition has not been discovered before that time.

■ **DIAGNOSTIC PROCEDURES** Observations during physical examination may suggest the diagnosis, but a positive **Ortolani's sign** will confirm the diagnosis. Ortolani's sign is the click felt when an examiner abducts (draws away from the body) and lifts the femurs of a supine (face upward) infant. The click indicates a partial or an incomplete displacement of the hip. X-ray may be used.

■ **TREATMENT** It is important for treatment to begin as soon as possible. Before 3 months of age, treatment requires closed reduction of the dislocation, followed by the use of a splint-brace or cast for 2 to 3 months. If the child is much older, open reduction followed by casting may be necessary.

ALTERNATIVE THERAPY: *No significant alternative therapy is indicated.*

TEACHING TIPS: Families need to be supported and taught how to care for an infant or a child with a cast or splint.

■ **PROGNOSIS** When treatment occurs before age 5, the prognosis is excellent. If not treated promptly, abnormal development of the hip and permanent disability may result.

■ **PREVENTION** There is no known prevention.

METABOLIC ERRORS

Cystic Fibrosis

■ **DESCRIPTION** Cystic fibrosis is a congenital disorder of the exocrine glands characterized by the production of copious amounts of abnormally thick mucus, especially in the bronchus, lungs, and pancreas.

■ **ETIOLOGY** The disease is caused by an underlying biochemical defect transmitted as an autosomal recessive trait. If both parents are carriers of the recessive gene, the offspring have a 25% chance of having the disease.

■ **SIGNS AND SYMPTOMS** The signs of cystic fibrosis may appear soon after birth or take some time to develop. Because all exocrine glands can be affected, the symptoms can be quite numerous. The sweat glands and respiratory and gastrointestinal functions are those most commonly affected. The sweat glands typically express increased concentrations of salt in sweat. Respiratory symptoms may include wheeze respirations, a dry cough, dyspnea, and tachypnea, all stemming from accumulations of thick secretions in the smaller passages conveying air with the lung (**bronchioles**) and the air sacs (**alveoli**) of the lungs. Gastrointestinal symptoms may include intestinal obstruction, vomiting, constipation, electrolyte imbalance, and the inability to absorb fats. Fibrous tissue and fat slowly replace the normal saclike swellings found in the pancreas, resulting in pancreatic insufficiency characterized by insufficient insulin production.

■ **DIAGNOSTIC PROCEDURES** The Cystic Fibrosis Foundation has developed the following criteria for a definitive diagnosis: two positive sweat tests using a sweat inducer and one from the following: obstructive pulmonary diseases, confirmed pancreatic insufficency or failure to thrive, and a family history of cystic fibrosis. DNA testing may be done prenatally to diagnose the disease. Chest x-rays and pulmonary function tests may be ordered to diagnose and evaluate respiratory function.

■ **TREATMENT** The treatment for cystic fibrosis is largely supportive and designed to help a child lead as normal a life as possible. Client management includes generous salting of food to replace salt lost in sweat, physical therapy to combat pulmonary dysfunction, loosening and removing mucopurulent secretions, and oxygen therapy. Vitamin and oral pancreatic supplements may be given. Both the family and the client require emotional support. A referral to the Cystic Fibrosis Foundation may be helpful.

ALTERNATIVE THERAPY: *No significant alternative therapy is indicated.*

TEACHING TIPS: Genetic counseling may be advisable in families known to be at risk.

■ **PROGNOSIS** The prognosis is poor. There is no cure for cystic fibrosis, but the average life expectancy has increased to 28 years or older. Cystic fibrosis is the most common fatal genetic disease. Death is usually due to complications such as shock and arrhythmias that may occur during hot weather due to profuse sweating. Serious, often fatal, respiratory complications include pneumonia, emphysema, and a collapsed lung (**atelectasis**). Gastrointestinal complications include rectal prolapse and malnutrition.

■ **PREVENTION** There is no known prevention.

Phenylketonuria

■ **DESCRIPTION** *Phenylketonuria (PKU)* is an autosomal recessive defect resulting in an error in phenylalanine metabolism.

■ **ETIOLOGY** During normal metabolic processes, the enzyme phenylalanine hydroxylase converts the amino acid phenylalanine to tyrosine, another amino acid. In PKU, this enzyme is not produced by the body, so phenylalanine accumulates in the blood and urine, and is toxic to the brain. Mental retardation results if the condition is not quickly corrected. The full extent of cerebral damage is complete by 2 or 3 years of age and is irreversible.

■ **SIGNS AND SYMPTOMS** The infant is typically asymptomatic until about 4 months of age, when signs and symptoms of mental retardation, such as hyperactivity, personality disorders, a smaller-than-normal head (**microcephaly**), and irritability, begin to appear. There often is a characteristic musty odor to the child's perspiration and urine due to the presence of phenylacetic acid, a metabolite of phenylalanine.

■ **DIAGNOSTIC PROCEDURES** The presence of an elevated blood phenylalanine level and an urine phenylpyruvic acid level after the infant has received dietary protein for 24 to 48 hours after birth confirms the diagnosis. A heelstick is generally used to obtain the blood sample. Repeated testing may need to be done and is likely to use the infant's urine to detect PKU.

■ **TREATMENT** Treatment consists of following a protein-restrictive diet for 3 to 6 years or, some authorities maintain, for life. Most natural proteins need to be restricted, because phenylalanine is a component of most proteins. Serum phenylalanine levels need to be monitored to determine the efficacy of the diet.

ALTERNATIVE THERAPY: *No significant alternative therapy is indicated.*

 TEACHING TIPS: Parents will need diet and nutritional assistance in maintaining a protein-restricted diet for their infant. The skills of a dietition can be beneficial.

■ **PROGNOSIS** The sooner the protein-restrictive diet is started, the better is the prognosis. If the disease is detected and treated before 2 years of age, the chances of the child achieving normal intelligence are good. The protein-restrictive diet will not reverse any existing mental retardation, but it will prevent further progression.

■ **PREVENTION** There is no known prevention.

Summary

In the introduction, it was stated that these diseases and disorders affect the entire family. Indeed, health-care professionals tend to the afflicted and the parents. There is a tendency, especially in congenital problems, for parents to blame themselves. Also, treatment and care are often arduous and lengthy. Referrals to appropriate support groups are especially helpful.

CASE STUDIES

■ Case Study 1

Nathan, who was born with a cleft lip and palate, is abandoned by his drug-dependent mother and unknown or unidentified father shortly after birth. Social services personnel place the infant in a foster home where the caregivers have experience with special needs children. In a short time, specialists rule that surgery is necessary. After three operations, Nathan's congenital defect is very difficult to detect.

Case Study Questions

1. What might have happened if Nathan's mother had kept him?
2. What future complications do Nathan's caregivers need to watch for?

■ Case Study 2

Alison and Jordan are considering having their first child. Close friends of theirs have a child who was born with serious heart defects. They have some fears about birth defects and the costs of any necessary treatment.

Case Study Questions

1. What resources could you recommend for them to read?
2. Would you advise that they speak to a specialist?
3. How might they research their health-care insurance coverage?

REVIEW QUESTIONS

True/False

Circle the correct answer:

T F   1. Spina bifida occulta is the least common neural tube defect.

T F   2. Hirschsprung's disease is called congenital aganglionic megacolon.

T F   3. In an infant with cryptorchidism, the testes generally will descend within the first
            year of life.

T F   4. The prognosis of pyloric stenosis is excellent after surgical repair.

T F   5. Hydrocephalus is defined as too little cerebrospinal fluid in the brain ventricles.

Matching

Match each of the following definitions with its correct term:

Spinal cord defects

_____ 1. Incomplete closure of one or more vertebrae   a. Meningomyelocele

_____ 2. Incomplete closure of vertebrae with protrusion of   b. Meningocele
         spinal fluid and meninges into the sac

_____ 3. External sac contains meninges, cerebrospinal fluid,   c. Spina bifida occulta
         and a portion of the cord and nerve roots

Congenital defects of the heart

_____ 4. Abnormal opening between the two atria   a. Ventricular septal defect

_____ 5. Failure of the fetal ductus arteriosus to completely close b. Atrial septal defect

_____ 6. Abnormal opening between the right and left ventricles   c. Coarctation of the aorta

_____ 7. Localized narrowing of the aorta   d. Patent ductus arteriosus

                                                                     e. Tetralogy of Fallot

Short Answer

1. The two different types of hydrocephalus are _____ and _____.

2. The characteristic symptom in pyloric stenosis is _____.

3. Another name for undescended testes is _____.

4. What does PKU stand for? _____. Describe it.

5. Name at least three congenital defects of the ureter, bladder, and urethra:

   a.

   b.

   c.

6. List the four most common forms of clubfoot or talipes:

   a.

   b.

   c.

   d.

7. List the three forms of congenital hip dysplasia:

   a.

   b.

   c.

Multiple Choice

Place a check next to the correct answers:

1. Select all the correct statements concerning CP:

   a. It is caused by central nervous system damage before birth.

   b. It may be spastic, athetoid, and ataxic.

   c. A neurologic assessment is the most common diagnostic tool.

   d. The condition is curable.

   e. a, b, c above.

2. Select all the correct signs and symptoms of cystic fibrosis:

   a. Intestinal obstruction

   b. Vomiting

   c. Constipation

   d. Wheezy respirations

   e. Dry cough

   f. Dyspnea

   g. Tachypnea

   h. Electrolyte imbalance

   i. Inability to absorb fats

   j. Deficient insulin

3. Cleft lip and palate

   a. Occurs 35 days after conception.

   b. Occurs in 1 in 10,000 births.

   c. Does not require any special feeding techniques.

   d. Is usually corrected in one surgery.

4. Congenital heart defects

   a. Can be broadly classified in three major groups: acyanotic, dyscyanotic, and cyanotic.

   b. Are generally caused by genetic anomalies.

   c. Do not respond well to surgical intervention.

   d. Are preventable through proper prenatal care.

5. Folic acid is recommended by alternative practitioners for the prevention of

   a. pyloric stenosis

   b. Hirschsprung's disease

   c. Congenital heart defects

   d. Neural tube defects

Discussion Questions/Personal Reflection

1. What can we do as individuals and/or families to help prevent congenital diseases? What is out of our control?

2. Focusing in on the nervous system diseases and metabolic diseases, what are some of the long-term effects of congenital diseases/disorders?

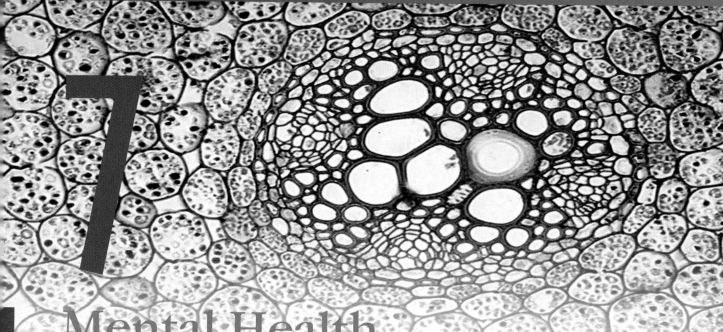

Mental Health Diseases and Disorders

CHAPTER OUTLINE

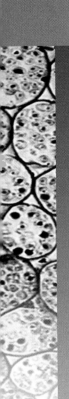

KEY WORDS

Decompensate (dē′kăm-pĕn•sāt)
Folate (fō′lāt)
Intromission (ĭn•trō-mĭ′shun)
Mutism (myŭ′•tĭ′•zĕm)

> *I will work in my own way, according to the light that is in me.*
>
> —LYDIA MARIA CHILD

LEARNING OBJECTIVES

Upon successful completion of this chapter, you will be able to:

- Discuss the use of the *Diagnostic and Statistical Manual of Mental Disorders (DSM-IV)*.
- Describe the difference between nature and nurture.
- Recall the influence of culture, age, and gender in mental disorders and diseases.
- Discuss the use of a mental health assessment tool.
- Name and define the three types of depression.
- Discuss the differences of depression in men and women and in adolescents and the elderly.
- State the alternative therapies of depression.
- Name and discuss the five different types of schizophrenia.
- Relate the possible etiologic factors of schizophrenia.
- Define the five different types of anxiety disorder.
- List the *DSM-IV* criteria for a diagnosis of Personality Disorder to be made.
- Discuss the alternative therapies for substance abuse.
- Recall incident rates for attention deficit-hyperactivity disorder (ADHD) and attention deficit disorder (ADD).
- Differentiate the four types of mental retardation.
- Recall the description of bulimia nervosa.
- Compare anorexia nervosa and bulimia nervosa.
- Relate teaching tips for anorexia nervosa.
- Compare and contrast sexual disorders between men and women.

In the not too distant past, medical doctors (physicians) and psychologists had little in common and often did not agree on treatment protocols for anyone with a mental health problem. There seemed to be a total separation of the body from the mind in determining the etiology and establishing a diagnosis. The result has been a proliferation of community and professional organizations that have established

121

family advocacy programs, substance abuse rehabilitation clinics, stress management seminars, bereavement counseling, and shelters for abused and battered women and an educational system that provides training and information.

Today, physicians and psychologists are more likely to have a working relationship with each other. Psychologists readily recommend a physical examination from a primary care physician before treating a client with a mental disorder. Physicians are more willing to refer a client to a mental health specialist in areas where counseling or psychotherapy is indicated. Specialists from the many community mental health resources are turning to both physicians and psychologists for guidance and assistance.

A serious economic crisis looms in the future; indeed, it may already have arrived. Decreased funding of mental health programs places the control of mental health services with state and local authorities—many of whom do not understand the issues involved and who do not have the training to make wise decisions. Further, fewer and fewer health insurance programs provide adequate coverage for mental health diseases and disorders.

Just as we have recommended that medicine combine the best modalities of nontraditional and traditional medicine and become integrated, there needs to be the same cooperation and integration among physicians, psychologists, and community mental health practitioners. The goal has to be the best care available for those who need it.

DIAGNOSTIC PROCEDURES

Diagnostic procedures identified in this chapter are brief and are not intended to provide specific procedures such as those detailed in the *Diagnostic and Statistical Manual of Mental Disorders, Fourth Edition (DSM-IV)*. This text, published by the American Psychiatric Association, provides a helpful guide with diagnostic criteria and classification that enable clinicians and investigators to diagnose, communicate about, study, and treat people with various mental disorders using a common foundation.

MENTAL HEALTH ASSESSMENT

Physicians, psychologists, mental health practitioners, and alternative therapy practitioners use a mental health evaluation in their assessment of a client with a suspected mental disorder. A portion of the evaluation is determined by observation and by being aware of a client's presentation.

The observation phase of the evaluation includes the following elements:

Appearance: Gender, age, ethnicity, apparent height and weight, any physical deformities, grooming, hygiene, gait and motor coordination, posture, noteworthy mannerisms, etc.

Manner and approach: Interpersonal characteristics and approach to evaluation; behavioral approval, speech, eye contact, expressive language, and whether English is the primary language; recall and memory

The orientation, alertness, and thought process portion of the evaluation that requires response from the client includes such questions as the following:

Orientation: Person, place, time, president, your name

Alertness: Sleepy, alert, dull and uninteresting

Coherence: Responses easy to understand, simple, and concrete

Concentration and attention: Count backward from 100 to 50 by sevens, name days of the week or months of the year in reverse order

Thought processes: Can or cannot recall plot of movies or books logically, difficult to follow line of reasoning, obsessions, confabulations, etc.

Hallucinations and delusions: Presence or absence, denied visual but admits to olfactory and auditory, shows signs during testing

Judgment and insight: Explanation of what happened and the expected outcome

Intellectual ability: Average, above average, and below average

Abstractory skills: Based on proverbs and sayings; ask the client to explain

Mood: Happy, sad, despondent, irritable, anxious

Rapport: Easy to establish, difficult, tenuous

Facial/emotional expressions: Relaxed, tense, smiles, tearful

Risk of violence: Fair, low, high, uncertain

Response to failure on test items: Unaware, frustrated, anxious

Impulsivity: Low, medium, high, affected by substance use

Anxiety: Level to be noted

Defense mechanisms: Any observed

NATURE VERSUS NURTURE

In the past decade, there has been increased research that points to a biological or genetic cause of many mental health illnesses. DNA research is still in its infancy, but there is increased evidence of the importance of genetics in many of the diseases and disorders presented here. That does not negate the importance of nurture, however. How a child is nurtured, what traumatic events that child experiences, and how those events are dealt with by family members have lasting effects on children. Children's minds are an open vessel for every event that comes their way. Events are recorded in their brain for future reference. For example, when a child is reared in an environment where there is a great deal of anxiety, the child also is likely to shows symptoms of stress and to express anxious behavior. *Nature* or *genetic makeup* is already determined and is still difficult or impossible to alter. *Nurture,* however, continually comes under the control of each of us. Close attention should be paid to its importance and to how we can nurture our children and each other to remain healthy.

CULTURE, AGE, AND GENDER

Probably more than in other diseases and disorders, culture and its influence are critical to individuals with mental health issues. Individuals with a mental health disease or disorder can benefit from individuals, including family members, who understand their ethnic background. Immigrants coming to the United States from another country often settle in clustered groups of similar populations. While this may be beneficial for support, it only delays their integration into the whole of society and can make any required treatment more difficult. Many of the diseases and disorders reflect gender bias; many afflict women more often than men. Age knows no limits in mental illness. Alcohol and drug problems are seen as early as age 8. Mental health issues in the elderly are often ignored in the beliefs that treatment would be difficult and that most elderly persons expect to have some mental health issues as they grow older.

65 DEPRESSION

■ **DESCRIPTION** Nearly 19 million U.S. adults have a depressive illness. The World Health Organization (WHO) predicts that by 2020, depression will be a leading cause of disability worldwide. The economic cost of depression is enormous, but the cost in human suffering cannot be estimated. Most people who suffer from depression do not seek treatment, but those who do, even those with severe depression, can be helped. Many years of fruitful research have introduced new medications and psychosocial therapies that help ease the pain of depression.

Depression affects the body, mood, and thoughts. It is not a passing "blue mood." It is not a sign of personal weakness, and people cannot merely pull themselves together. This disorder is a syndrome of symptoms that comes in different forms—major depression, dysthymia, and bipolar disorder.

Major depression causes individuals to have feelings of worthlessness, guilt, and hopelessness. They have difficulty in working, studying, sleeping, and enjoying life's pleasures. Major depression occurs in up to 17% of adults and affects all racial and ethnic groups, and both genders. About one half of depressed clients have only a single episode of depression; the rest have more than one occurrence. Major depression can profoundly affect all facets of one's life. The most serious consequence of this form of depression is suicide. Suicide occurs when the feelings of despair are so great that an individual believes there is no longer a reason to go on living.

Dysthymia is a less-severe form of depression that involves long-term, chronic symptoms that do not disable but keep a person from feeling good or from functioning well. Many people with this form of depression also suffer major depressive episodes at some time in their lives.

Bipolar disorder, also called *manic-depressive disorder*, is not as prevalent as the other forms of depression. It is characterized by cycling mood changes from severe highs (mania) to severe lows (depression). Sometimes the mood switches are dramatic, but more often they are gradual. When in the depression cycle, an individual can have all of the symptoms of a depressive disorder. In the manic cycle, the individual may be overactive, talk too much, and have enormous energy. Mania can affect thinking, judgment, and social behavior in ways that can cause serious problems and embarrassment. For instance, the individual in this phase may make unwise business decisions or create grand schemes that are difficult to fulfill. Untreated, mania may worsen to a psychotic state.

■ **ETIOLOGY** There are many possible causes of depression. Bipolar depression tends to run in families. Major depression is often associated with changes in brain structure and brain function and seems to occur generation after generation, possibly with a genetic connection. Research has shown that a gene that helps to regulate *serotonin*, a chemical messenger in the brain, is known to play a role in depression. Other possibilities include biochemical, physical, psychological, and social causes. Depression may be secondary to a medical condition such as those seen with metabolic disturbances, endocrine disorders, nervous disorders, cancers, cardiovascular disorders, and many chronic and/or degenerative diseases. Some prescription drugs can cause depression. Alcohol and substance abuse can also cause depression.

■ **SIGNS AND SYMPTOMS** The primary symptom is a predominantly sad mood and a loss of interest in pleasurable activities that last more than several days. Individuals may seem unhappy and apathetic, have difficulty concentrating, and be unable to finish tasks. Fatigue and insomnia can occur. Some individuals lose their appetite; others may want to eat all the time. Symptoms of mania include abnormal elation, unusual irritability, decreased need for sleep, grandiose notions, racing thoughts and increased talking, increased sexual desire, increased energy, poor judgment, and inappropriate social behavior.

■ **DIAGNOSTIC PROCEDURES** The *DSM-IV* identifies the criteria for diagnosing major depression. At least five of the following symptoms must be present during a 2-week period and must represent a change from previous functioning.

- Persistent, sad, anxious or depressed mood
- Diminished interest or pleasure in most all activities
- Significant weight loss or weight gain
- Insomnia or excessive sleep nearly every day
- Agitated or reduced psychomotor activity
- Fatigue or loss of energy
- Inappropriate guilt feelings or feelings of worthlessness, hopelessness
- Diminished ability to concentrate, make decisions, remember
- Thoughts of death or suicide
- Persistent physical symptoms that do not respond to treatment

Depression in Women

Women experience depression about twice as often as do men; hormonal factors are thought to contribute to this increased rate. Menstrual cycle changes, pregnancy, miscarriage, postpartum period, premenopause, and menopause are considered contributing factors.

Depression in Men

Men are less likely to admit to depression. The rate of suicide in men is four times that of women, and is even higher after age 70, reaching its peak after age 85. Depression in men is often masked by the use of alcohol and drugs or by socially acceptable habits such as working excessively long hours. Men are more likely to exhibit symptoms of irritability, anger, and being discouraged.

Depression in Adolescents

Depression in this age group can be a response to many situations and stresses. Conflict with parents, fluctuating hormones, reaction to a disturbing event, feelings of low self-esteem, and feelings of no control in his or her life or that "life sucks" can be triggers to a depressive mood.

Depression in the Elderly

Diagnosis is difficult because some ordinary symptoms of depression, such as fatigue, loss of appetite, and sleep difficulties, may not represent depression but rather symptoms associated with the normal aging process. Depression in the elderly, however, is a widespread problem and often goes undiagnosed and frequently untreated.

■ **TREATMENT** Depression is difficult to treat, especially in children, adolescents, and the elderly. A good diagnostic evaluation is necessary to determine the presence of depression and its appropriate treatment; this includes a complete physical examination and a review of client history and any symptoms presented. Treatment choice depends on the evaluation, but the primary treatments are drug therapy, psychotherapy, and, in some cases, electroconvulsive therapy (ECT).

The primary medications used are antidepressants: selective serotonin reuptake inhibitors (SSRIs), tricyclic antidepressants (TCAs), and monoamine oxidase inhibitors (MAOIs). The SSRIs have fewer side effects than the TCAs, however, SSRIs need to be used with caution due to recent research that indicates a higher risk of suicide rates among those taking SSRIs. Sometimes it takes a variety of antidepressants before an effective medication is found to treat the disorder. Sometimes dosages need to be increased; in general, antidepressants must be taken regularly for 3 to 6 weeks before the full therapeutic effect occurs. Often individuals take themselves off the medication too soon, either because they are feeling better or because they think the drug is not working. Antidepressants should be taken and stopped only under the direct supervision of a physician.

Individuals with depression may do well with psychotherapy or a combination of antidepressants and psychotherapy. Many therapists believe that the best results are achieved with a combination of individual, family, and group therapy. "Talking" therapies help individuals gain insight into and resolve their own problems through verbal exchanges with the therapist or with others. Behavioral therapists help individuals learn how to obtain more satisfaction and rewards through their own actions and how to unlearn the behavioral patterns that contribute to or result from their depression.

ECT is useful for individuals whose depression is severe or life threatening or who cannot take antidepressants. In recent years, ECT has been much improved. A muscle relaxant is given to the client and the ECT is administered under brief anesthesia. Electrodes are placed at precise locations on the head to deliver electrical impulses. The stimulation causes about 30 seconds of seizure within the brain. The person receiving ECT does not consciously experience the electrical stimulus. Typically, several sessions of ECT are given at the rate of three per week.

ALTERNATIVE THERAPY: *St. John's wort is an herb that has been used extensively in the treatment of mild to moderate depression in Europe. The National Institutes of Health (NIH), in conjunction with the National Institute of Mental Health (NIMH) and the National Center for Complementary and Alternative Medicine, recently conducted a study of the use of St. John's wort in clients with major depression. The study included three groups: individuals on St John's wort, individuals on an SSRI medication, and individuals on a placebo. The research showed there was no significant difference in the rate of response for depression, but the scale for overall functioning was better for the antidepressant than for either St. John's wort or the placebo. The NIH is supporting research to examine a possible role for St. John's wort in the treatment of milder forms of depression. It should be noted, however, that the Food and Drug Administration has issued a Public Health Advisory that St. John's wort is contraindicated for any individuals who are taking medications for such conditions as AIDS, heart disease, depression, seizures, certain cancers, and rejection of transplants. Any herbal supplement should be taken only after consultation with your physician.*

TEACHING TIPS: Appropriate diagnosis and treatment are important. Individuals should be encouraged to continue with their treatment until symptoms abate. Regular follow-up care should be provided so that adjustments can be made in treatment as necessary. Individuals suffering from depression need understanding, patience, affection, and encouragement. A depressed person may need diversion or companionship, but too many demands can increase feelings of failure.

■ **PROGNOSIS** Good results can be obtained with the proper treatment of mild and moderate depression. Major depression may require long-term or life-long treatment, but improved quality of life is possible. Suicide is an ever-present risk, especially in severe cases, and all precautions should be taken to prevent such an act.

■ **PREVENTION** Some episodes of depression can be avoided by practicing effective stress management techniques; avoiding drugs, alcohol, and caffeine; exercising regularly; and maintaining good sleep habits. Many episodes of depression are not preventable. Treatment, including medications and psychiatric intervention, may prevent recurrences.

SCHIZOPHRENIA

■ **DESCRIPTION** Schizophrenia is an altered sensory perception disorder with physical and psychological changes that affect brain functioning, behavior patterns, and all five senses. In the United

States, approximately 2.2 million adults have schizophrenia. It is the most chronic and disabling of the severe mental illnesses. People with schizophrenia often experience frightening symptoms such as hearing internal voices or believing that others are controlling their thoughts or plotting to harm them. Schizophrenia generally is diagnosed during adolescence or in the early 20s or 30s. Overall, men and women are affected with equal frequency; however, schizophrenia appears at an earlier age in men than in women. It is rarely diagnosed in children.

The five types of schizophrenia are as follows:

- *Paranoid*: Persons have persecutory or grandiose delusions, often organized around a theme; or auditory hallucinations that generally are related to the delusional theme. They have intense interpersonal relationships and express a superior and often patronizing manner.
- *Disorganized*: Persons generally have disorganized thoughts or behaviors, confusion, and a flat affect. They show an inability to perform daily life tasks, and they exhibit other odd behaviors.
- *Catatonic*: Persons have extreme negativism, **mutism** (not speaking), and excessive motor activity that does not make sense or have purpose and is not necessarily influenced by any external stimuli. They experience *echolalia*, which is a pathologic, senseless repetition of a word or phrase just spoken; it is a parrot-like repetition. During some periods, this person will need close supervision because he or she can harm himself or herself or others.
- *Undifferentiated*: Persons will show pronounced delusions, disorganized thought processes and behavior, and hallucinations.
- *Residual*: Persons exhibit at least one episode of schizophrenia, but the course of the disorder may be time limited or it can present continuously for many years. Usually there is the absence of hallucinations or delusions.

■ **ETIOLOGY** Possible etiologic theories of schizophrenia include the following:

- *Genetic theory:* The actual genetic defect has not been identified, but it is believed that a potential location is on chromosomes 13 and

6. Predisposing genetic factors include intrauterine starvation, viral infections, and perinatal complications. Studies of families, twins, and adoptive parents show increased risk for the disease in people with first-degree relatives (biological parents and siblings) with schizophrenia. In fact, a person with a parent or sibling with schizophrenia has an approximately 10% risk of developing the disorder compared with a 1% risk for a person with no family history.

- *Psychodynamic neurobiological theory:* Research studies of living and postmortem brains of people with schizophrenia show decreased brain volume and abnormal functioning. Neurochemical studies reveal alterations in neurotransmitter systems. In neurodevelopment, studies have shown that there are functional, structural, and chemical brain deviations in those with schizophrenia, and such deviations can be found long before the diagnosis is made. It is unknown if these are either genetic or environmental in nature or a combination of both.
- *Diathesis stress theory:* This theory states that symptoms develop based on a relationship between the amount of stress a person experiences and the individual's internal stress tolerance. Schizophrenia is a disorder that both causes stress and can be exacerbated by stress.

■ **SIGNS AND SYMPTOMS** Two or more of the following signs and symptoms must be present for at least 1 month, allowing for a significant amount of time for the diagnosis of schizophrenia to be made. The signs and symptoms are classified as both *positive,* those that are excessive or distortions of normal functions, and *negative,* those that reflect a loss of or decrease in normal functions. Positive symptoms include hallucinations, delusions, and disorganized speech, whereas negative symptoms include flat affect, **alogia** (inability to speak owing to a mental condition or symptoms of dementia), attention deficit, and **avolition** (decreased motivation).

■ **DIAGNOSTIC PROCEDURES** A good genetic and family history is required to aid in the diagnosis. Computed tomography (CT) scans of the head and other imaging techniques may identify some changes associated with the disorder and may rule out other neurophysiologic disorders. A psychiatric evaluation and interview with the person and family are necessary.

■ **TREATMENT** Treatment includes psychotropic medications, psychotherapy, and counseling. Newer medications, called atypical antipsychotics, are effective in the treatment of psychosis, including hallucinations and delusions. Medication levels and dosages will have to be carefully monitored every 1 to 2 weeks. Long-term psychotherapy may be needed. Counseling focuses on educating clients on their disorder as well as on how they cope. Stress and crisis management is essential, as is social skill development. Persons may identify an agent (a trusted person) to act on their behalf when they **decompensate** (failure or inability to act appropriately in acute episodes of mental illness) or are hospitalized.

An advanced directive may be formed with the client and caregivers so that clients, while at a maximum level of psychological health and well-being, can have a say in their course of treatment. Such directives are individual care plans for people with schizophrenia and are an effective way to not only involve clients in self-care but also provide the motivation for clients to continue with their care plan.

In the treatment of persons with schizophrenia, it is imperative that there is collaboration between medical and mental health practitioners. All health practitioners must focus on clients' rights while providing care that addresses the clients' diverse communities and lifestyles.

ALTERNATIVE THERAPY: *Acupuncture has proved useful in paranoid schizophrenia. In fact, in one study, hospital stays decreased after the initiation of acupuncture. Biofeedback, relaxation, and guided imagery have proved helpful in reducing stress associated with schizophrenia. If histamine levels are low, alternative therapists prescribe* **folate** *(a form of vitamin B complex) and nutrients. If the histamine levels are high, calcium is given to help release excess histamine from body cells.*

TEACHING TIPS: Teaching is dependent on the type of schizophrenia. It is important that you teach your client the importance of strict adherence to the treatment regimen, especially taking the medications as prescribed. Clients may do well in a support group or daycare treatment. Encourage families to become involved in the client's care and treatment. Because of the chronic nature of the condition, it is important to educate clients about their illness, possible complications, and their specific treatment plan.

■ **PROGNOSIS** Recognizing the early signs and symptoms of schizophrenia improves prognosis. The prognosis varies; most improve with medication, but many experience functional disability and are at risk for repeated acute episodes. When a client with the paranoid type of schizophrenia is working, the prognosis is generally better.

■ **PREVENTION** Some persons refuse to take their medications because of side effects or discontinue them because they believe they are able to cope without the medicine. It is important to monitor the medication dosage and to encourage the client to continue the medication as prescribed. The latter is the best prevention. Continued participation in community support groups and vocational counseling is definitely beneficial. Some persons remain too disabled to live independently, requiring group homes or other long-term structured living situations.

ANXIETY DISORDERS

Anxiety disorders are a very common mental health problem, affecting about 19 million adults in America. Anxiety disorders can be terrifying and crippling. These disorders are highly treatable, yet only about one-third of those with the disorder receive treatment. Singly or in combination, psychotherapy, cognitive-behavioral therapy (CBT), and medication therapy are effective treatments. Treatment success varies with the individual. Some clients also have depression, substance abuse, or both, which further complicates treatment.

■ **DESCRIPTION** The following are types of anxiety disorders:

* *Generalized anxiety disorder (GAD):* Excessive and unrealistic worry lasting 6 months or longer with accompanying physical symptoms that might include gastrointestinal upset, heart palpitations, headaches, etc. Women are two

more times as likely to be afflicted than are men.

- *Obsessive-compulsive disorder (OCD):* Persistent, recurring thoughts that reflect exaggerated fear. Some thoughts are violent; others include worrying about contamination with dirt, germs, or feces. Some perform ritualistic, repetitive, involuntary, and compulsive behaviors such as counting, touching, handwashing, and repeated "checking" to make certain something is in place. Women are two more times as likely to be afflicted than are men.
- *Panic disorder:* Recurrent episodes of intense apprehension, terror, or impending doom. This is anxiety in its most severe form. Heart palpitations, chest pain, sweating, trembling, and a feeling of choking are a few of the symptoms. Women are two more times as likely to be afflicted than are men.
- *Posttraumatic stress disorder (PTSD):* Psychological consequences that persist for at least 1 month after a traumatic event outside the realm of usual human experiences. Examples of traumatic events include events of war, terror attacks, serious accident, physical assault, and rape. Individuals suffer (1) flashbacks or nightmares, (2) avoidance of place related to the trauma, and (3) emotional numbing or detachment from others. Women are more likely to be afflicted than are men.
- *Phobias:* A persistent and irrational fear of an object, an activity, or a situation that compels a client to avoid the perceived hazard. Individuals know the fear is irrational but are unable to control the fear. Phobias represent one of the most common psychiatric disorders. There are three types: *agoraphobia,* fear of being alone or in open spaces, more common in women; *social,* fear of embarrassing oneself in public (men and women are afflicted equally); and *specific,* fear of a single specific object or situation (women are twice as likely to be afflicted than are men).

Severe anxiety is reported when a client is confronted with the feared object or situation. Some clients report dizziness, loss of bladder or bowel control, tachypnea, feelings of pain, and shortness of breath.

■ **ETIOLOGY** The causes may be unknown, but some theorists believe that conflict, whether intrapsychic, sociopersonal, or interpersonal, promotes an anxious state. Distressful events and major depression may also be causes.

■ **TREATMENT** The goal of treatment is to help individuals function effectively. Antianxiety drugs and antidepressants may help to relieve symptoms.

ALTERNATIVE THERAPY: *Practicing meditation and deep breathing exercises may be helpful. Hypnotherapy is often beneficial. (See previous Alternative Therapy note within Depression regarding St. John's wort.)*

 TEACHING TIPS: It is helpful if a partner or close friend is supportive and encouraging of the person with an anxiety disorder. It is not helpful to tease or poke fun at an anxious individual. Recognize the anxiety as real and approach the person unhurriedly. Encourage active diversion through activities such as whistling or humming to divert unwanted thoughts.

■ **PROGNOSIS** The prognosis is good when clients are able to learn to cope with their anxiety.

■ **PREVENTION** There is no known prevention other than avoidance of the stimuli.

PERSONALITY DISORDERS

■ **DESCRIPTION** Personality Disorders are a set or pattern of behaviors and experiences that prevent a person from maintaining healthy relationships with others and from adapting to the everyday situations in their environment. There is a persistent inability to cope with the demands and expectations of self, others, and life. The pattern is pervasive and continuous rather than episodic or of short duration. Its onset is generally in adolescence or early adulthood. In the general population, 10% to 18% have a personality disorder. The *DSM-IV* lists 10 specific types of Personality Disorders. Four of the more common ones found in ambulatory care are presented, as follows:

- *Antisocial Personality Disorder:* Pattern showing disregard for rights of others and violating those rights; lying, seduction, and manipulation.

- *Borderline Personality Disorder:* Patterns of attention seeking and excessive emotions; self-destructive behavior; profound mood shifts.
- *Narcissistic Personality Disorder:* Pattern of lack of empathy; need for admiration and grandiosity.
- *Avoidant Personality Disorder:* Pattern of feeling of inadequacies; hypersensitivity to negative criticism; social inhibition.

ETIOLOGY It is unclear what causes Personality Disorders; however, it is thought to be a multifactorial approach. The etiologic theories are (1) neurobiological factors, (2) developmental factors, and (3) sociocultural factors. Many researchers believe that there is a genetic susceptibility or inherited biological link, especially in some of the more severe Personality Disorders. One study shows some structural brain dysfunction; other studies have shown a link to alcohol and drug abuse. The developmental factors indicate that early separation from parents, disturbed parental involvement, and child abuse may predispose a child to develop a Personality Disorder; however, child abuse and neglect by itself is not sufficient to invoke a diagnosis. In fact, theories of family impact on Personality Disorders are highly controversial. It is known that sociocultural factors can influence a person's ability to establish and maintain relationships. Immigrants who move to another country may experience loneliness and alienation. Sometimes people form their own close-knit groups to help form relationships but may, in fact, put up barriers to the outside world, further alienating themselves.

SIGNS AND SYMPTOMS Persons are inflexible and maladaptive in their environment and have very few strategies in forming and maintaining relationships. Their patterns of behavior and communication evoke negative reactions from others. They lack resilience in day-to-day life and are often unable to adapt to changes in their world. As a consequence, they experience loneliness, withdraw, and become dependent on their jobs and their homes for their solace. Each specific type of Personality Disorder has its unique set of signs and symptoms in addition to those listed here.

DIAGNOSTIC PROCEDURES For a diagnosis to be made, the person must exhibit a marked devia-

tion in at least two of the following areas: (1) cognitive, (2) affectivity, (3) impulse control, and (4) interpersonal functioning. After a complete physical examination, an evaluation of the long-term patterns of functioning must be investigated and evaluated. Such an evaluation may need to be done over time and in different situations to glean a true picture of the person's disorder. A person's ethnic, cultural, and social background must be taken into account when diagnosing the disorder to ensure the patterns are indeed markedly deviant. In children younger than 18 years, the signs and symptoms must be present for at least 1 year for a diagnosis to be made.

TREATMENT Treatment is difficult and requires a trusting relationship among client, physician, and therapist. The type of treatment is dependent on the client's signs and symptoms and their severity. In general, clients come for treatment for depression, anxiety, alcoholism, or difficulties at work or in their relationships. Medication is prescribed only for the more acute signs and symptoms rather than on a long-term basis. The goal of treatment is to help clients change their behavior and thinking that result from their personality traits or patterns. Whatever the treatment, it needs to be consistent and structured. The treatment will encourage expression of feelings, self-analysis of behavior, and accountability for actions. Family will need to be involved to address the maladaptive social responses. In some forms of Personality Disorder, the client will need protection from harming himself or herself. It is hoped that the client will report improvement of quality and quantity of interpersonal relationships.

ALTERNATIVE THERAPY: *Some nutrients may be deficient; hence, alternative therapy practitioners may supplement those nutrients in consultation with the physician. Biofeedback, relaxation, and guided imagery may prove useful to address the stress that clients experience.*

 TEACHING TIPS: Family members will need to be involved in the treatment of the client. It is important to provide a supportive atmosphere and encourage the client to follow the individualized plan. Watch for signs of suicide or self-harm, and seek appropriate medical attention as needed.

■ **PROGNOSIS** The prognosis depends on the type and severity of the Personality Disorder. Some Personality Disorders diminish as the person ages, whereas for others, lifelong treatment is required. Most clients with Personality Disorder also have depression, substance abuse disorder, or both, so the incidence of suicide is high.

■ **PREVENTION** There is no known prevention.

SUBSTANCE ABUSE

■ **DESCRIPTION** Addictions to alcohol and to psychoactive drugs are both serious and chronic diseases that can be life threatening. Both interfere with physical and mental health, family and social relationships, and occupational responsibilities. Addiction cuts across all social and economic groups, involves both genders, and occurs at all stages of the life cycle, beginning as early as elementary school. Table 7.1 provides a list of addictive substances.

- *Alcohol dependence:* Drinking is most prevalent between the ages of 21 and 34, but about 19% of 12- to 17-year-olds have a serious drinking problem. Men are five times more likely to abuse alcohol than are women. Alcohol abuse is a factor in approximately 60% of all automobile accidents.
- *Psychoactive drug addiction:* Experimentation with drugs can occur at any age but commonly occurs in adolescence or even earlier. Drug abuse can lead to either physical or psychological dependence, or both.

The most dangerous form of any addiction or abuse is when users mix multiple drugs simultaneously—including alcohol.

Table 7.1

COMMONLY ABUSED SUBSTANCES

Opiates and Narcotics	Powerful painkillers with sedative and euphoric qualities.	Heroin Opium Codeine Meperidine Demerol Hydropmorphone (Dilaudid) Oxycontin Fentanyl
Central Nervous System Stimulants	Stimulating effects and can produce tolerance.	Amphetamines Cocaine Dextroamphetamine Methamphetamines (meth, speed, crank) Methylphenidate (Ritalin) Caffeine Nicotine Crack cocaine (crack)
Central Nervous System Depressants	Produce a soothing sedative and anxiety-reducing effect and can lead to dependence. Includes many prescription drugs.	Barbiturates (amobarbital, pentobarbital, secobarbital) Benzodiazepine (Valium, Ativan, Xanax) Chloral hydrate Paraldehyde Alcohol Ephedrine Nitrous oxide Halothane Flunitrazepam (Rohypnol) Gamma Hydroxyl Butyrate (GHB) Amyl nitrate Methaqualone

(Continued on the following page)

Hallucinogens	Hallucinogenic properties and can produce psychological dependence.	Lysergic acid diethylamide (LSD) Mescaline Psilocybin/psilocin Phencyclidine (PCP or "angel dust") MDMA (ecstasy) Ketamine
Anabolic Steroids	Any drug or hormonal substance chemically and pharmacologically related to testosterone (other than estrogens, progestins, and corticosteroids) that promote muscle growth.	Boldenone Fluoxymesterone Methandriol Methyltestosterone Oxandrolone Oxymetholone Trenbolone
Tetrahydrocannabinol (THC)	Although used for their relaxing properties, THC-derived drugs can also lead to paranoia and anxiety.	Cannabis Marijuana Hashish

■ **ETIOLOGY** Numerous biological, psychological, and sociocultural factors appear to be involved in alcohol and psychoactive drug abuse. Biological factors may include genetic or biochemical abnormalities, nutritional deficiencies, endocrine imbalances, and allergic responses. It is estimated that about 50% to 60% of the variance in alcohol dependence is due to genetic factors. Alcohol-dependent persons are six times more likely than are nonalcoholic persons to have blood relatives who are alcohol dependent. Psychological factors may include the urge to drink or experiment with drugs to reduce anxiety or avoid the responsibilities of family, life, and work situations. There is also the desire to experience the temporary euphoria or "feel good" state that allows individuals to feel pleasure. Individuals with addiction to alcohol and psychoactive drugs may have low self-esteem, peer pressure, and inadequate coping skills. Individuals tend to hide their dependence on either alcohol or drugs and may temporarily maintain function in their lives only to gradually have that ability disappear as dependence becomes greater.

■ **SIGNS AND SYMPTOMS**

• *Alcohol dependence*: Individuals are unable to control their drinking even when it becomes the underlying cause of serious harm, including medical disorders, marital difficulties, job loss, and automobile accidents. A person dependent on alcohol develops a craving that must be satisfied. They experience impaired control and have an inability to stop drinking once they start. When they stop drinking after a period of heavy use, they experience unpleasant physical ailments from withdrawal that include nausea, sweating, shaking, and anxiety. They drink to stop these symptoms and thereby develop a greater tolerance for alcohol.

• *Psychoactive drug dependence:* Signs and symptoms of drug dependence depend on the particular drug. Symptoms of opiate and narcotic dependence can include needle marks, scars from skin abscesses, rapid heart rate, constricted pupils, and a relaxed or euphoric state. Symptoms of nervous system stimulant dependence are similar except the pupils are dilated and the individual may be restless and hyperactive. Symptoms of hallucinogen dependence include anxiety, frightening hallucinations, paranoid delusions, blurred vision, dilated pupils, and tremor.

■ **DIAGNOSTIC PROCEDURES** Toxicology screens on blood and urine can confirm the presence of alcohol and drugs in the body. In regular users, some drugs can be detected in urine up to 28 days. A client history may reveal past substance abuse.

■ **TREATMENT** Total abstinence from alcohol and the drug or drugs of choice is the only effective treatment. There are many programs aimed at detoxification, rehabilitation, and aftercare that can be helpful to both the client and the involved family. Long-term successful treatment will also depend on individuals in recovery filling the place that alcohol or the abused substance once occupied in their life with something constructive.

ALTERNATIVE THERAPY: *Recent research in the field of addiction suggests that excessive craving for any substance indicates an allergic condition in relation to that substance. Therefore, abstinence is advised. Acupuncture has proved effective in treating cocaine, heroin, and crack addictions. It is most effective when used in conjunction with other therapies, including psychological counseling. Biofeedback and neurofeedback may be useful to bring about significant behavioral changes in the addictive personality. Some herbal medications may be useful in treating the symptoms of withdrawal.*

TEACHING TIPS: Substance abuse affects the entire family. Perhaps the best advice that can be given is to have everyone receive as much information as possible on substance abuse, its possible causes, and treatments. Blame and guilt only worsen the problem.

■ **PROGNOSIS** Clients can recover with total abstinence from alcohol and drugs, but there is no cure. Only 15% of those with alcohol dependence seek treatment for this disease. Relapse after treatment is common, so it is important to maintain support systems to cope with any slips and to ensure that they do not turn into complete reversals. Treatment programs have varying success rates, but many people with alcohol and psychoactive drug dependency have a full recovery.

■ **PREVENTION** Abstinence from alcohol and drugs and replacement of the substance with constructive activities are essential. Support and encouragement of family members and a support group can be helpful, but ultimately a person in recovery knows that he or she alone is responsible for abstinence.

DISORDERS GENERALLY DIAGNOSED DURING CHILDHOOD OR ADOLESCENCE

Mental Retardation

■ **DESCRIPTION** Mental retardation is a condition of subaverage intellectual functioning with concurrent deficits in adaptive behavior that exhibits itself generally before 8 years of age. The IQ is approximately 70 or below on an individually administered test. It is estimated that 1% to 3% of the general population have mental retardation to some degree. According to the *DSM-IV*, there are four types of mental retardation, defined by their degree of severity, as follows:

- *Mild mental retardation:* Eighty-five percent of those with mental retardation fall into this category. Usually these children develop their communication and social skills during preschool. On graduating from high school, they usually achieve at the sixth-grade level. This mental retardation generally will be noticed in elementary grade schools. As adults, they can work but will need support to address social and economic stresses.
- *Moderate mental retardation:* Ten percent of mentally retarded persons are in this category. They achieve second-grade level in education. Moderate supervision is required for persons to take care of their personal needs, and additional support is needed for vocational training. They have difficulty in social and relationship situations. In adulthood, they can function in supervised settings.
- *Severe mental retardation:* From 3% to 4% of those with mental retardation fall into this category. During their early childhood years, they acquire little to no communication skills. In school, they learn elementary skills to care for themselves and learn to talk. In adult life, they live in group homes or with their families.
- *Profound mental retardation:* From 1% to 2% of mentally retarded individuals fall into this category. They generally have a neurologic disorder that accounts for their mental retardation. They display sensory motor function deficiencies in early childhood and require a caregiver and constant supervision.

■ **ETIOLOGY** The exact cause of mental retardation is known only in a small percentage of people. For example, in profound mental retardation, there is a neurologic problem responsible, whereas in the others forms, it may be a combination of factors. Other possible causes include prenatal causes such as hydrocephalus; chromosomal abnormalities such as in Down syndrome; metabolic causes such as phenylketonuria (PKU) or Tay-Sachs disease;

environmental causes such as cultural-familial retardation or poor nutrition; gestational causes such as prematurity; infection and intoxication such as lead poisoning; congenital rubella; psychiatric disorders such as autism; or trauma such as mechanical injury.

■ **SIGNS AND SYMPTOMS** In general, the child's delay in development is noted by the parents or pediatrician. The child may show deviations in adaptive behaviors, experience learning disabilities, or have severe cognitive and motor skill impairment. Parents may be frustrated and exhausted with the child's lack of progress and development in communication, sensory, and motor skill development.

■ **DIAGNOSTIC PROCEDURES** There are no laboratory tests to detect mental retardation other than tests for the suspected neurologic problem causing the retardation. A psychological evaluation is needed as well as an adaptive behavior evaluation. The child needs to be deficient in any two of the following areas for diagnosis: self-care, home living, communication, social/interpersonal skills, use of community resources, self-direction, functional academic skills, work, leisure, health, and safety. The diagnosis generally is given before the child reaches 18 years of age.

■ **TREATMENT** Treatment requires a team approach that builds on the client's strengths. The focus of treatment is in skill development in the following areas: adaptive skills, communication, social, and motor areas. Special education classes are available, and there are many resources in the community that will benefit families who have a child with mental retardation.

ALTERNATIVE THERAPY: *No significant alternative therapy is indicated.*

TEACHING TIPS: Parents may be overwhelmed with caring for a mentally retarded child, so support of the parents is essential. They also may need financial resources. If the child has an associated disability, special education may be necessary and a referral should be made when the disability is first noted. The earlier education and training are available, the better is the prognosis, in most cases. If the child is severely retarded, the family may need counseling and support for the home care required for the child.

■ **PROGNOSIS** The prognosis depends on the client's degree of mental retardation, motivation and skill level, availability of training opportunities, and any associated neurologic problems. Many people with mental retardation live productive, happy lives.

■ **PREVENTION** Prenatal screening and genetic counseling are advised for high-risk families. Where the cause is unknown, there is no known prevention.

Attention-Deficit/Hyperactivity Disorder and Attention Deficit Disorder

■ **DESCRIPTION** Attention-deficit/hyperactivity disorder (ADHD) is the most common neurobiological disorder in children. It occurs in adults as well, although there is limited research on adult ADHD. The person with ADHD is inattentive, impulsive, and hyperactive and will have difficulties with gratification. People with ADHD are on a roller coaster due to their impulsiveness and emotional overarousal. Many times they receive more negative reinforcement and feedback because of their behavioral patterns.

ADHD is found in about 5% to 8% of the general population. Unfortunately, it is estimated that fewer than one half of these individuals are appropriately diagnosed. In the general population, the disorder is 3 to 10 times more common in males than in females; in children, ADHD is 4 times more common in boys than in girls. About 50% to 80% of children with ADHD carry their symptoms into adulthood.

The difference between ADHD and ADD is mainly one of terminology. ADHD is also the "official term" for attention deficit disorder (ADD). ADD is more commonly used in the general population for all types of ADHD and may be used among professionals as well. However, ADHD is used here.

There are three types of ADHD: (1) attention-deficit/hyperactivity disorder, a combined type; (2) attention deficit/hyperactivity disorder: predominantly inattentive; and (3) attention deficit/hyperactivity disorder, predominately hyperactive or impulsive. A general discussion of all three is given.

■ **ETIOLOGY** It is believed that environmental factors such as lead poisoning, genetic factors, socioeconomic factors, and prenatal and perinatal complications all play a part in the development of the disorder. Most support a neurobiological basis as well. In ADHD, the brain areas that control attention use less glucose, indicating that they are less active. The conclusion is that a lower level of activity in the brain may cause inattention and other ADHD symptoms. Research has shown that ADHD does run in families. For the general population, the risk of ADHD is 4% to 6%, whereas when one person in the family has ADHD, there is a 25% to 35% risk that any other family member also will have ADHD. Contrary to popular belief, ADHD is not caused by bad parenting, poor teachers, family problems, food allergies, or too much sugar. The family may experience conflict and parenting problems, although the latter may be a result of the child's behavior rather than be a causative factor.

■ **SIGNS AND SYMPTOMS** The classic symptoms include distractibility, impulsivity, and hyperactivity. These symptoms must be excessive and long term, occur before the age of 7, and continue at least 6 months. The behaviors must create a real handicap in at least two of the following three areas: home, school, or social settings.

The person does not listen, avoids difficult tasks, talks excessively, is careless, and has difficulty following through. In general, the person will be forgetful, be fidgety, and have a difficult temperament. Many times people with ADHD will refuse to wait to speak until a sentence is finished and do not like waiting for their turn.

■ **DIAGNOSTIC PROCEDURES** Many times the diagnosis of ADHD is not made until the child starts school, as parents tend to tolerate the expressed behaviors better than do others. In school, the behaviors interfere with the child's academic performance and peer relationships. Many earlier indicators generally are present, however. A physical examination is completed first to rule out any other problems that require treatment. This is followed by a comprehensive evaluation that includes a complete individual and family history, ability tests, achievement tests, and a collection of observations of those closest to the individual. Other disorders need to be evaluated through a comprehensive psychological screening.

■ **TREATMENT** Obviously, the treatment of the disorder encompasses the client and the entire family. Treatment includes medication to improve brain function. Most of the time psychotropic medications are stimulants, but antidepressants, antihypertensives, or tricyclic antidepressants may be prescribed. Adjusting the medication dosage is a challenge in children because they metabolize and eliminate drugs more rapidly than do adults.

Behavior management, social skill development, and cognitive therapy are initiated to help the child learn problem-solving and communication skills. Parents are educated about the disorder and the child's individual treatment plan. Art therapy, children's games, and storytelling help children deal with their feelings, relieve their distress, and teach them new coping skills. Children may need continued counseling with or without their family. It is imperative that the treatment plans continue, and children may require day treatment programs as well as intensive in-home programs.

In adults, medication is prescribed, along with behavior management and cognitive therapy. Work may pose challenges requiring mental health counseling.

ALTERNATIVE THERAPY: *Some practitioners recommend that the client eat every 2 hours and restrict foods high in sugar to combat symptoms of hypoglycemia. Others recommend that clients take high-potency nutritional supplements with the approval of the primary care physician. If food allergies are a problem, avoid the allergens. Any herbal tea that has a calming or relaxing effect may be tried.*

 TEACHING TIPS: Those closest to the individual with ADHD need to provide a supportive environment, teaching the person organizational, study, and memory skills. Basic time management and learning how to be self-aware need to be reinforced. Whether at work or at school, it is important to investigate what kind of environment best suits them so that they can be productive. Proper diet and sleep are essential, especially due to the side effects of some medications that might be prescribed.

■ **PROGNOSIS** By the time the child is diagnosed with ADHD, other mental health problems may have surfaced, such as low self-esteem and poor socialization. If the child has associated mental health problems, the prognosis is not as good. In fact, personality and social adjustment problems will continue. ADHD will continue into adulthood in one half to one third of those affected. Obviously, this affects their job, family, and social relationships. ADHD is recognized as a disability under the Americans with Disabilities Act and as such requires reasonable accommodation in school and at work. This helps ADHD clients to live more productive lives.

■ PREVENTION There is no known prevention.

EATING DISORDERS

Anorexia Nervosa

■ DESCRIPTION *Anorexia nervosa* is a complex psychogenic eating disorder. The key feature is self-imposed starvation and an irrational fear of gaining weight, even when the individual is already emaciated. It is also marked by weight loss, clinical evidence of semistarvation, amenorrhea, and an alteration in body image. The disorder, primarily affecting young women, occurs in 5% to 10% of the population around the age of puberty. White women from middle-class backgrounds are affected most frequently. The reported incidence of anorexia in men is low.

■ ETIOLOGY The cause of anorexia nervosa is not known, although most health professionals believe it is essentially a psychiatric disorder. Some theorists believe the refusal to eat is a subconscious effort to exert control over one's life. Attitudes in society that equate slimness with beauty play some role in provoking the disorder. A client's socioeconomic status, family background, and cultural conditioning may be predisposing factors in development of the condition.

■ SIGNS AND SYMPTOMS A loss of at least 25% of original body weight, in the absence of any detectable underlying medical disorder, may suggest a diagnosis of anorexia nervosa. Evidence of food avoidance, vomiting, and excessive exercise also suggest the diagnosis. In severe cases, a host of secondary symptoms may be evident as a result of metabolic and hormonal disturbances resulting from malnutrition. The affected individual also may tend to deny feelings of hunger and will typically claim to be overweight despite physical evidence to the contrary.

■ DIAGNOSTIC PROCEDURES Careful interpretation of clinical data is important to rule out other disorders that cause physical wasting. No specific diagnostic tests exist for anorexia nervosa, but blood testing may reveal associated nutritional anemia and vitamin or mineral deficiencies. The *DSM-IV* relies on the symptoms for its diagnosing criteria.

■ TREATMENT Medical treatment of anorexia nervosa is aimed at reversing the effects of malnutrition and controlling the individual compulsion to binge and purge. Noncooperation on the part of the affected individual, however, typically makes treatment of this disorder difficult. Aggressive medical management, nutritional counseling, and individual and family psychotherapy are recommended. Hospitalization may be required in the event of severe weight loss and malnutrition.

ALTERNATIVE THERAPY: *For both anorexia nervosa and bulimia nervosa, hypnotherapy may be beneficial. Some practitioners believe the absence of zinc may be a contributing factor in the disease; any zinc supplement should be given only under the supervision of a qualified practitioner. A well-balanced diet high in fiber should be established.*

TEACHING TIPS: It may be necessary to stay with the individual during and after meals and to give rewards for satisfactory weight gain. Referring the client and family members to the American Anorexia/Bulimia Association for additional information and support can be beneficial.

■ PROGNOSIS The prognosis varies. Relapses are frequent. Death may occur from malnutrition and complications such as hypothermia and cardiac disturbances in as many as one-fourth of diagnosed cases, especially when the person is not anxious to overcome the disorder.

■ PREVENTION There is no known specific prevention, but it seems helpful that an individual develop a sense of self-esteem that is not dependent on the thin, "model-like" body image so prized in today's society.

Bulimia Nervosa

■ DESCRIPTION *Bulimia nervosa* is a psychogenic eating disorder characterized by repetitive gorging with food, followed by self-induced vomiting. The condition also may involve laxative abuse, the use of diuretics, and fasting. The individual with anorexia nervosa seems obsessed with becoming even thinner, the person with bulimia has a morbid fear of becoming fat. Other behavioral abnormalities include obsessive secrecy about the condition and sometimes food stealing. The disorder principally affects young women and may occur simutaneously with anorexia nervosa.

■ **ETIOLOGY** The cause of bulimia is not known. Psychosocial factors such as family conflict, sexual abuse, and a cultural overemphasis on physical appearance may be contributing factors. There may be a struggle for self-identity and a history of depression, anxiety, phobias, and obsessive-compulsive disorder (OCD).

■ **SIGNS AND SYMPTOMS** Most persons with bulimia hide the behavioral evidence of their condition, and they are often of normal weight or even slightly overweight on diagnosis. They may still exhibit signs of malnutrition, however, because the "binge" diet of a bulimic individual is often wildly unbalanced, usually consisting of "junk" foods such as donuts, ice cream, and candy. Owing to the high sugar content of the binge diet and the subsequent reflux of gastric juices during vomiting, the bulimic person typically has a high incidence of dental decay. Reflux of gastric secretions also can produce a chronic sore throat. Menstrual irregularities are much less common in bulimia than in anorexia nervosa.

■ **DIAGNOSTIC PROCEDURES** Chronic depression, low tolerance for frustation, anxiety, self-consciousness, and difficultly expressing feelings, such as anger, are common. The client is apt to possess an exaggerated sense of guilt and have difficulty controlling impulses. Serum electrolyte studies may reveal the diagnosis. Other tests may reveal cardiac arrhythmias or evidence of renal dysfunction.

■ **TREATMENT** Long-term psychotherapy is usually indicated. The bulimic person knows that the eating patterns are abnormal but is unable to control them. As with the anorexic person, noncooperation on the part of the bulimic client generally makes treatment difficult and frustrating. Treatment concentrates on interrupting the binge-purge cycle and helping the client regain control over eating behavior.

ALTERNATIVE THERAPY: *See Anorexia Nervosa.*

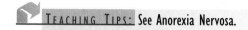 **TEACHING TIPS:** See Anorexia Nervosa.

■ **PROGNOSIS** The prognosis is guarded unless the client responds to therapy. Bulimic persons have twice as high an incidence of suicide as do anorexics. Other complications may include pneumonia, rupturing of the esophagus or stomach, and pancreatitis.

■ **PREVENTION** There is no known specific prevention.

SEXUAL DISORDERS

Sexual disorders are characterized by physiologic and psychological changes that disturb the sexual desire and the sexual response cycle and cause difficulties among sexual partners. The three major categories and their disorders are as follows:

- Sexual pain disorder, including dyspareunia
- Sexual arousal disorder, including male erectile disorder and female sexual arousal disorder
- Orgasmic disorder, including premature ejaculation

Etiologic factors generally are believed to be psychological factors and a medical condition that may contribute to but not necessarily be sufficient by itself to cause the disorder. In the diagnosis and treatment phases, it is important to consider the individual's ethnic, cultural, religious, and social backgrounds, all of which may affect the client's attitude, perception, desire, and expectations about performance.

An important consideration in the treatment of any sexual disorder is a sensitivity to open communication about the problem. Both the client and the physician may have difficulty raising questions regarding sexual functions. If this occurs, disorders may go undetected and untreated.

All health-care professionals need to be alert to an individual's signals and questions that may indicate a sexual concern. Clients often feel more comfortable raising a question with someone other than the physician; therefore, it is important that the physician include a detailed sexual history as part of the medical history. All health professionals need to feel comfortable initiating questions about sexual function. Health care in which the total person is treated cannot ignore the human sexual response and its function or dysfunction.

Sexual Pain Disorder/Dyspareunia

■ **DESCRIPTION** A sexual pain disorder, *dyspareunia* (painful intercourse), refers to pain that is associated with sexual intercourse. It may occur in men or women during, before, or after sexual intercourse.

■ **ETIOLOGY** The cause of the pain may be anatomic or physiologic, including, but not limited to, lesions of the vagina, retroversion of the uterus, urinary tract infection, lack of lubrication, scar tissue, or abnormal growths. More commonly the cause may be psychosomatic, which can include fear of pain or injury, feelings of guilt or shame, ignorance of sexual anatomy and physiology, and fear of pregnancy.

■ **SIGNS AND SYMPTOMS** For a diagnosis to be made, the person must experience persistent genital pain. The disturbance causes interpersonal difficulty and marked distress. The individual may experience mild to severe discomfort before, during, or after intercourse.

■ **DIAGNOSTIC PROCEDURES** A physical examination will be performed and diagnostic tests ordered to detect any underlying anatomic or pathologic causes of the dyspareunia. A detailed sexual history is important to help reveal any psychological factors that may be causing the disorder.

■ **TREATMENT** Individuals may be instructed to use creams or water-soluble jellies for lubrication before intercourse. Medications may be prescribed if any infections are detected. Excision of any scars and gentle stretching of the vaginal orifice may be needed. Education about the sexual response and counseling or short-term psychotherapy may be indicated.

ALTERNATIVE THERAPY: *No significant alternative therapy is indicated.*

 TEACHING TIPS: Sexual partners need to listen to one another, learn foreplay techniques, and be patient. Open communication is important.

■ **PROGNOSIS** The prognosis is good with adequate treatment, proper education, and sensitivity on the part of both sexual partners.

■ **PREVENTION** Preventive measures include prompt treatment of any infections or inflammatory diseases of the genitourinary tract.

Sexual Arousal Disorder/Male Erectile Disorder

■ **DESCRIPTION** A sexual arousal disorder, *erectile disorder* is the inability of a man to achieve or sustain an erection sufficient to complete sexual intercourse.

■ **ETIOLOGY** Erectile disorder may be psychological or physiologic in cause. Psychological causes account for 50% to 60% of the cases and include anxiety or depression, feelings of inadequacy, and rejection of others. Physiologic causes include certain pharmacologic agents, drug and alcohol abuse, diabetes mellitus, surgical complications, spinal cord and disc injuries, and neurologic, endocrine, or urologic disorders.

■ **SIGNS AND SYMPTOMS** Erectile disorder may occur when a person is unable to achieve any erection, is able to achieve an initial erection and then loses it, or is able to achieve an erection only during self-masturbation.

■ **DIAGNOSTIC PROCEDURES** The diagnostic procedures will help to differentiate between physiologic and psychological causes of the erectile disorder. They typically include a physical examination, medical history, and detailed sexual history.

■ **TREATMENT** The aim of treatment of erectile disorder is to correct any underlying physiologic disorders and counseling or psychotherapy to alleviate psychological problems. The surgical implantation of a penile prosthesis is a treatment option for individuals when erectile dysfunction is due to untreatable neurologic or vascular disorders. The drug sildenafil (Viagra) has proved successful in some men with erectile disorder. The drug enhances the effect of nitric oxide, the chemical released into the penis during sexual arousal, allowing the increased blood circulation necessary for an erection. Sildenafil should be taken while the client is in the care of a physician, who will need to determine the appropriate dosage.

ALTERNATIVE THERAPY: *Alternative health-care practitioners identify Arginino supplements that work like Viagra to improve a man's ability to have an erection. The supplement should not be taken without a physician's supervision. Ginkgo biloba boosts circulation to the penis, thus helping to reverse erectile disorder. The branch of yoga known as Tantra teaches techniques for improving sexual performance. Two methods are "holding the wand" and "tapping into pleasure." These methods involve grasping the penis, manipulating it as if it were a wand, gently rubbing the head across the clitoris, and tapping the penis against the lips of the vagina and the clitoris.*

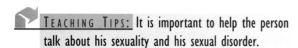

TEACHING TIPS: It is important to help the person talk about his sexuality and his sexual disorder.

■ **PROGNOSIS** The prognosis is variable, depending on how long the client has suffered from the disorder and its severity.

■ **PREVENTION** Prompt treatment of any physiologic cause is important.

Sexual Arousal Disorder/Female Sexual Arousal Disorder

■ **DESCRIPTION** A sexual arousal disorder, *female sexual arousal disorder* is an inability to achieve orgasm. Female arousal disorder is characterized by the lack of desire for sexual activity and arousal.

■ **ETIOLOGY** Female arousal disorder may be caused by physiologic factors, especially diseases that produce nerve damage, such as diabetes mellitus or multiple sclerosis. Drug reactions, pelvic infections, and vascular disease also may be the cause. More commonly, however, arousal disorder is due to psychological factors such as anxiety, depression, stress, and fatigue; sexual misinformation; inadequate or ineffective stimulation; and early traumatic sexual experiences. The prevalence of female sexual arousal disorder is probably more common in younger women; however, once a woman reaches orgasm, she is not likely to lose it, unless she has a traumatic experience or a relationship conflict.

■ **SIGNS AND SYMPTOMS** A woman with arousal dysfunction may express a loss of sexual desire or report slow sexual arousal. She may lack the vaginal lubrication and vasocongestive response of sexual arousal. The woman with orgasmic disorder has an inability to achieve orgasm totally or under certain circumstances.

■ **DIAGNOSTIC PROCEDURES** A physical examination, a medical history, and a detailed sexual history are needed to differentiate physiologic causes from psychological causes.

■ **TREATMENT** The treatment of arousal disorder is directed toward correcting underlying physiologic disorders or alleviating any psychological problems. The latter may involve sex therapy for both partners. The goal of treatment for orgasmic disorder is to eliminate involuntary inhibition of the orgasmic reflex. Treatment may include short-term psychotherapy or behavior modification.

ALTERNATIVE THERAPY: *No significant alternative therapy is indicated.*

TEACHING TIPS: It is important that the woman understand her sexuality and experiences surrounding it. Counseling with a sexual partner is helpful.

■ **PROGNOSIS** In the absence of nerve damage, the prognosis is good if the woman has had some pleasurable sexual arousal previously. Psychological causes require more lengthy treatment.

■ **PREVENTION** Early treatment of any physiologic or psychological problem is the best prevention.

Orgasmic Disorder/ Premature Ejaculation

■ **DESCRIPTION** An orgasmic disorder, *premature ejaculation* is the persistent or recurrent onset of orgasm and expulsion of seminal fluid before complete erection of the penis. It generally occurs immediately after the beginning of sexual intercourse or before the person wishes to ejaculate.

■ **ETIOLOGY** Psychological factors of premature ejaculation include anxiety or guilt feelings about sex. Negative sexual relationships, such as may exist when a man unconsciously dislikes women or seeks to deny his partner's need for sexual gratification, also may induce premature ejaculation. Pathologic factors are rare, but they may be linked to degenerative neurologic disorders, urethritis, or prostatitis.

■ **SIGNS AND SYMPTOMS** Ejaculation during foreplay, before complete erection of the penis, or as soon as **intromission** (insertion of one part into another) occurs is a classic symptom.

■ **DIAGNOSTIC PROCEDURES** Physical examination and laboratory tests may be ordered to rule out any pathologic causes. A detailed sexual history is important to adequately assess this disorder. The disorder must cause marked distress or interpersonal difficulty.

■ **TREATMENT** An intensive program of sex therapy may be necessary. It is important that both partners be involved in the treatment to learn the technique of delaying ejaculation and that they understand that the condition is reversible.

ALTERNATIVE THERAPY: *Practitioners recommend the scrotal pull. During self-stimulation, the man gently pulls down on his scrotal sac before orgasm. During the sexual act, either partner may pull on the scrotal sac. Eventually the pull is no longer needed. Another technique is an exercise wherein the person squeezes the muscles in the anal area as if trying to stop the flow of urine. The exercise is repeated several times. This exercise strengthens the muscles used during sexual intercourse, especially those used during ejaculation.*

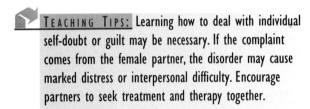

TEACHING TIPS: Learning how to deal with individual self-doubt or guilt may be necessary. If the complaint comes from the female partner, the disorder may cause marked distress or interpersonal difficulty. Encourage partners to seek treatment and therapy together.

■ **PROGNOSIS** The prognosis is excellent with proper treatment and understanding on the part of both partners. A positive self-image should be encouraged by explaining that premature ejaculation is a disorder that does not reflect on one's masculinity.

■ **PREVENTION** There is no known prevention.

CASE STUDIES

■ Case Study 1

Laura Henderson is a 17-year-old who has been diagnosed with anorexia nervosa. She is a long-distance runner and a straight A student in high school and is very popular. After initial treatment and family and individual therapy, she has been doing fairly well. Then Laura's sister caught her sticking her fingers in her mouth to induce vomiting after dinner. Her mother discussed the incident with Laura and found laxatives in her drawer. The family already sits with her at dinner and tries to stay with her for at least an hour after dinner, but it is difficult. Since Laura can no longer easily purge what she has eaten, her desire is to bolt from the chair to go out to run for several miles, an exercise that she hopes will "run off" the calories she has eaten..

Case Study Questions

1. Discuss the implications this case has on each family member.
2. What long-term consequences are there in this situation?

(Continued on the following page)

Continued

■ Case Study 2

Pat Schnell is more withdrawn than usual. She is usually active in her children's activities, attends church regularly, and walks for exercise. Lately, however, she has an unrealistic fear of being in public places. She refuses to go to the grocery store even with her husband.

Case Study Questions

1. What might be the mental health issue Pat is experiencing?
2. What treatment might be suggested?
3. Will Pat be able to return to her previous pattern of functioning?

■ Case Study 3

Earl and Suzie have been married for a number of years and have three children. There is unhappiness, however, in their lives. Earl has premature ejaculation every time sexual intercourse is attempted, and Suzie is nonorgasmic. Suzie refuses to seek counseling. Earl is embarrassed and does not like the idea that there might be something "abnormal" about his sexual performance, but he would like to correct the problems.

Case Study Questions

1. What recommendations might be made to Earl and Suzie?
2. Discuss the meaning of sexual health.

REVIEW QUESTIONS

True/False

Circle the correct answer:

T   F   1. The major cause of mental retardation is a neurologic disease.

T   F   2. There is adequate funding for mental health from community, state, and federal funding.

T   F   3. Age and gender have little to do with mental illnesses.

T   F   4. By the year 2010, according to the World Health Organization, depression will be a leading cause of disability.

T   F   5. Bipolar disorder is not as prevalent as other forms of depression.

Matching

Match the following by placing the correct letter in the column:

_____ 1. Persons have persecutory delusions

_____ 2. Senseless repetition of words or phrases

_____ 3. Confused thoughts or behaviors

_____ 4. Posttraumatic stress disorder

_____ 5. Fear of being alone or in open spaces

a. Paranoid schizophrenia

b. Disorganized schizophrenia

c. Catatonic schizophrenia

d. Echolalia

e. PTSD

f. Agoraphobia

Short Answer

1. The primary antidepressants are _____, _____, and _____.

2. Persons might receive _____ for depression if they cannot take antidepressants and their depression is severe and life threatening.

3. The incidence of schizophrenia in the United States is _____.

4. The Personality Disorder that does not respect the rights of others is _____.

5. Substance abuse programs are aimed at _____, _____, and _____.

Multiple Choice

Place a checkmark next to the correct answer:

1. Anorexia nervosa is (a)

    a. Personality Disorder.

    b. Morbid fear of becoming fat.

    c. Disorder that affects young males more than females.

    d. Self-imposed starvation.

2. ADHD is

    a. Found in about 20% of the general population.

    b. More common in females than in males.

    c. Exhibited in three types.

    d. Easily preventable.

3. Sexual disorders are identified by

    a. Pain disorder.

    b. Arousal disorder.

    c. Orgasmic disorder.

    d. All of the above.

4. Subaverage intellectual functioning with current deficit adaptive behaviors is known as

    a. ADHD.

    b. Personality Disorder.

    c. Schizophrenia

    d. Mental retardation.

5. Which of the following statements is false?

    a. The *DSM-IV* is published by the American Psychiatric Association.

    b. Major depression affects all ethnic groups and both genders.

    c. Dysthymia is a severe form of depression.

    d. St. John's wort is contraindicated with some mental disorder medications.

Discussion Questions/Personal Reflection

1. Discuss the implications on the family when a family member is diagnosed with one of the schizophrenia disorders.

2. Brainstorm and identify possible socially acceptable activities that replace the time and the energy put into abusing alcohol or drugs.

8

Urinary System Diseases and Disorders

CHAPTER OUTLINE

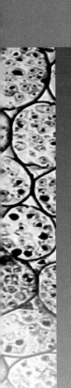

Antiemetic (ăn•tĭ•ē•mĕt′ĭk)
Antipyretic (ăn•tĭ•pī•rĕt′ĭk)
Ascites (ă•sī′tēz)
Azotemia (ā•zō′tē•mē•ă)
Calyx (kā′lĭks)
Creatinine (krē•ăt′ĭn•ĭn)
Cystectomy (sĭs•tĕk′tō•mē)
Dysuria (dĭs•ū′rē•ă)
Electrolyte (ē•lĕk′trō•līt)
Hematuria (hē•mă•tū′rē•ă)
Hyperkalemia (hī•pĕr•kă•lē′mē•ă)
Hyperlipemia (hī•pĕr•lĭp•ē′mē•ă)
Hyperparathyroidism (hī•pĕr•păr•ă•thī′
    roy• dĭzm)
Hypertension (hī•pĕr•tĕn′shun)
Hypoalbuminemia (hī•pō•ăl•bū •mĭn•
    ē′mē•ă)
Insidious (ĭn•sĭd′ē•ŭs)
Ischemia (ĭs•kē′mē•ă)
Lipiduria (lĭp•ĭ•dū′rē•ă)
Micturition (mĭk•tū•rĭ′shŭn)
Nocturia (nŏk•tū′rē•ă)
Oliguria (ŏl•ĭg•ū′rē•ă)
Pallor (păl′ŏr)
Polyuria (pŏl•ē•ū′rē•ă)
Proteinuria (prō•tē•ĭn•ū′rē•ă)
Pyuria (pī •yū r•ē•ă)
Transurethral resection (trăns•ū •re′thrăl rē•
    sĕk′shŭn)
Urea (ū •rē′ă)
Uremia (ū •rē′mē•ă)
Urolith (ū′rō•lĭth)

> *Everything is funny as long as it hap-*
> *pens to somebody else.*
>
> —WILL ROGERS

LEARNING OBJECTIVES

Upon successful completion of this chapter, you will be able to:

- Identify the major diseases of the kidney.
- Name the most common diagnostic procedures used to detect kidney and kidney-related diseases.
- List at least three characteristics common to polycystic kidney disease.
- Identify complications of kidney-related diseases.
- Compare and contrast pyelonephritis and glomerulonephritis.
- Recall infectious precursors to kidney-related diseases.
- Explain why women are more prone to urinary tract infections.
- List the characteristics unique to nephrotic syndrome.
- Name at least three causes of end-stage renal disease.
- Distinguish between the three types of kidney dialysis.
- Describe how acute tubular necrosis occurs.
- Discuss the complications of renal calculi.
- Identify possible treatments for hydronephrosis.
- Repeat the common signs and symptoms of lower urinary tract infections.
- Describe the prognosis of lower urinary tract infections.
- Define neurogenic bladder.
- Recall the major cause of tumors of the bladder.
- List at least four common complaints of the urinary system.

The urinary system is responsible for the production and elimination of urine. The former is the function of the kidneys, whereas the rest of the system is responsible for the elimination of urine. The organs of this system include two kidneys, two ureters, the urinary bladder, and the urethra. Figure 8.1 illustrates the urinary system in relationship to the body, and Figure 8.2 illustrates the interior and exterior features of the urinary system organs.

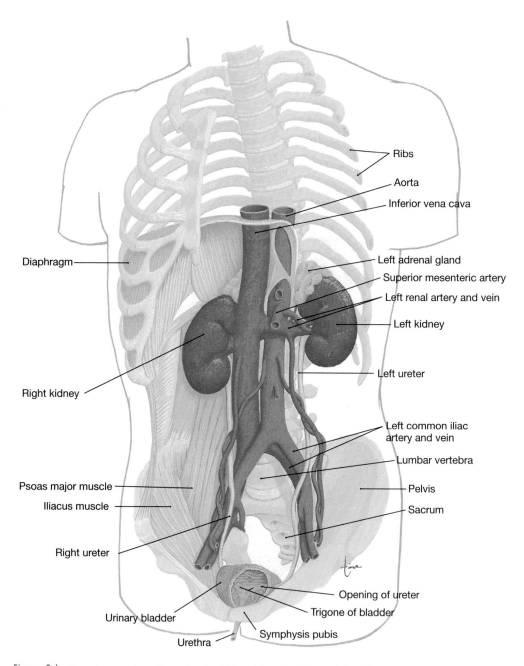

Figure 8.1 The urinary system. (From Scanlon, VC, and Sanders, T: Essentials of Anatomy and Physiology, ed 4. FA Davis, Philadelphia, 2003, p 399, with permission.)

The kidneys help to regulate the water, **electrolyte** (ionized salt), and acid-base content of the blood and selectively filter out the waste products of metabolism. They also play an important role in regulating blood pressure. Each kidney contains more than 1 million nephrons (Fig. 8.3), which are the principal functional units of the kidney. It is here that the three-part process of selective filtration of wastes, reabsorption of vital minerals and fluid, and secretion of waste products and other substances takes place.

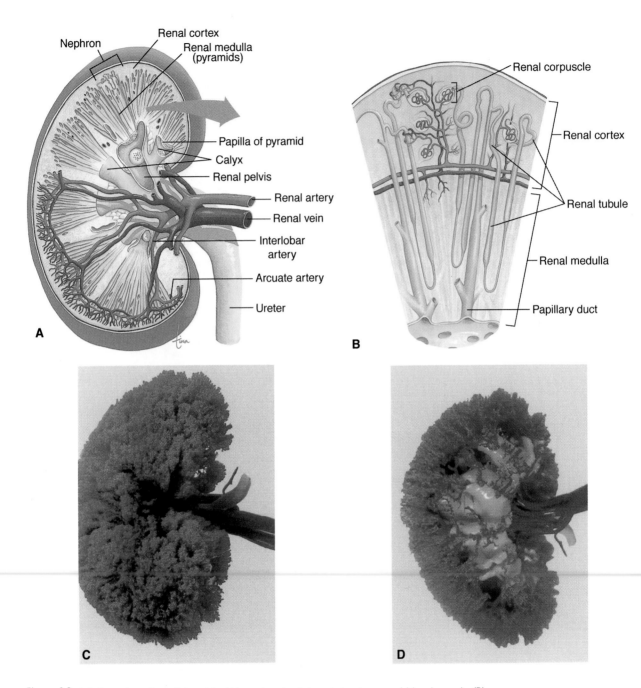

Figure 8.2 (A) Frontal section of the right kidney showing internal structures and blood vessels. (B) Magnified section of the kidney shows several nephrons. (From Scanlon, VC, and Sanders, T: Essentials of Anatomy and Physiology, ed 4. FA Davis, Philadelphia, 2003, p 401, with permission.) (C) Vascular cast of a kidney in lateral view. Red plastic fills the blood vessels. (D) Vascular cast in medial view. Blood vessels have been removed; yellow plastic fills the renal pelvis. (C,D: Photographs by Dan Kaufman.)

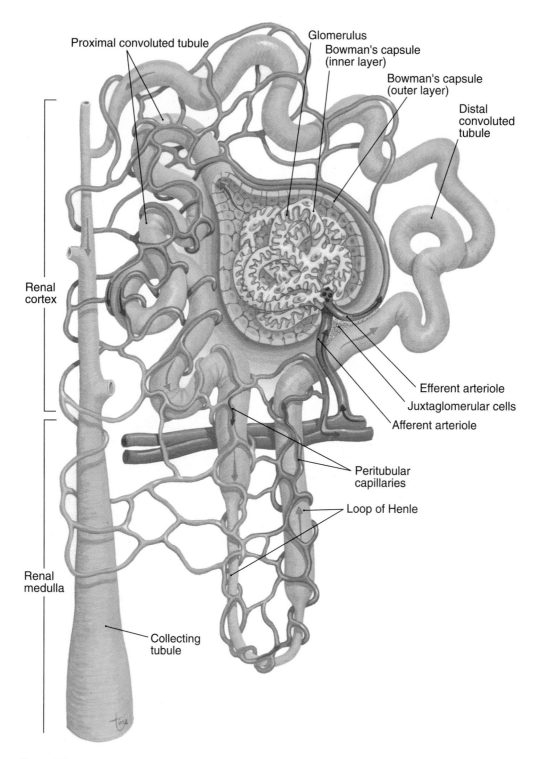

Figure 8.3 Nephron with associated blood vessels. Arrows, direction of blood flow and the flow of renal filtrate. (From Scanlon, VC, and Sanders, T: Essentials of Anatomy and Physiology, ed 3. FA Davis, Philadelphia, 1999, p 406, with permission.)

It is worth emphasizing the reabsorption process of the kidneys' nephrons. Were it not for this process, the body would rapidly be depleted of its fluid. Typically, only 1% of the fluid passing through a nephron is excreted as urine.

A routine diagnostic test for suspected urinary disease is a urinalysis, which includes testing the specific gravity, pH, presence of protein, blood, sugar, and ketones. It includes a microscopic examination for the presence of white and red blood cells, casts, bacteria, and crystals. Normal urine is amber in color with a slightly acid reaction, has a peculiar odor, and frequently deposits a precipitate of phosphates when fresh. The specific gravity varies from 1.005 to 1.030. The greater the rate of urine excretion, the lower is the specific gravity. Refer to Table 8.1, Significance of Changes in Urine, as you read the chapter, noting possible abnormalities and their significance to the disease in question.

KIDNEY DISEASES AND DISORDERS

Polycystic Kidney Disease

■ DESCRIPTION *Polycystic kidney disease* is a developmental defect of the collecting tubules in the cortex of the kidneys. Groups of tubules that fail to empty properly into the renal pelvis slowly swell into multiple, grapelike, fluid-filled sacs or cysts. The pressure from the expanding cysts slowly destroys adjacent normal tissue, progressively impairing kidney function. Both kidneys are usually affected and are grossly enlarged. Polycystic kidney disease is one of the most common hereditary diseases in the United States, affecting more than 500,000 people.

■ ETIOLOGY There are two forms of the disease, each due to a genetic defect. The more common adult form, usually manifested during midlife, is an autosomal dominant defect. The much less common infant and childhood forms, manifested at birth or during childhood, are autosomal recessive defects. The following discussion pertains to the more frequently occurring adult form. The majority of the adult cases are inherited as an autosomal dominant trait, and the remainder are spontaneous mutations.

■ SIGNS AND SYMPTOMS The disease is usually asymptomatic until midlife. Then the client may complain of colic and lumbar pain or mention seeing blood in the urine or passing renal calculi. The pain is generally from the enlarging cysts. The onset is **insidious,** or occurs slowly with few or unnoticable symptoms.

■ DIAGNOSTIC PROCEDURES The history may reveal a family tendency toward renal disease. The physical examination may reveal palpably enlarged kidneys and **hypertension,** which is persistently high arterial blood pressure. The physician may order an excretory urography, ultrasound examination, or computed tomography (CT) scan to detect enlarged kidneys and the presence of cysts. Ultrasonography and CT scans have largely replaced excretory urography due to the fact that the former are able to detect small cysts. Urinalysis may be ordered to evaluate renal function and to detect **hematuria** or blood in the urine.

■ TREATMENT No treatment will stop the course of the disease; however, treatment attempts to minimize the symptoms. Treatment goals include guarding against or managing urinary tract infections and controlling secondary hypertension. Urine cultures should be performed at regular intervals to detect infection. In the event of renal failure, renal dialysis or kidney transplantation may be attempted to prolong life.

ALTERNATIVE THERAPY: *No significant alternative therapy is indicated.*

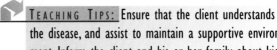

TEACHING TIPS: Ensure that the client understands the disease, and assist to maintain a supportive environment. Inform the client and his or her family about kidney dialysis and transplantation.

■ PROGNOSIS The prognosis is variable yet poor as there is no cure. Kidney function is progressively impaired, leading to renal failure, a toxic condition, or **uremia** (creatinine and urea in the blood), and eventual death, usually within 10 years.

■ PREVENTION No prevention is known. Genetic counseling is indicated for first-degree relatives of infected persons or for families at risk.

Pyelonephritis (Acute)

■ DESCRIPTION *Pyelonephritis,* also called *infective tubulointerstitial nephritis,* is inflammation

■ Table 8.1

SIGNIFICANCE OF CHANGES IN URINE

	NORMAL	ABNORMAL	SIGNIFICANCE
Quantity	1000 to 1500 mL (approx. 95% H_2O)		Depends on water and fluid, foods consumed, exercise, temperature, kidney function
		High (polyuria)	Diabetes mellitus, diabetes insipidus, nervous diseases, certain types of chronic nephritis (kidney disorder), diuretics (e.g., caffeine, digitalis) causing increased urinary excretion
		Low (oliguria)	Acute nephritis, heart disease, fever, eclampsia, diarrhea, vomiting, inadequate fluid intake
		None (anuria)	Uremia (nitrogenous wastes in blood), acute nephritis, metal poisoning (e.g., due to bichloride of mercury), complete obstruction of urinary tract
Color	Yellow to amber		Depends on concentration of pigment (urochrome)
		Pale	Diabetes insipidus; due to a very dilute urine
		Milky	Fat globules, pus in genitourinary infections
		Reddish	Blood pigments, drugs, or food pigments
		Greenish	Bile pigment, associated with jaundice
		Brown-black	Poisoning (mercury, lead, phenol), hemorrhage
Transparency	Clear		Normal
	Cloudy on standing		Precipitation of mucin from urinary tract; not pathologic
	Turbid		Precipitation of calcium phosphate; not pathologic
		Milky	Presence of fat globules; pathologic
		Turbid	Presence of pus due to inflammation of urinary tract; pathologic
Odor	Faintly aromatic		Normal
		Pleasant (sweet)	Acetone, associated with diabetes mellitus
		Unpleasant	Decomposition or ingestion of certain drugs or foods
	Peppermint		Menthol ingestion
	Acrid		Asparagus in diet
	Spicy		Ingestion of sandalwood oil or saffron
Proteinuria	Albumin and globulin		Excretion of 10 to 100 mg every 24 hours is normal, but this amount is not detected by usual tests.

(Continued on following page)

	NORMAL	ABNORMAL	SIGNIFICANCE
		Albumin	Evidence of altered renal function; may be due to renal pathology or a systemic disease such as diabetes mellitus
		Globulin	Bence-Jones proteins associated with multiple myeloma and diseases of globulin metabolism; other types of globulins may be present in acute and chronic pyelonephritis
Specific Gravity	1.010 to 1.025; can vary in absence of pathology		Ordinary; specific gravity inversely proportional to volume
		Low (chronic)	Dilution if volume is large; otherwise nephritis
		High (chronic)	Acute nephritis; concentrated if volume is small; otherwise, if light colored and volume is large, diabetes mellitus
Acidity	Acid (slight)		Diet of acid-forming foods (meats, eggs, prunes, wheat) overbalances the base-forming foods (vegetables and fruits)
		High acidity	Acidosis, diabetes mellitus, many pathological disorders (fevers, starvation)
		Alkaline	Vegetarian diet changes urea into ammonium carbonate; infection or ingestion of alkaline compounds

Source: Venes, D (ed): Taber's Cyclopedic Medical Dictionary, ed 19. FA Davis, Philadelphia, 2001, pp 2188–2189, with permission.

of the kidney and renal pelvis due to infection. One or both kidneys may be affected. The infection can result in the destruction or scarring of renal tissue, impairing kidney function. It is the most common type of kidney disease and is far more common in women than in men. The higher incidence of acute pyelonephritis in women may be due in part to the anatomic difference between men and women. Because the female urethra is shorter and the urinary meatus is closer to the rectum in women, bacteria have less distance to travel to reach the bladder.

■ **ETIOLOGY** Pyelonephritis is most commonly due to infection by the bacteria *Escherichia coli. E. coli* is a normal intestinal bacteria that grows rapidly. It is found in fecal matter. *Proteus, pseudomonas, Staphylococcus,* and *Enterococcus* bacteria are less frequent agents of infection. The bacteria typically ascend to the kidneys from the lower urinary tract, but they also may enter the kidneys through the blood or lymph.

Women are most at risk, particularly those who are pregnant or practice poor genital hygiene. In men, pyelonephritis may arise as a complication of prostate enlargement. Any catheterization of the urinary tract also increases the likelihood of infection.

■ **SIGNS AND SYMPTOMS** The individual experiencing acute pyelonephritis may complain of nausea, vomiting, diarrhea, chills, fever, and lumbar pain. These symptoms may be accompanied by pus in the urine (**pyuria**), difficult or painful urination (**dysuria**), and excessive urination at night (**nocturia**). The client often looks quite ill and reports that the symptoms appeared rapidly.

■ **DIAGNOSTIC PROCEDURES** The physical examination may reveal tenderness during palpation of abdominal or lumbar areas. Culture and sensitivity tests are performed on a clean-catch urine specimen, which may appear cloudy and have a "fishy" odor. Urinalysis also may reveal casts, white blood cells, bacteria, and hematuria. X-ray studies of the kidney, ureter, and bladder may be done; however, an ultrasound or CT scan study is more frequently used to detect any obstruction in the urinary tract.

■ **TREATMENT** Antibiotic therapy, appropriate to the infecting organism, is the treatment of choice. **Antipyretics** may be ordered to decrease the fever. An increase in liquids is helpful. It is important that the client is kept hydrated and strictly adheres to taking all the ordered medication. Generally, a follow-up culture is done 2 weeks after the person has finished the antibiotic therapy to ensure that the infection is gone.

ALTERNATIVE THERAPY: *No signficant alternative therapy is indicated.*

 TEACHING TIPS: Individuals should practice proper genital hygiene to avoid introducing bacteria into the urinary tract. If the disease recurs, it would be helpful to determine any factor that might predispose a person to recurrent infection.

■ **PROGNOSIS** The prognosis is variable but usually good with proper treatment and follow-up care. Acute pyelonephritis frequently subsides in a few days, even without treatment with antibiotics. Reinfection is likely, however, for persons of high risk, such as those with prolonged use of an indwelling catheter. Repeated infection may lead to a chronic form of the disease, causing sufficient destruction of kidney tissue to produce renal failure.

■ **PREVENTION** The best prevention is avoidance of any infection and the use of proper hygiene.

Glomerulonephritis (Acute)

■ **DESCRIPTION** *Glomerulonephritis*, which is the allergic inflammation of the glomeruli in the kidney's nephrons, is also known as *acute poststreptococcal glomerulonephritis* (APSGN). It usually follows a streptococcal infection of the respiratory tract. The rate of filtration of the blood is reduced, causing retention of water and salts. Resulting injury to the glomeruli may allow red blood cells and serum protein to pass into the urine. Both kidneys are affected.

■ **ETIOLOGY** The disease is caused by circulating antigen-antibody complexes that become trapped within the network of the capillaries of a glomerulus. The complexes are produced as a consequence of an infection elsewhere in the body, most frequently following an infection of the upper respiratory tract or the middle ear by streptococcal bacteria. Other bacteria, however, and certain viruses and parasites, such as impetigo, mumps, Epstein-Barr virus, and hepatitis B, also may induce glomerulonephritis. The interval between the original infection and the glomerulonephritis may be 2 weeks or longer. This suggests that it is an immunologic inflammatory response, as described in Chapter 1. The disease also may arise as a consequence of various multisystem diseases such as lupus erythematosus (see Chapter 15).

■ **SIGNS AND SYMPTOMS** The primary presenting sign is hematuria, and the urine may be cola in color due to the red blood cells and casts. Usually the disease has an abrupt onset. There may be headaches from secondary hypertension; puffy eyes due to edema from leaky, inflamed capillaries; pain in the lumbar region from swollen kidneys; and reduced urine secretion (**oliguria**) due to the nephron damage. There also may be malaise, anorexia, and a low-grade fever.

■ **DIAGNOSTIC PROCEDURES** A detailed medical history is important and may reveal a recent streptococcal infection of the upper respiratory tract. Blood tests may show elevated blood urea nitrogen, a nitrogen-based compound called **creatinine**, and a rapid sedimentation rate. The nitrogen and creatinine are present in the blood because these final products of decomposition cannot be excreted in normal amounts. Urine may also be described as "bloody," "coffee-colored," or "smoky." Urinalysis will show hematuria and **proteinuria** (excessive levels of serum protein in the urine). A renal biopsy is necessary to confirm the diagnosis. Immunofluorescent analysis of the immune mechanism is used to identify the nature of the lesion. Electron microscopy is helpful in distinguishing among different forms of glomerulonephritis.

■ **TREATMENT** Treatment goals are generally supportive. The physician may prescribe diuretics to control edema and hypertension. Bed rest is usually indicated. Dietary restrictions on salt, protein, and fluid intake may be advised. If an underlying streptococcal infection can be confirmed, antibiotics may be prescribed.

ALTERNATIVE THERAPY: *No significant alternative therapy is indicated.*

> **TEACHING TIPS:** Refer to a dietitian to provide a diet high in calories and low in protein and sodium. Remind the client that follow-up examinations may be necessary to prevent chronic glomerulonephritis.

■ **PROGNOSIS** The prognosis is generally good. Most clients with acute glomerulonephritis experience a resolution of symptoms within a few weeks of onset. Children generally recover more rapidly than adults. A few cases, though, may progress into a chronic form of the disease. Repeated acute attacks also may induce the onset of chronic glomerulonephritis.

■ **PREVENTION** Prompt treatment of any streptococcal pharyngitis or other upper respiratory tract infection is important. Careful attention to any other disease that might cause glmerulonephritis is also important.

Nephrotic Syndrome

■ **DESCRIPTION** *Nephrotic syndrome* is a condition or a complex of signs and symptoms (syndrome) of the basement membrane of the glomerulus. (The basement membrane surrounds each of the many fine capillaries comprising a glomerulus.) The disease is characterized by severe proteinuria, often to the extent that the body cannot keep up with the protein loss (**hypoalbuminemia**). The disease is further characterized by excessive levels of fatlike substances called lipids in the blood (**hyperlipemia**), lipids in the urine (**lipiduria**), and generalized edema.

■ **ETIOLOGY** Nephrotic syndrome may result from a variety of disease processes having the capacity to damage the basement membrane of the glomerulus. Between 70% and 75% of the cases of nephrotic syndrome result from some form of glomerulonephritis. The syndrome also may arise as a consequence of diabetes mellitus, systemic lupus erythematosus, neoplasms, or reactions to drugs or toxins. The disease is occasionally idiopathic in origin.

■ **SIGNS AND SYMPTOMS** Edema is the most common symptom, and it may be either slow in onset or sudden. As body fluid accumulates, the client may experience shortness of breath and anorexia. Abnormal accumulation of fluid in the peritoneal cavity (**ascites**), hypertension, paleness (**pallor**), and fatigue may result.

■ **DIAGNOSTIC PROCEDURES** Nephrotic syndrome may be difficult to diagnose. Urinalysis may reveal proteinuria and increased waxy, fatty, granular casts. Blood serum tests may show decreased albumin levels and increased cholesterol. Renal biopsy is important to reach a definitive diagnosis.

■ **TREATMENT** Treatment is symptomatic and supportive and preserves renal function. The physician will attempt to manage the edema and hyperlipemia. High-protein diets, vitamin supplementation, and salt restriction may be prescribed. Any underlying disease or condition determined to be responsible for the nephrotic syndrome must be treated as well. Corticosteroids may be prescribed. Some people will recover spontaneously.

ALTERNATIVE THERAPY: *No significant alternative therapy is indicated.*

> **TEACHING TIPS:** It is important to encourage the client to routinely check the urine protein level. A dietitian referral should be encouraged to help with a high-protein, low-sodium diet. High activity and exercise should be stressed, as well as good skin care, especially during the edema phase.

■ **PROGNOSIS** The prognosis varies according to the underlying cause and the age of the client. The prognosis is good for children. With adults, nephrotic syndrome is frequently a manifestation of a serious, progressive kidney disorder or of a disorder elsewhere in the body leading to renal failure. Renal vein thrombosis is a complication that significantly worsens the prognosis.

■ **PREVENTION** Nephrotic syndrome is sometimes avoided through prompt diagnosis and treatment of underlying disorders with the capacity to produce this syndrome.

End-Stage Renal Disease

■ **DESCRIPTION** *End-stage renal disease (ESRD),* sometimes referred to as *chronic renal failure (CRF),* is the gradual, progressive deterioration of kidney function. As the kidney tissue is progressively destroyed, the kidney loses its ability to excrete the nitrogenous end products of metabolism such as **urea** and creatinine, which accumulate in the blood, eventually reaching toxic levels. As kidney function diminishes, every organ in the body is affected, and dialysis or kidney transplantation is eventually needed for survival.

■ **ETIOLOGY** Causes include diabetes mellitus (leading cause), hypertension, chronic glomerulonephritis, pyelonephritis, obstruction of the urinary tract, congenital anomalies such as polycystic kidneys, vascular disorders, infections, medications, and toxic agents.

■ **SIGNS AND SYMPTOMS** The early signs and symptoms are oliguria and the presence of nitrogenous compounds in increased amounts in the blood (**azotemia**); then electrolyte imbalance and metabolic acidosis follow. The client may complain of progressive weakness and lethargy, weight loss, anorexia, diarrhea, hiccups, pruritus, and excessive formation and discharge of urine (**polyuria**). The individual with ESRD also may appear mentally confused and have skin that is pallid and scaly. The severity of signs and symptoms varies depending on the extent of the renal damage and remaining function, any other underlying conditions, and the person's age.

■ **DIAGNOSTIC PROCEDURES** The history may reveal a previous renal disease or other predisposing disorder. The physical examination may reveal one or more of the presenting signs and symptoms, along with hypertension. Blood testing typically reveals elevated serum creatinine, blood urea nitrogen, and potassium levels, along with decreased hemoglobin and hematocrit. Urinalysis may reveal proteinuria and urine that is highly diluted. Other tests include ultrasonography and renal scan.

■ **TREATMENT** Treatment is generally directed at relieving symptoms, retarding deterioration of remaining renal function, assisting the body in compensating for the existing impairment, and guarding against complications. Dietary restrictions of protein, sodium, and potassium intake may be attempted. Drugs that prevent or stop vomiting (**antiemetics**) may be prescribed for nausea. Hypertension must be controlled. Dialysis or kidney transplantation is attempted to prolong life.

Dialysis

The blood of an individual experiencing acute or chronic renal failure typically contains high concentrations of metabolic waste products. Dialysis may be attempted to remove these wastes. In its broadest sense, dialysis is a process in which water-soluble substances diffuse across a semipermeable membrane. Most clients undergo 9 to 12 hours of dialysis per week, equally divided among several sessions. Factors determining the amount of dialysis include the client's size, dietary intake, illnesses, and remaining renal function. Three methods are currently used to dialyze the blood: *peritoneal dialysis, hemodialysis,* and *continuous renal replacement therapy (CRRT).*

■ **PERITONEAL DIALYSIS** This process uses a person's own peritoneum as the dialyzing membrane. A plastic tube is inserted through the client's abdomen into the peritoneal cavity and sutured in place. A dialyzing fluid is passed through the tube into the person's peritoneal cavity and left there for a prescribed period. During this time, wastes diffuse across the peritoneal membrane into the fluid. The contaminated fluid is then drained and replaced with fresh solution. This process can be performed manually or automatically by machine; generally, it is repeated three times a week or as often as required. This type of dialysis may be continuous or intermittent and is easier than hemodialysis for individuals to perform themselves.

■ **HEMODIALYSIS (EXTRACORPOREAL HEMODIALYSIS)** In this process, blood is drawn outside the person's body for dialysis in an artificial kidney, or *dialyzer,* and then returned to the individual via tubes connected to the person's circulatory system. This form of dialysis treatment takes from 3 to 5 hours, about half the time of peritoneal dialysis. It is the most common form and the preferred dialysis method in cases of acute renal failure.

■ **CONTINUOUS RENAL REPLACEMENT THER-APY** There are several types of CRRT, which are generally used in critical care units. It is used in persons who are unstable clinically and can be started quickly in hospitals with dialysis machines. An extremely porous blood filter containing a semipermeable membrane is used in all methods.

Kidney Transplantation

Kidney transplantation has become the treatment of choice for ESRD. The donor of a kidney can be either a close relative of the person receiving the kidney or a recently deceased person (cadaver donor). If the donor and recipient are related, the graft has a better chance of survival.

Every transplanted kidney contains antigens foreign to the recipient, unless it is donated by an identical twin. Once the donor antigens are in the recipient, a rejection process begins, in which the recipient's immune system produces antibodies that lead to the destruction of the tissue of the transplanted kidney. Immunosuppressive drugs may be administered to combat this process. Still, some recipients may reject the kidney. Once rejection occurs, the donated kidney is removed, and the client must resume dialysis.

For those persons who do not reject the donor kidney, life can seem relatively normal. Immunosuppressive drugs must be continued indefinitely, however, making the person more susceptible to infections and other diseases. Sometimes, too, the underlying disease process that destroyed the original kidney will destroy the donor kidney.

ALTERNATIVE THERAPY: *No significant alternative therapy is indicated.*

TEACHING TIPS: A dietitian will provide useful information on a high-calorie, low-sodium, low-protein, low-potassium diet with vitamin supplements. Giving emotional support to the client and family is paramount. Ensure that the living environment is safe and free of hazards.

■ **PROGNOSIS** The prognosis is guarded even with transplantation because of the alteration in function of virtually every organ system in the body. A variety of complications often cause death before complete kidney failure occurs. Chief among these are infections; others include a spectrum of cardio-vascular, blood, and gastrointestinal abnormalities.

■ **PREVENTION** No prevention is known, other than prompt treatment of underlying disorders that may eventually lead to ESRD.

Acute Tubular Necrosis

■ **DESCRIPTION** *Acute tubular necrosis (ATN)* is the rapid destruction or degeneration of the tubular segments of nephrons in the kidneys. ATN is characterized by a sudden deterioration in renal function, with resulting accumulation of nitrogenous wastes in the body. Impaired or interrupted renal function from ATN is considered reversible.

■ **ETIOLOGY** The majority of cases of ATN are due to renal **ischemia**, or the interruption or impairment of blood flow in and out of the kidneys. ATN is the most common cause of acute renal failure in critically ill persons. Although there can be numerous causes for such impairment, renal ischemia leading to ATN is most frequently produced by severe bodily trauma or as a complication following surgery. The renal tubules also can be damaged in other ways. ATN may be toxin induced (as a result of exposure to solvents, heavy metals, or certain antibiotics), may be caused by transfusion reactions, or may arise as a complication of pregnancy.

■ **SIGNS AND SYMPTOMS** Because renal failure affects the function of nearly every organ in the body, the individual with ATN may have a host of widely distributed symptoms. Principal symptoms include oliguria and an excessive amount of potassium in the blood or **hyperkalemia**. Other generalized symptoms include weakness, mental confusion, and edema. ATN has four phases: (1) onset, or initiating, phase, (2) oliguria, or anuric, phase, (3) diuretic phase, and (4) recovery, or convalescent, phase. The onset phase is from the precipitating event until tubular injury results. The oliguira phase, with decreased urine output and increased fluid retention, lasts generally 10 to 14 days. The diuretic phase is when the nephrons recover to the point where urine excretion is possible. Then, during the recovery phase, renal function slowly recovers. Some kidney damage may persist.

■ **DIAGNOSTIC PROCEDURES** A history of chronic and debilitating illness, trauma, surgery, transfusion, or pregnancy complications may indicate a risk for ATN. The physician also may seek to determine if the individual could have been exposed to any toxins or was taking certain antibiotics. The physician will attempt to eliminate any underlying kidney diseases or urinary tract obstructions as possible causes for the renal failure. Diagnostic tests ordered may include urinalysis, which for ATN reveals dilute urine with red blood cells and casts. Blood tests will often indicate increased blood urea nitrogen and creatinine or reveal disturbances in the electrolyte balance of the blood. Most of the time, diagnosis occurs when the disease is more advanced.

■ **TREATMENT** The main goal of treatment is to identify and correct the underlying cause. The physician will generally attempt to promote proper renal circulation if the ATN is due to ischemia. If the ATN is toxin induced, dialysis may be attempted to cleanse the blood. Otherwise, treatment is largely supportive until kidney function increases. Supportive treatment may include dietary modifications and careful control of fluid intake. Dialysis may be indicated to allow the kidneys to rest and to improve conditions for regeneration.

ALTERNATIVE THERAPY: *No significant alternative therapy is indicated.*

> **TEACHING TIPS:** Maintaining proper fluid and electrolyte balance is important. Providing emotional support for the client and family is helpful.

■ **PROGNOSIS** The prognosis is guarded. Before adequate renal function resumes (highly variable period), many individuals with ATN die from complications, which may include cardiovascular complications, gastrointestinal disorders, blood abnormalities, and infections.

■ **PREVENTION** Prevention includes avoiding exposure to toxins and careful monitoring of individuals known to be at risk, especially those with diabetes.

Renal Calculi (Uroliths or Kidney Stones)

■ **DESCRIPTION** *Renal calculi* are the most common cause of urinary obstruction. A renal calculus is a concentration of various mineral salts in the renal pelvis or the cuplike extension of the renal pelvis called the **calyx** of the kidney or elsewhere in the urinary tract (Fig. 8.4). Most stones develop in the kidney and are from calcium salts, uric acid, cystine, and struvite, in descending order of frequency.

■ **ETIOLOGY** Renal calculi form as a result of a disturbance in the kidney's delicate balancing act of preventing water loss while at the same time eliminating water-soluble mineral wastes. Many factors, such as prolonged dehydration or immobilization, can upset this balance. The balance also may be upset by underlying diseases such as gout, **hyperparathyroidism** (disease caused by oversecretion of the parathyroid glands), Cushing's syndrome, or urinary tract infections and neoplasms. A person may develop renal calculi because of an excessive intake of vitamin D or dietary calcium. The condition appears to be genetic for certain types of stones, with men much more commonly affected than women. In many instances, no specific cause can be pinpointed.

■ **SIGNS AND SYMPTOMS** A person having renal calculi may remain asymptomatic for long periods. If a stone or calculus fragment lodges in a ureter, however, the individual may complain of intense flank pain and urinary urgency. Classic ureteral colicky pain is manifested by acute, intermittent, and excruciating pain in the flank and upper outer quadrant of the abdomen on the affected side. If calculi are in the renal pelvis and calyces, the pain is duller and more constant. Back pain and severe abdominal pain may occur. Other presenting symptoms include nausea, vomiting, chills and fever, hematuria, and abdominal distention.

■ **DIAGNOSTIC PROCEDURES** The history may reveal a familial tendency toward the formation of kidney stones. A urinalysis may be ordered to detect elevated levels of red or white blood cells in the urine or to check for the presence of protein, pus, and bacteria. CT scan, abdominal x-ray, excretory urography, retrograde urography, ultrasonography, and magnetic resonance imaging may be ordered to determine the locations of calculus formation. Blood testing may be helpful in confirming imbalances of minerals in the blood or the existence of other metabolic disorders.

■ **TREATMENT** Treatment is directed at clearing obstructive stones and preventing the formation of new ones. Increased fluid intake (>3 L/day) may enhance elimination of stones in some cases, but

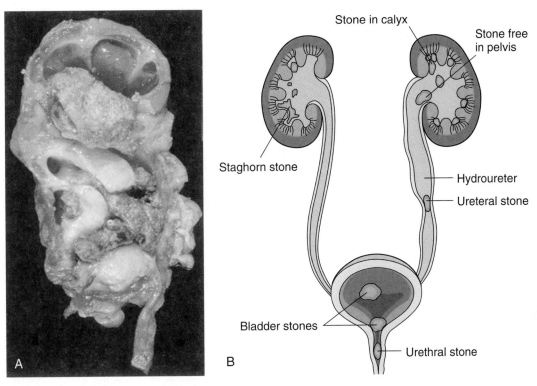

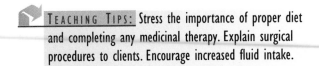

Figure 8.4 (A) Staghorn calculi; the kidney shows hydronephrosis and stones that are casts of the dilated calyces. (From Rubin, E, and Farber, JL [eds]: Pathology, ed 3. Lippincott-Raven, Philadelphia, 1999, p 909, with permission.) (B) Location of calculi in the urinary tract. (From Williams, LS, and Hopper, PD [eds]: Understanding Medical-Surgical Nursing. FA Davis, Philadelphia, 1999, p 691, with permission.)

large stones may require surgical intervention, especially if renal function is threatened. Ureteroscopic removal with the use of fluoroscopic guidance may be used to dilate the ureter to grasp and remove the stone. Techniques such as ultrasonic percutaneous lithotripsy and extracorporeal shock wave lithotripsy pulverize stones in place, allowing them to be passed in the urine or removed by suction. Lithotripsy via a ureteroscope can also be used to remove urethral stones. Antibiotics may be prescribed if it is determined that the calculus buildup is due to bacterial infection. Analgesics may be necessary for the relief of intense pain.

ALTERNATIVE THERAPY: *Alternative therapists recommend drinking eight or more glasses of water per day and eating a diet high in fiber and low in fat, with reduction of red meat consumption. Vitamin and minerals may be helpful especially when coordinated with the primary care physi-*

cian. Relaxation techniques may be beneficial to deal with the pain.

TEACHING TIPS: Stress the importance of proper diet and completing any medicinal therapy. Explain surgical procedures to clients. Encourage increased fluid intake.

■ **PROGNOSIS** The prognosis is good if urinary tract obstruction is prevented, and underlying disorders are promptly treated. However, about 60% of people who have a calcium stone have further stone formation later.

■ **PREVENTION** An adequate daily fluid intake is the best way to minimize the chance of stone formation, especially among individuals at risk. Fruit juices, especially cranberry juice, help acidify urine and may help prevent the formation of renal calculi.

Hydronephrosis

■ **DESCRIPTION Hydronephrosis** is the distention of the renal pelvis and calyces of a kidney due to pressure from accumulating urine. The pressure impairs, and may eventually interrupt, kidney function. One or both kidneys may be affected.

■ **ETIOLOGY** Hydronephrosis is caused by a urinary tract obstruction. The ureters and renal pelvis dilate proximal to, or behind, the obstruction. This swelling causes the hydronephrosis with resultant destruction of functional tissue. In children, the obstruction is usually the result of some congenital defect in urinary tract structure. In adults, the obstruction is more often acquired, resulting from blockage by neoplasms or **uroliths**, commonly called kidney stones. Urinary tract obstruction in men may be produced by benign or malignant enlargement of the prostate. Women may experience urinary tract obstruction as a complication of pregnancy. Underlying disorders, such as neurogenic bladder, also may allow urine to accumulate to the extent that it produces hydronephrosis.

■ **SIGNS AND SYMPTOMS** The signs and symptoms depend on the site of obstruction, the cause, and the rapidity with which the condition developed. If the obstruction is above the opening of the bladder, only one kidney may be affected and the person may be asymptomatic for a prolonged period ("silent" hydronephrosis). Symptoms may be severe, however, especially if both kidneys are affected. The person may complain of intense flank pain, nausea, vomiting, oliguria or anuria, and hematuria.

■ **DIAGNOSTIC PROCEDURES** Palpation and percussion of the abdomen may reveal distention of the kidney or urinary bladder. A history of changes in urinary volume, difficulty in voiding, and pain may be found. Ultrasound may be ordered to visualize obstructions. An excretory urogram, CT scan, and renal scan may be ordered to further define the site of obstruction. Urinalysis may reveal hematuria, pus, and bacteria and may be helpful in determining the extent of any impairment of renal function.

■ **TREATMENT** Treatment goals include removing the obstruction, preventing complications, and treating underlying disorders. Catheterization may be attempted for the immediate relief of urinary pressure. Analgesics may be prescribed. Antibiotics are required if infection occurs. Surgery is sometimes required to dilate a ureteral stricture. Treatment procedures for renal stones were discussed in the preceding section.

ALTERNATIVE THERAPY: *No significant alternative therapy is indicated.*

> **TEACHING TIPS:** Encourage regular medical checkups, and explain symptoms of hydronephrosis so that the client can report as necessary.

■ **PROGNOSIS** The prognosis is variable, depending on whether one or both kidneys are affected, whether the obstruction can be removed, and whether permanent renal damage has occurred.

■ **PREVENTION** There are no specific preventative measures.

LOWER URINARY TRACT DISEASES AND DISORDERS

Cystitis and Urethritis

■ **DESCRIPTION** *Cystitis*, or inflammation of the bladder, and *urethritis*, or inflammation of the urethra, are common lower urinary tract infections (UTIs). Together these diseases account for the majority of physician visits by individuals experiencing urinary tract problems. In fact, after upper respiratory tract infections, UTIs are the most common type of bacterial infection seen by physicians.

■ **ETIOLOGY** Infection by the bacteria *Escherichia coli* accounts for most cases of cystitis and urethritis. Other causative organisms can include *Proteus, Klebsiella, Enterobacter,* and *Serratia* bacteria. These organisms typically ascend the urinary tract from the opening of the urethra, but they also may be introduced as a result of urinary tract catheterization. Urethritis also may be caused by sexually transmitted organisms such as *Chlamydia trachomatis* and *Neisseria gonorrhoeae* (the agents of chlamydia and gonorrhea, respectively).

Women are 10 times more susceptible to ascending UTIs than are men (except for men older than 50 years). This is due in part to the shorter urethra in women and the comparative ease with which fecal contaminants can be spread from the anus to the opening of the vagina. Women who are sexually active are more predisposed to cystitis, because sexual intercourse enhances the bacterial transfer from the urethra into the bladder. Finally, both women and men are more at risk of contracting a lower UTI as a complication of any disorder that obstructs normal urinary flow.

■ **SIGNS AND SYMPTOMS** Signs and symptoms cannot be relied on for the diagnosis or localization of a UTI. Some individuals may present with few symptoms, yet have significant bacteriuria. The person presenting with cystitis may complain of dysuria, urinary frequency and urgency, and pain above the pubic region. Cloudy, bloody, or foul-smelling urine also may be noted. The individual with urethritis will typically present with similar symptoms, with the exception that the quality of the urine is often not affected. Any other symptoms, such as fever, nausea, vomiting, and low back pain, may indicate a simultaneous upper UTI such as pyelonephritis.

■ **DIAGNOSTIC PROCEDURES** The medical history may reveal past UTIs, recent catheterization, or a change in sexual partners. A urine culture is necessary to identify the organism responsible for the infection. The presence of red and white blood cells in the urine sample is also an indicator. Sensitivity tests are necessary to prescribe the appropriate antimicrobial agent. X-ray, ultrasonography, CT, and renal scans may be necessary to identify contributing factors such as an obstruction.

■ **TREATMENT** Antibiotics or sulfa drugs appropriate to combat the particular causative organisms may be prescribed. Fluid intake may be increased to promote urinary outflow. Analgesics may be prescribed for short-term pain relief. The physician may also prescribe urinary antiseptics and antispasmodics for the relief of bladder spasms.

ALTERNATIVE THERAPY: *The client should abstain from ingesting alcohol, caffeine, or high concentrations of sugar (such as in soft drinks). Diluting fruit juices is recommended because the sugar content is too high. Herbal teas are good. Urinating after intercourse may help by flushing out any bacteria that was introduced.*

TEACHING TIPS: Explain the purpose and course of the medication. Advise your clients to drink plenty of water. Some fruit juices may be helpful.

■ **PROGNOSIS** If no complications arise, the prognosis for complete recovery from cystitis and urethritis is quite good. If the disease is uncomplicated, infections of the lower urinary tract usually respond to short courses of therapy, whereas those of the upper urinary tract require a longer course of treatment. Reinfection in susceptible individuals is likely.

■ **PREVENTION** Preventive measures include complete emptying of the bladder and avoiding "holding urine." Proper feminine hygiene, including wiping the perineum from front to back and cleansing well after a bowel movement, will lessen the chance of introducing disease-causing microorganisms into the urethra. Women with a history of lower UTI also may be placed on a long-term course of antibiotics. Fruit juices, especially cranberry or blueberry juice, may help acidify urine. Most bacteria grow poorly in an acid environment.

Neurogenic Bladder

■ **DESCRIPTION** *Neurogenic bladder* refers to any loss or impairment of bladder function caused by central nervous system injury or by damage to nerves supplying the bladder. Impaired bladder function may be manifested as either loss of voluntary control of urination (or **micturition**) or loss of the autonomic reflex, producing the sensation that the bladder is full.

■ **ETIOLOGY** Neurogenic bladder may present in one of the following two ways: (1) specific bladder dysfunction where the neurologic lesions are above S2-4 or (2) flaccid bladder dysfunction where the lesions are below S2-4. Physical trauma to the spinal cord is a frequent cause of neurogenic bladder. Other causes can include nerve damage as a consequence of chronic alcoholism or heavy-metal poisoning. Metabolic disorders (e.g., diabetes mellitus or hypothyroidism) and collagen diseases (e.g., systemic lupus erythematosus) may cause this disorder. Neurogenic bladder may arise as a consequence of multiple sclerosis, dementia, and Parkinson's disease.

■ **SIGNS AND SYMPTOMS** An individual with neurogenic bladder may complain of mild to severe urinary incontinence or the inability to control the passage of urine, inability to empty the bladder completely, difficulty in starting or stopping voiding, and bladder spasms.

■ **DIAGNOSTIC PROCEDURES** Neurogenic bladder often is difficult to diagnose. A detailed history and a physical examination that includes a neurologic evaluation are essential. Special tests that may be ordered include a cystourethrograph to evaluate bladder function, a urine flow study to assess urine flow, and a sphincter electromyelograph to evaluate how well the bladder and urinary sphincter muscles work together.

■ **TREATMENT** Treatment goals include preventing complications from UTIs and controlling incontinence through learning special bladder evacuation techniques. The physician may recommend one of two common methods of evacuation to clients who are unable to empty the bladder completely. In *Credé's method*, the client presses on the lower abdomen while voiding. The second method, *intermittent self-catheterization*, requires the client to insert a catheter into his or her bladder through the urethra.

Any underlying diseases that are detected will be treated. Various forms of drug therapy or surgery may be attempted to restore bladder function.

ALTERNATIVE THERAPY: *Biofeedback may be useful for teaching some aspects of bladder control.*

 TEACHING TIPS: Teach the client and family bladder evacuation techniques. Provide emotional support for both the client and the family.

■ **PROGNOSIS** The prognosis depends on whether the damage to the nerves supplying the bladder is reversible. Such complications as UTIs and the formation of renal calculi worsen the prognosis. If the disorder is of the form in which sensation of a full bladder is lost, urine may back up, causing **hydronephrosis** and possible renal failure.

■ **PREVENTION** There is no specific prevention other than prompt treatment of diseases that may produce the nerve damage that leads to neurogenic bladder.

TUMORS OF THE BLADDER

■ **DESCRIPTION** *Tumors of the bladder* arise from the epithelial cell membrane lining the bladder interior. These neoplasms are almost always malignant, and they metastasize readily. Bladder tumors are staged according to their depth of penetration.

■ **ETIOLOGY** The cause of bladder tumors is unknown; however, cigarette smoking is thought to be the predominant cause. Predisposing factors may include exposure to certain types of industrial chemicals. Individuals with chronic cystitis also seem prone to develop bladder tumors. The disease affects men three times more frequently than women and generally occurs between the ages 50 and 70 years. Bladder cancer is the fourth most common cancer in men.

■ **SIGNS AND SYMPTOMS** Many persons are asymptomatic until advanced stages of the disease. For those presenting with symptoms, however, painless, gross hematuria is the most common indicator. Less frequently, the individual may complain of dysuria, urinary frequency and urgency, or nocturia. A UTI is a common complication.

■ **DIAGNOSTIC PROCEDURES** The history may reveal occupational exposure to certain industrial chemicals. A complete physical examination and a urinalysis to detect hematuria will be performed. Cystoscopy and biopsy of the suspected lesions are usually required to reach a definite diagnosis. A bone scan will help determine possible metastases. A CT scan may be ordered to help diagnose the tumor. Ultrasound, excretory urography, and bimanual examination with the person anesthetized may be ordered.

■ **TREATMENT** The choice of treatment is based on the extent of the disease. If the disease is superficial, an endoscopic resection may be all that is necessary. If it is invasive, further surgery is required. The tumor may be surgically removed through fulguration (electrical destruction) or **transurethral resection**, a surgical procedure in which a portion of the prostate is removed using an instrument passed through the urethra. For advanced cases, removal of the urinary bladder or radical **cystectomy** may be required, followed by radiation or chemotherapy treatment.

ALTERNATIVE THERAPY: *No significant alternative therapy is indicated.*

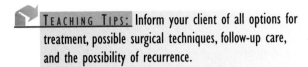

TEACHING TIPS: Inform your client of all options for treatment, possible surgical techniques, follow-up care, and the possibility of recurrence.

■ **PROGNOSIS** The prognosis varies, depending on the depth of penetration of the tumor. Although the immediate prognosis for an individual with a superficial bladder tumor may be good, there is still a great likelihood of recurrence within 3 years. When the tumor penetrates the bladder more deeply or has metastasized, the prognosis is poor, with a low 5-year survival rate.

■ **PREVENTION** The best prevention is to minimize risk factors by protecting oneself from exposure to industrial chemicals and by not smoking.

COMMON SYMPTOMS OF URINARY SYSTEM DISEASES AND DISORDERS

Individuals may present with the following common complaints, which deserve attention from health professionals:

- Any change in normal urinary patterns, such as nocturia, hematuria, pyuria, proteinuria, dysuria, or urgency and frequency
- Pain in the lumbar region or flank pain, varying from slight tenderness to intense pain
- Fever
- Nausea and vomiting or anorexia
- Malaise, fatigue, and lethargy

Serious urinary system diseases also may produce circulatory system and respiratory system symptoms. These symptoms might include hypertension, edema, ascites, and shortness of breath.

CASE STUDIES

■ Case Study 1

A 27-year-old man named Carlos Santiago comes into an ambulatory care facility complaining of extreme flank pain and frequent urination. The physician asks if Carlos has noted any difference in the color or appearance of his urine, and Carlos reports that he has noted some bits that look like sand in his urine. Carlos also says he recently was treated for a urinary tract infection.

Case Study Questions

1. What diagnostic tests might the physician order?
2. What are some effective preventative measures for urinary disease?

■ Case Study 2

Trang Ngoc, a 35-year-old woman, reports pain on urination, pain in the pubic area, and the need for frequent urination. Trang also says that the need to urinate is urgent and that her urine is foul smelling.

Case Study Questions

1. When this person comes to the ambulatory care setting, what questions will you ask?
2. What tests do you think the physician will order for this person?
3. What preventative measure could this person take in the future?

REVIEW QUESTIONS

True/False

Circle the correct answer:

T F 1. Women are at the greatest risk for pyelonephritis.

T F 2. Pyuria means painful urination.

T F 3. End-stage renal disease may indicate dialysis and/or transplantation.

T F 4. Lithotripsy is a type of treatment for kidney stones.

T F 5. Cigarette smoking is thought to be a predominant cause of bladder cancer.

Matching

Match the following by placing the correct letter in the column:

_____ 1. Nocturia

_____ 2. APSGN

_____ 3. Ascites

_____ 4. Uremia

_____ 5. Micturition

_____ 6. Pruritus

_____ 7. Pyuria

_____ 8. Oliguria

_____ 9. Hematuria

a. Acute poststreptotocccal glomerulonephritis

b. Accumulation of serous fluid in abdominal cavity

c. Blood in urine

d. Urination

e. Excessive urination at night

f. Scanty urine

g. Urine in the blood

h. Pus in urine

i. Itching

Short Answer

1. A disease that exhibits multiple, grapelike, fluid-filled sacs or cysts in the kidney cortex is _____.

2. When the body cannot keep up with the loss of protein in the urine, the result is _____.

3. Chronic renal failure is referred to as _____.

4. Intense pain with urinary frequency, nausea, vomiting, fever, hematuria, and flank pain may indicate _____.

5. A disorder, often difficult to diagnose, that is related to some kind of nerve dysfunction of the bladder is _____.

6. The most common type of kidney disease is _____.

7. Headaches from secondary hypertension and puffy eyes due to edema from leaky capillaries may indicate _____.

8. UTI refers to _____.

Multiple Choice

Place a checkmark next to the correct answer:

1. The kidney is responsible for
   a. Regulation of body fluids.
   b. Filtration of wastes from blood.
   c. Regulation of blood pressure.
   d. All of the above.
   e. Only a and b.

2. Of the fluid that passes through the nephron, what percent becomes urine?
   a. 1%
   b. 5%
   c. 10%
   d. 50%
   e. 98%

3. Urinary tract infections
   a. Are more common in males.
   b. Usually are characterized by dysuria, urgency, and frequency.
   c. Commonly are caused by a virus.
   d. Do not respond to antibiotic therapy.
   e. Have a poor prognosis.

4. The three forms of dialysis are
   a. Peritoneal, hemodialysis, and CRRT.
   b. Perineal, hemodialysis, and ESRD.
   c. Peritoneal, extracorporeal, and CRRT.
   d. Perineal, extracorporeal, and ATN.

5. The inability to control urine excretion is called
   a. Incontinence.
   b. Micturition.
   c. Ischemia.
   d. Anuria.
   e. Nocturia.

Discussion Questions/Personal Reflection

1. Discuss the anatomic differences of the male and the female urethra as they relate to urinary diseases and disorders.

2. Discuss the differences and similarities of the three types of dialysis and when a particular type would be chosen. If the client had a choice, which one would be chosen? Although not discussed in the text, what would the client do when traveling?

Notes

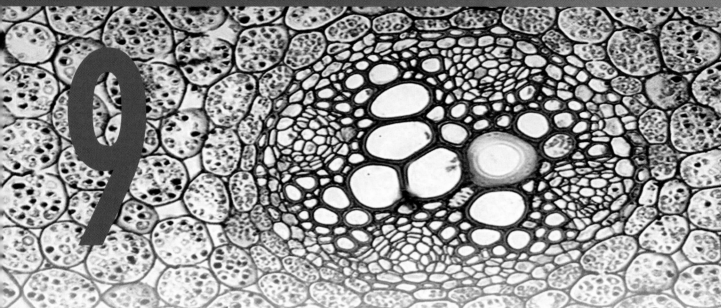

9

Reproductive System Diseases and Disorders

CHAPTER OUTLINE

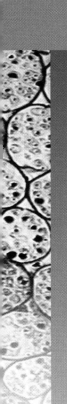

KEY WORDS

Alopecia (ăl•ō•pē′shē•ă)
Anuria (ĕ•nyŭr′•ē•a)
Azoospermia (ă•zō•ō•spĕr′mē•ă)
Cervicitis (sĕr•vĭ•sī′tĭs)
Chancre (shăng′kĕr)
Conization (kŏn•ĭ•zā′shŭn)
Corpus luteum (kŏr′pŭs lū′tē•ŭm)
Dilation and curettage (D&C) (dī•lā′•shŭn
  ănd kū′rĕ•tăzh)
Ectopic (ĕk•tŏp′ĭk)
Effacement (ē•fās′mĕnt)
Endometrium (ĕn•dō•mē′trē•ŭm)
Gonorrheal ophthalmia neonatorum
  (gŏn•ŏ•rē′ăl ŏf•thăl′mē•ă nē•ō•nă•tŏr′ŭm)
Hysterosalpingography (hĭs•tĕr•ō•săl•pĭn•
  gŏg′ră•fē)
Leiomyoma (lī•ō•mī•ō′mă)
Menarche (mĕn•ăr′kē)
Metrorrhea (me′trō•rē′ă)
Nystagmus (nĭs•tăg′mŭs)
Oligomenorrhea (ŏl•ĭ•gō•mĕn•ō•rē′ă)
Oligospermia (ŏl•ĭ•gō•spĕr′mē•ă)
Orchidectomy (ŏr•kĭ•dĕk′tō•mē)
Panhysterosalpingo-oophorectomy
  (păn•hĭs•tĕr•ō•săl•pĭng•gō ō•ŏf•ĕr•ĕk′ tō•
  mē)
Papilloma (păp•ĭ•lō′mă)
Papillomatosis (păp•ĭ•lō•mă•tō′sĭs)
Papillomavirus (păp•ĭ•lō•mă•vī′rŭs)
Parity (păr′ĭ•tē)
Parturition (păr•tū•rĭsh′ŭn)
Primigravida (prī•mĭ • grăv′ĭ•dă)
Prostaglandin (prăs′tĕ•glăn•dĕn)
Purulent (pū r′ū•lĕnt)
Rhonchus (pl. **rhonchi**) (rŏng′kŭs)
Septicemia (sĕp•tĭ•sē′mē•ă)
Teratoma (tĕr•ă•tō′mă)
Varicocele (văr′ĭ•kō•sēl)

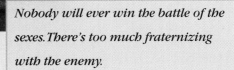

> *Nobody will ever win the battle of the sexes. There's too much fraternizing with the enemy.*
>
> —HENRY A. KISSINGER

LEARNING OBJECTIVES

Upon successful completion of this chapter, you will be able to:

- List the factors that contribute to both female and male fertility.
- Describe the necessity for a complete sexual history when obtaining a client's medical history.
- List seven sexually transmitted diseases (STDs).
- Contrast the causes of STDs.
- Identify the diseases related to the prostate gland.
- Discuss the complications of prostate-related disorders.
- Restate the common causes of epididymitis.
- List the characteristic signs and symptoms of ovarian cysts or tumors.
- Define *endometriosis*.
- Identify a primary complication of endometriosis.
- List the causes of pelvic inflammatory disease.
- Discuss the signs and symptoms of menopause.
- Describe ovarian cancer and its signs and symptoms.
- Recall treatment protocols for breast cancer.
- Recall the possible causes of spontaneous abortion.
- Define *ectopic pregnancy*.
- Compare preeclampsia with eclampsia.
- Compare placenta previa with abruptio placentae.
- Define *premature rupture of membranes* (PROM).
- Recall at least six common symptoms of the reproductive system diseases and disorders.

The only mammals known to express caring and loving in the sexual act are human beings. For males and females, the function of sexuality is twofold—reproduction and the enhancement of caring and pleasure.

The World Health Organization identifies *sexual health* as a state of physical, emotional, mental, and social well-being related to sexuality; it is not merely

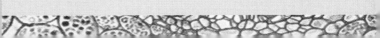

the absence of disease, dysfunction, or infirmity. Sexual health requires a positive and respectful approach to sexuality and sexual relationships, as well as the possibility of having pleasurable and safe sexual experiences, free of coercion, discrimination, and violence. For sexual health to be attained and maintained, the sexual rights of all persons must be respected, protected, and fulfilled.

The reproductive system functions to continue the human species; hence, the organs of the system are usually classified into two groups: gonads (testes and ovaries), which produce germ cells, and hormones with their duct system for the transportation of the germ cells. Cell division called **meiosis** produces gametes or the sperm and the ovum. The gametes each contain half the number of chromosomes necessary to produce an offspring. If fertilization occurs, the nuclei of the sperm and ovum fuse and produce a zygote with the full chromosome complement. The ductal system of the female transports, nourishes, and grows the fertilized ovum.

The male reproductive system consists of the testes and a series of ducts and glands. During ejaculation, the sperm is transported through the epididymis, ductus deferens, ejaculatory duct, and urethra. The male reproductive glands—the seminal vesicles, prostate gland, and bulbourethral glands—produce fluid secretions that become part of the semen. The urethra is the final duct through which the semen passes, and its longest portion is enclosed within the penis, an external genital organ.

The female reproductive system consists of the paired ovaries and fallopian tubes, the uterus, the vagina, and the external genital structures. The egg cells, the ova, are produced in the ovaries and travel though the fallopian tubes to the uterus, where a fertilized ovum implants and grows. The ovaries produce hormones necessary for the secondary sex characteristics and for maintenance of pregnancy. The breasts are accessory organs of the reproductive system, and they provide milk for the infant.

MALE AND FEMALE INFERTILITY

■ **DESCRIPTION** *Infertility* is diagnosed as the failure to become pregnant after 1 year of regular, unprotected intercourse, even after one or more pregnancies. According to the Centers for Disease Control and Prevention, 2.1 million couples experience infer-

tility or other conditions that impair their ability to have children. Female fertility normally peaks at 24 years of age and diminishes after 30, with pregnancy occurring rarely after the age of 50. Hormonal balances, the ovulation cycle, and vaginal secretions determine female fertility. A female is most fertile within 24 hours of ovulation.

Male fertility peaks usually at age 25 and declines after age 40. Sperm count, semen composition, and bodily hormonal changes affect male fertility. The greatest fertility for a male occurs when he has sexual intercourse four times a week.

■ **ETIOLOGY** Causes of infertility in females include hormonal problems, nutritional deficiencies, infections, tumors, and anomalies of the reproductive organs, such as cervical mucous problems, uterine cavity abnormalities, and tubal factors. In males, persistent infertility may be caused by sperm deficiencies, congenital abnormalities, endocrine imbalances, surgical intervention, and infections and chronic inflammation of the testes, epididymis, or vas deferens. In both males and females, advancing age is a factor in fertility. The causes are equally divided among males and females. In 10% of the cases, the cause remains unknown.

■ **SIGNS AND SYMPTOMS** Inability to conceive after 1 year of regular, unprotected intercourse.

■ **DIAGNOSTIC PROCEDURES** In a female, a complete medical, surgical, and gynecologic history and physical examination are essential. The laboratory studies ordered may include urinalysis, complete blood cell count, blood hormone levels, and immunologic or antibody testing that detects spermicidal antibodies in the serums of the female. X-rays to visualize the uterus and fallopian tubes (**hysterosalpingography**) may be necessary to detect uterine or tubal abnormalities. Endoscopy of the uterus, its lining (the **endometrium**), the fallopian tubes, ovaries, and abdominal and pelvic areas may be done. One test that may be done is an analysis of cervical mucus within 1 hour after coitus to check for motile sperm cells. This test is called the *Huhner test*. Vaginal smears or an endometrial biopsy may be required. A laparoscopy may be ordered to detect abnormalities of the abdominal and pelvic areas.

In a male, a complete ejaculate following sexual abstinence for 4 days should be examined within 1 to 2 hours of collection. A complete physical examina-

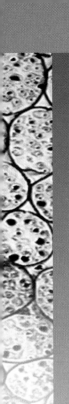

Alopecia (ăl•ō•pē′shē•ă)

Anuria (ĕ•nyŭr′•ē•a)

Azoospermia (ă•zō•ō•spĕr′mē•ă)

Cervicitis (sĕr•vĭ•sī′tĭs)

Chancre (shăng′kĕr)

Conization (kŏn•ĭ•zā′shŭn)

Corpus luteum (kŏr′pŭs lū′tē•ŭm)

Dilation and curettage (D&C) (dī•lā′•shŭn ănd kū′rĕ•tăzh)

Ectopic (ĕk•tŏp′ĭk)

Effacement (ē•fās′mĕnt)

Endometrium (ĕn•dō•mē′trē•ŭm)

Gonorrheal ophthalmia neonatorum (gŏn•ŏ•rē′ăl ŏf•thăl′mē•ă nē•ō•nă•tŏr′ŭm)

Hysterosalpingography (hĭs•tĕr•ō•săl•pĭn•gŏg′ră•fē)

Leiomyoma (lī•ō•mī•ō′mă)

Menarche (mĕn•ăr′kē)

Metrorrhea (me′trō•rē′ă)

Nystagmus (nĭs•tăg′mŭs)

Oligomenorrhea (ŏl•ĭ•gō•mĕn•ō•rē′ă)

Oligospermia (ŏl•ĭ•gō•spĕr′mē•ă)

Orchidectomy (ŏr•kĭ•dĕk′tō•mē)

Panhysterosalpingo-oophorectomy (păn•hĭs•tĕr•ō•săl•pĭng•gō ō•ŏf•ĕr•ēk′ tō•mē)

Papilloma (păp•ĭ•lō′mă)

Papillomatosis (păp•ĭ•lō•mă•tō′sĭs)

Papillomavirus (păp•ĭ•lō•mă•vī′rŭs)

Parity (păr′ĭ•tē)

Parturition (păr•tū•rĭsh′ŭn)

Primigravida (prī•mĭ•grăv′ĭ•dă)

Prostaglandin (prăs′tĕ•glăn•dĕn)

Purulent (pū r′ū•lĕnt)

Rhonchus (pl. **rhonchi**) (rŏng′kŭs)

Septicemia (sĕp•tĭ•sē′mē•ă)

Teratoma (tĕr•ă•tō′mă)

Varicocele (văr′ĭ•kō•sēl)

> *Nobody will ever win the battle of the sexes. There's too much fraternizing with the enemy.*
>
> —HENRY A. KISSINGER

LEARNING OBJECTIVES

Upon successful completion of this chapter, you will be able to:

- List the factors that contribute to both female and male fertility.
- Describe the necessity for a complete sexual history when obtaining a client's medical history.
- List seven sexually transmitted diseases (STDs).
- Contrast the causes of STDs.
- Identify the diseases related to the prostate gland.
- Discuss the complications of prostate-related disorders.
- Restate the common causes of epididymitis.
- List the characteristic signs and symptoms of ovarian cysts or tumors.
- Define *endometriosis*.
- Identify a primary complication of endometriosis.
- List the causes of pelvic inflammatory disease.
- Discuss the signs and symptoms of menopause.
- Describe ovarian cancer and its signs and symptoms.
- Recall treatment protocols for breast cancer.
- Recall the possible causes of spontaneous abortion.
- Define *ectopic pregnancy*.
- Compare preeclampsia with eclampsia.
- Compare placenta previa with abruptio placentae.
- Define *premature rupture of membranes* (PROM).
- Recall at least six common symptoms of the reproductive system diseases and disorders.

The only mammals known to express caring and loving in the sexual act are human beings. For males and females, the function of sexuality is twofold—reproduction and the enhancement of caring and pleasure.

The World Health Organization identifies *sexual health* as a state of physical, emotional, mental, and social well-being related to sexuality; it is not merely the absence of disease, dysfunction, or infirmity. Sexual health requires a positive and respectful approach to sexuality and sexual relationships, as well as the possibility of having pleasurable and safe sexual experiences, free of coercion, discrimination, and violence. For sexual health to be attained and maintained, the sexual rights of all persons must be respected, protected, and fulfilled.

The reproductive system functions to continue the human species; hence, the organs of the system are usually classified into two groups: gonads (testes and ovaries), which produce germ cells, and hormones with their duct system for the transportation of the germ cells. Cell division called **meiosis** produces gametes or the sperm and the ovum. The gametes each contain half the number of chromosomes necessary to produce an offspring. If fertilization occurs, the nuclei of the sperm and ovum fuse and produce a zygote with the full chromosome complement. The ductal system of the female transports, nourishes, and grows the fertilized ovum.

The male reproductive system consists of the testes and a series of ducts and glands. During ejaculation, the sperm is transported through the epididymis, ductus deferens, ejaculatory duct, and urethra. The male reproductive glands—the seminal vesicles, prostate gland, and bulbourethral glands—produce fluid secretions that become part of the semen. The urethra is the final duct through which the semen passes, and its longest portion is enclosed within the penis, an external genital organ.

The female reproductive system consists of the paired ovaries and fallopian tubes, the uterus, the vagina, and the external genital structures. The egg cells, the ova, are produced in the ovaries and travel though the fallopian tubes to the uterus, where a fertilized ovum implants and grows. The ovaries produce hormones necessary for the secondary sex characteristics and for maintenance of pregnancy. The breasts are accessory organs of the reproductive system, and they provide milk for the infant.

MALE AND FEMALE INFERTILITY

■ **DESCRIPTION** *Infertility* is diagnosed as the failure to become pregnant after 1 year of regular, unprotected intercourse, even after one or more pregnancies. According to the Centers for Disease Control and Prevention, 2.1 million couples experience infer-

tility or other conditions that impair their ability to have children. Female fertility normally peaks at 24 years of age and diminishes after 30, with pregnancy occurring rarely after the age of 50. Hormonal balances, the ovulation cycle, and vaginal secretions determine female fertility. A female is most fertile within 24 hours of ovulation.

Male fertility peaks usually at age 25 and declines after age 40. Sperm count, semen composition, and bodily hormonal changes affect male fertility. The greatest fertility for a male occurs when he has sexual intercourse four times a week.

■ **ETIOLOGY** Causes of infertility in females include hormonal problems, nutritional deficiencies, infections, tumors, and anomalies of the reproductive organs, such as cervical mucous problems, uterine cavity abnormalities, and tubal factors. In males, persistent infertility may be caused by sperm deficiencies, congenital abnormalities, endocrine imbalances, surgical intervention, and infections and chronic inflammation of the testes, epididymis, or vas deferens. In both males and females, advancing age is a factor in fertility. The causes are equally divided among males and females. In 10% of the cases, the cause remains unknown.

■ **SIGNS AND SYMPTOMS** Inability to conceive after 1 year of regular, unprotected intercourse.

■ **DIAGNOSTIC PROCEDURES** In a female, a complete medical, surgical, and gynecologic history and physical examination are essential. The laboratory studies ordered may include urinalysis, complete blood cell count, blood hormone levels, and immunologic or antibody testing that detects spermicidal antibodies in the serums of the female. X-rays to visualize the uterus and fallopian tubes (**hysterosalpingography**) may be necessary to detect uterine or tubal abnormalities. Endoscopy of the uterus, its lining (the **endometrium**), the fallopian tubes, ovaries, and abdominal and pelvic areas may be done. One test that may be done is an analysis of cervical mucus within 1 hour after coitus to check for motile sperm cells. This test is called the *Huhner test*. Vaginal smears or an endometrial biopsy may be required. A laparoscopy may be ordered to detect abnormalities of the abdominal and pelvic areas.

In a male, a complete ejaculate following sexual abstinence for 4 days should be examined within 1 to 2 hours of collection. A complete physical examination including rectal and genital palpation is essential. The laboratory studies ordered may include a sperm count, complete blood cell count, reproductive hormones, and urine 17-ketosteroid levels to measure testicular function. A testicular biopsy may be performed if **azoospermia** (absence of sperm in the semen) or **oligospermia** (deficient quantity of sperm in the semen) is determined. Cystoscopy and catheterization of ejaculatory ducts may be ordered to detect any occlusion or stenosis of the tubes. Vasography and seminal vesculography may be necessary.

■ **TREATMENT** The treatment of infertility is dependent on the cause. In a female, treatment may include any of the following:

- Salpingostomy
- Lysis of adhesions
- Removal of ovarian abnormalities
- Correction of endocrine imbalance
- Alleviation of inflammation of the cervix (**cervicitis**)
- Hormone therapy
- Microsurgical excision of tubal obstructions

In males, treatment may include any of the following:

- Surgical correction of any abnormality
- Correction of testicular hypofunction secondary to hypothyroidism
- Surgical correction of hydrocele or **varicocele,** which is a dilation of the complex network of veins that comprise part of the spermatic cord to form a palpable swelling within the scrotum
- Hormone therapy

Assisted reproductive technology (ART) may be tried. The technologies include in vitro fertilization (IVF) (the most common method), gamete intrafallopian transfer (GIFT), zygote intrafallopian transfer (ZIFT), and tubal embryo transplant (TET). All of these procedures stimulate the eggs, combine the eggs with sperm, and return the eggs to the female's body. (See the Glossary for definitions of each of the different types of ART.)

ALTERNATIVE THERAPY: *Traditional Chinese medicine can work in conjunction with traditional medicine by designing acupuncture treatments that complement and support other medical procedures. Acupuncture treatment may be help-ful to females who have just been artifically inseminated.*

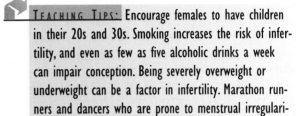

TEACHING TIPS: Encourage females to have children in their 20s and 30s. Smoking increases the risk of infertility, and even as few as five alcoholic drinks a week can impair conception. Being severely overweight or underweight can be a factor in infertility. Marathon runners and dancers who are prone to menstrual irregularities may have problems getting pregnant.

■ **PROGNOSIS** About 50% of the couples who are treated for infertility achieve pregnancy. About 5% of couples undergoing infertility treatment need ART; the remainder of the cases are untreatable.

■ **PREVENTION** Prevention of infertility in females and males generally involves avoiding the causative factors leading to acquired infertility, such as infections, drugs and alcohol, trauma, and environmental agents. Infertile couples may suffer loss, and they may experience guilt and anger. They need information and emotional support.

SEXUALLY TRANSMITTED DISEASES

Gonorrhea

■ **DESCRIPTION** *Gonorrhea* is a contagious bacterial infection of the epithelial surfaces of the genitourinary tract in males and females. It is currently one of the most prevalent sexually transmitted (venereal) diseases (STDs) in the United States. One of every 700 Americans is infected.

■ **ETIOLOGY** Gonorrhea is caused by the bacterium *Neisseria gonorrhoeae.* The disease is transmitted during sexual intercourse with an infected partner or through other forms of intimate sexual contact. Infants born of infected mothers can contract gonorrhea during vaginal delivery, and the bacteria may infect the conjunctivae, respiratory tract, or anal canal.

■ **SIGNS AND SYMPTOMS** The signs and symptoms of gonorrhea vary according to the site and duration of the infection, the particular characteristics of the infecting strain, and whether the infection remains localized or becomes systemic. It is worth emphasizing, however, that many cases of gonorrhea, especially in females, are asymptomatic or produce symptoms that are so slight that they are ignored by the infected individual.

The presenting symptoms of an infected male are typically those of acute urethritis: pus or **purulent** urethral discharge, pain, and urinary frequency. A purulent discharge from the pharynx or rectum with accompanying pain may be the presenting symptoms among infected homosexual males.

The symptoms of an infected female are typically those of acute cervicitis: purulent greenish-yellow discharge from the cervix, urinary frequency, and itching and burning pain. Other symptoms may include pelvic pain with muscular rigidity or abdominal tenderness and distention.

In the newborn, **gonorrheal ophthalmia neonatorum** may result. This is a severe, hyperacute inflammation of the membrane lining the inner surface of the eyelids and covering the white of the eye. Gonorrheal ophthalmia neonatorum may produce a purulent discharge from the eyes 2 to 3 days after birth. Eyelid edema may be evident as well.

■ **DIAGNOSTIC PROCEDURES** Bacterial cultures from the site of infection will generally establish the diagnosis.

■ **TREATMENT** Antibiotics will be given, but increasing numbers of strains are resistant to penicillin; therefore, a large number of new and very potent antibiotics are necessary, including ceftriaxone, cefixime, and ciprofloxacin. Clients are advised to have a second culture 1 to 2 weeks after the first and an additional culture in about 6 months to ensure that they no longer have the disease.

ALTERNATIVE THERAPY: *Emphasize treating the disease and stimulating the immune system. Elimination of fatty foods, sugar, white flour, salt, and caffeine will help to boost the immune system. Vitamins and herbal supplements may be recommended.*

▶ TEACHING TIPS: Practicing safer sex should be advised. Remind individuals to take all of their medications and to return for follow-up cultures.

■ **PROGNOSIS** The prognosis is good with prompt diagnosis and treatment of localized gonorrheal infections. Systemic gonorrheal infections may produce joint destruction or life-threatening complications such as meningitis or endocarditis. Pelvic inflammatory disease (PID) is a serious complication of gonorrheal infection among females, producing fever, nausea, vomiting, and tachycardia.

■ **PREVENTION** The use of condoms, avoidance of multiple partners, and the tracing of the sexual contacts of an infected individual can prevent the spread of gonorrhea. Instillation of a 1% silver nitrate solution in the eyes of the newborn has reduced the incidence of gonorrheal ophthalmia neonatorum.

Genital Herpes

■ **DESCRIPTION** *Genital*, or *venereal*, *herpes* is a highly contagious viral infection of the male and female genitalia. Unlike other STDs, genital herpes tends to recur spontaneously. The disease has two stages. During the active stage, characteristic skin lesions and other accompanying symptoms may occur. During the latent stage, the individual is asymptomatic. The incidence of genital herpes is steadily increasing in the United States.

■ **ETIOLOGY** Genital herpes is caused by the herpes simplex virus (HSV). Two strains of the virus—designated HSV-1 and HSV-2—may produce the disease. Most cases of genital herpes, however, are attributable to HSV-2. The disease is transmitted through direct contact with infected bodily secretions. Infection typically occurs during sexual intercourse, oral-genital sexual activity, kissing, and hand-to-body contact. A particularly life-threatening form of the disease can occur in infants infected by the virus during vaginal birth.

■ **SIGNS AND SYMPTOMS** During the active phase of the disease, males and females may present with characteristic skin lesions on their genitals, mouth, and/or anus. These appear as multiple, shallow ulcerations, pustules, or erythematous vesicles. The diffuse redness of the skin or erythema is caused by dilation of the superficial capillaries. The vesicles tend to rupture, causing acute pain and consequent itching. Other generalized symptoms may include fever, headache, malaise, muscle pain, anorexia, and dysuria. Leukorrhea may be a further symptom in females.

■ **DIAGNOSTIC PROCEDURES** Physical examination for evidence of the characteristic lesions is usually sufficient for diagnosis. Scraping and biopsy of the ulceration with evidence of HSV-2 may be required to confirm the diagnosis.

■ **TREATMENT** Acyclovir is an effective treatment for genital herpes. Newer agents include famiciclovir and valacyclovir. These drugs, however, will not eradicate the virus but when taken as soon as an outbreak occurs it can shut down virus production. Secondary infections need to be prevented or speedily managed. Topical medications may be ordered to reduce edema and pain. The individual should be encouraged to keep any lesions clean and dry.

ALTERNATIVE THERAPY: *Alternative therapy aims to diminish discomfort and hasten recovery. An ice pack applied to sores at the beginning of eruptions can help. Cool compressions or baking soda also soothes lesions. A topical cream made from the Prunella vulgaris plant has shown promise in reducing skin lesions.*

TEACHING TIPS: Your clients may be embarrassed about their disease, so reassure them that they can lead a sexually healthy life so long as they adhere to proper precautions.

■ **PROGNOSIS** Genital herpes cannot be cured. The prognosis varies according to the individual's age, the severity of the infection, the promptness of treatment, and the individual's immunologic response. It is estimated that as many as 80% of individuals with primary genital herpes infections will experience a recurrence within 12 months. Very serious complications can result if the virus spreads systemically. The virus is also associated with cervical cancer.

■ **PREVENTION** No proven method of prevention among adults has been established other than avoiding sexual intercourse with infected individuals and using condoms during all sexual exposure. Transmission of the disease to infants can be minimized through cesarean delivery when it is known that the mother is infected.

Genital Warts

■ **DESCRIPTION** *Genital warts* are circumscribed, elevated skin lesions, usually seen on the external genitalia or near the anus. These **papillomas** have fibrous tissue overgrowth from the dermis and a thickened epithelium. They are the most common of the STDs. They are uncommon before puberty and after menopause.

■ **ETIOLOGY** Genital warts are caused by more than 60 types of human **papillomaviruses** (HPVs). They are typically spread from person to person during intimate sexual contact. These warts have a prolonged incubation period of 1 to 6 months and grow rapidly in the presence of heavy perspiration, poor hygiene, or pregnancy.

■ **SIGNS AND SYMPTOMS** The client may be asymptomatic or experience tenderness in the area of the wart. Genital warts appear as solitary or clustered lesions. In males, the warts typically occur at the end of the penis, but they may appear anywhere along the penis as well. They also may appear in the perianal area. In females, the warts typically appear near the opening of the vagina, and they commonly spread to the perianal area. The warts start as tiny pink or red swellings and grow to 3 or 4 inches in diameter.

■ **DIAGNOSTIC PROCEDURES** The characteristic appearance and location of the lesions are usually sufficient for diagnosis. Dark-field scrapings from wart cells may help in confirming the diagnosis.

■ **TREATMENT** The goal of treatment is to eradicate genital infections. Topical medication may be applied, or carboxdioxide laser treatment, cryosurgery, electrocautery, or débridement may be attempted. Some cases are treated with injections of interferon. Small warts may require no treatment.

ALTERNATIVE THERAPY: *An ointment made of vitamin A and herbs may be topically applied. Encourage your clients to know the sexual histories of their partners, to limit the number of sexual partners, and to avoid exchanges of bodily fluids, especially blood and semen.*

TEACHING TIPS: Encourage handwashing after the application of topical treatments. Recommend the use of condoms. Sexually active females should have annual Pap tests.

■ **PROGNOSIS** The prognosis is variable. Spontaneous "cures" are rare, and the remainder of cases may be unresponsive to any form of treatment. Relapses are common. Genital warts may cause Pap smear abnormalities.

■ **PREVENTION** There is no known prevention other than avoiding sexual intercourse with infected individuals and regular washing of the genitalia with soap and water.

Syphilis

■ **DESCRIPTION** *Syphilis* is a highly infectious, chronic STD characterized by lesions that may involve any organ or tissue. After a brief decline in cases in the late 1990s, cases have again begun to rise.

■ **ETIOLOGY** Syphilis is caused by the bacterium *Treponema pallidum*. The bacteria are transmitted via direct contact with infected lesions, typically through sexual intercourse or through contact with infected bodily fluids. Syphilis also may be contracted as a consequence of transfusion with infected blood (a rare occurrence). In pregnant females, *T. pallidum* can cross the placenta and infect the fetus, causing serious fetal damage.

The bacteria rapidly penetrate skin or mucous membranes. From the point of infection, they spread into the lymphatic system and the blood, producing a systemic infection. Typically, the bacteria will have been carried throughout the body long before the first clinical symptoms appear.

■ **SIGNS AND SYMPTOMS** When untreated, syphilis typically progresses through three clinical stages, each with characteristic signs and symptoms. Note, however, that some infected individuals will be asymptomatic or present with symptoms that are not readily evident on casual inspection.

Primary syphilis, which has an incubation period of about 3 weeks, is characterized by the appearance of a distinctive, red, ulcerated, painless lesion, called a **chancre**, at the point of infection. In males, the chancre typically appears on the penis. The chancre also may appear on the anus or within the rectum of homosexual males. Among females, the lesion typically appears on the labia of the vagina or within the vagina or cervix. Among both males and females, chancres also may appear on the lips, tongue, fingers, or nipples. The appearance of the chancre also may be accompanied by regional lymphadenopathy, a disease of the lymph nodes, usually manifested as swelling of the nodes. It must be emphasized that the chancres are *highly contagious*. During this stage, the chancre usually heals within 3 to 12 weeks without treatment.

Secondary syphilis can produce a host of symptoms, many of which may be mistaken as symptoms of other diseases. Most frequently, however, individuals at this stage of the disease present with a rash characterized by uniform macular, papular, pustular, or nodular lesions. These typically, but not exclusively, appear on the palms or soles. In moist areas of the body, these lesions can erode and become contagious. Various general or systemic manifestations may accompany the rash, including headache, malaise, gastrointestinal upset, sore throat, fever, **alopecia** (commonly called baldness), and brittle nails. This stage generally lasts 3 to 6 months.

After the manifestations of secondary syphilis subside, a *latent* stage of the disease begins in which the infected individual is generally asymptomatic. The bacteria may remain latent indefinitely. In roughly half of untreated individuals with latent syphilis, manifestations of the final, or *tertiary*, stage of the disease begin to appear 2 to 7 years after the initial infection. However, some cases may not appear until 20 years after the initial infection. In tertiary syphilis, the *Treponema* bacteria may cause life-threatening damage to the aorta of the heart, the central nervous system, or the musculoskeletal system; no organ system is immune from damage. Consequently, the symptoms of tertiary syphilis mimic the symptoms of other organ system diseases, making diagnosis difficult.

■ **DIAGNOSTIC PROCEDURES** The most sensitive test available for detecting syphilis is the *fluorescent treponemal antibody-absorption (FTA-ABS) test*. A rapid plasma reagin (RPR) test, a Venereal Disease Research Laboratories (VDRL) test, and cerebrospinal fluid (CSF) examination also may be performed.

■ **TREATMENT** Penicillin, intramuscularly or intravenously, is the antibiotic of choice for the treatment of all stages of syphilis. Doxycycline may be used in the event of allergic reaction to penicillin. Any lesions should be kept as dry and clean as possible. An RPR or the VDRL test typically accompanies the drug therapy to ensure the *Treponema* bacteria have been eradicated.

ALTERNATIVE THERAPY: *Alternative therapists recommend sitz baths and may prescribe a mixture of herbs to enhance the immune system.*

TEACHING TIPS: The use of condoms is highly recommended. The client must limit and know his or her sexual partners, especially their sexual history. The client must be screened frequently for STDs if the client or the client's partner is at risk for STDs.

■ **PROGNOSIS** The prognosis varies with the age of the affected individual and with the stage at which the disease is detected and treated. The prognosis for complete recovery is very good for adults treated for primary and secondary syphilis. Although tertiary syphilis also can be successfully treated, any organ system damage that may have occurred to that point is generally irreversible. Untreated, the disease may lead to life-threatening cardiac, central nervous system, or musculoskeletal disorders. The prognosis is poor for a fetus infected with syphilis, with spontaneous abortion or stillbirth occurring in nearly 20% of cases.

■ **PREVENTION** The use of condoms during sexual intercourse can reduce the possibility of transmitting or acquiring syphilis, but contact tracing of intimate partners and serologic screening remain the most important methods in limiting the spread of this disease. Sexual partners should be evaluated and treated even if they show no symptoms.

Trichomoniasis

■ **DESCRIPTION** *Trichomoniasis* is a protozoal infestation of the vagina, urethra, or prostate.

■ **ETIOLOGY** *Trichomonas vaginalis*, a motile protozoan, is the cause of trichomoniasis. The disease usually is transmitted via sexual intercourse and affects 10% to 15% of sexually active persons. Women may increase their susceptibility to *Trichomonas* infection by using vaginal sprays and over-the-counter douches. These preparations may change the natural flora of the vagina such that a more hospitable environment for the parasite is created.

■ **SIGNS AND SYMPTOMS** From 10% to 25% of the females with trichomoniasis are asymptomatic. When symptoms occur, they are usually those of acute vaginitis: a strong-smelling, greenish yellow, frothy vaginal discharge, possibly accompanied by itching, swelling, dyspareunia, and dysuria. Symptoms may persist for several months if untreated.

In most males, the disease is asymptomatic. When symptoms are present, they are typically those of urethritis, such as dysuria and urinary frequency.

■ **DIAGNOSTIC PROCEDURES** The diagnosis of trichomoniasis is facilitated by wet-mount microscopic examination of vaginal or seminal discharges. The disease also may be detected through urinalysis.

■ **TREATMENT** The treatment of choice is oral metrononidazole (Flagyl). Alcohol should be avoided during and for 24 to 48 hours after treatment because of its adverse reaction with Flagyl. Treatment of both partners with antiparasitic drugs usually cures trichomoniasis. After treatment, both sexual partners should have a follow-up examination.

ALTERNATIVE THERAPY: *The client should practice abstinence, especially during the periods of infection and treatment. In addition, the client should limit his or her sexual partners and know their sexual histories.*

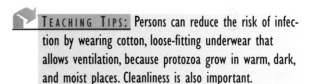

TEACHING TIPS: Persons can reduce the risk of infection by wearing cotton, loose-fitting underwear that allows ventilation, because protozoa grow in warm, dark, and moist places. Cleanliness is also important.

■ **PROGNOSIS** The prognosis is good with proper treatment, although reinfection may occur.

■ **PREVENTION** Over-the-counter douches and vaginal sprays should be avoided; abstinence from intercourse or the use of condoms is recommended.

Chlamydial Infections

■ **DESCRIPTION** *Chlamydial infection* is a sexually transmitted infection that is now highly prevalent and among the most potentially damaging of all the STDs in the United States.

■ **ETIOLOGY** Chlamydial infection is caused by the bacterium *Chlamydia trachomatis*. Transmission is usually through sexual intercourse, rectal intercourse, or genital-oral contact with an infected person.

■ **SIGNS AND SYMPTOMS** An individual may be asymptomatic or present with very mild symptoms; this disease is sometimes called the "silent" STD because symptoms are often absent. Sexual transmission occurs unknowingly. Clinical manifestations in many females may resemble those of gonorrhea and include itching and burning in the genital area, mucopurulent vaginal discharge, and cervicitis. In males, there will be discharge from the penis with a burning sensation on urination. The scrotum may be swollen.

■ **DIAGNOSTIC PROCEDURES** Diagnosis can be confirmed by cytologic and serologic studies, which reveal *C. trachomatis* in infected body fluids.

■ **TREATMENT** The recommended treatment is an antibiotic such as tetracycline or erythromycin. Both partners should be treated simultaneously.

ALTERNATIVE THERAPY: *See Trichomoniasis.*

 TEACHING TIPS: Remind clients to refrain from sexual activity during known active infection and to take all prescribed medication.

■ **PROGNOSIS** The prognosis is good if treatment is instituted early. If left untreated, complications include disease of the fallopian tubes, pelvic inflammatory disease or PID, and infertility in females. Males may suffer from epididymitis and become sterile.

■ **PREVENTION** The use of condoms during sexual intercourse can reduce the possibility of transmitting or acquiring chlamydial infection, but contact tracing of intimate partners and serologic screening remain the most important methods of limiting the spread of this disease.

Common Symptoms of Sexually Transmitted Diseases (STDs)

Individuals with STDs may present with the following common symptoms, which deserve attention from health professionals:

- Dysuria, hematuria, urinary frequency or incontinence, purulent discharge, or burning and itching on urination
- Pelvic or genital pain
- Any skin ulcerations, especially in the genital area
- Fever and malaise
- Dyspareunia

MALE REPRODUCTIVE DISEASES AND DISORDERS

ALTERNATIVE THERAPY: *The alternative therapy is so similar for all the male reproductive diseases that it is presented here rather than with each disease. Alternative therapy most often includes nutritional and diet recommendations, herbal medicines, homeopathy, natural hormone therapy, acupuncture, traditional Chinese medicine, and Ayurvedic medicine. Integrative medicine may be the best way to look at underlying causes and to treat as needed using the best of both traditional and alternative therapy to provide longer and lasting overall health.*

Benign Prostatic Hyperplasia

■ **DESCRIPTION** *Benign prostatic hyperplasia (BPH)* is the overproliferation of cells within the inner portion of the prostate. The condition is common in males older than 50 years, and the incidence increases with age. It is only clinically significant if the enlarging, hyperplastic portion of the prostate obstructs urinary outflow.

■ **ETIOLOGY** The etiology of BPH is not well understood, but it seems to be due to metabolic and hormonal changes associated with aging. In clinically significant BPH, the gland compresses the urethra or the neck of the bladder, obstructing urinary flow.

■ **SIGNS AND SYMPTOMS** The individual may report symptoms of urinary obstruction, such as difficulty in initiating urination or in completely emptying the bladder in the first stage. As the obstruction increases in size, symptoms may include nocturia, dribbling, urinary frequency, and weak urine stream.

■ **DIAGNOSTIC PROCEDURES** Symptomatology of the individual and a rectal examination are usually sufficient for diagnosis, but urinalysis, urine culture, and/or excretory urography may be ordered for confirmation. Prostatic biopsy may be required to ensure that prostatic carcinoma is not causing the enlargement. The distended bladder may be palpable.

■ **TREATMENT** Symptomatic treatment may include prostatic massage, catheterization, and sitz baths. Various medications that act to shrink the prostate or relax the muscles in the prostate show moderate success. A new treatment is under study, a nonsurgical option is called *transurethral thermoablation therapy* (T3). T3 uses microwave energy to heat and destroy the constricting tissue while preserving the urethra and nonprostatic tissues. Various surgical

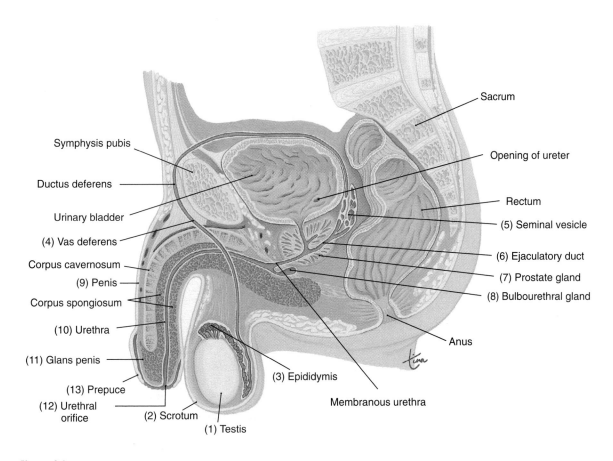

Symphysis pubis

Ductus deferens

Urinary bladder

(4) Vas deferens

Corpus cavernosum

(9) Penis

Corpus spongiosum

(10) Urethra

(11) Glans penis

(13) Prepuce

(12) Urethral orifice

(2) Scrotum

(1) Testis

(3) Epididymis

Membranous urethra

Anus

Sacrum

Opening of ureter

Rectum

(5) Seminal vesicle

(6) Ejaculatory duct

(7) Prostate gland

(8) Bulbourethral gland

Figure 9.1 Male reproductive system. (From Scanlon, VC, and Sanders, T: Essentials of Anatomy and Physiology, ed 4. FA Davis, Philadelphia, 2003, p 438, with permission.)

procedures, such as transurethral prostate resection (TURP), may be performed to remove urinary tract obstruction.

ALTERNATIVE THERAPY: *The client should avoid prostatic irritants such as caffeine, alcohol, tobacco, and red pepper and should take 30 g of zinc picolinate daily. A herbal remedy made from saw palmetto products may be beneficial. The client should add soy to the diet and increase consumption of tomatoes for their content of lycopene.*

TEACHING TIPS: Remind clients of the importance of regular follow-up examinations and surgical choices while in the "watchful" stage of the disorder. Men are sensitive to their sexuality and will need to discuss their fear of impotence and/or incontinence if surgery is a choice.

■ **PROGNOSIS** Prognosis is good with proper intervention. There is a surgical success rate of 80% to 90%. Impotence or incontinence is usually not a problem. There may be retrograde ejaculation, but this does not affect sexual pleasure for either partner. If untreated, infections may ascend to the kidney, or various urinary obstructive disorders may result. Complications include cystitis, dilation of the ureters, hydronephrosis, pyelonephritis, and uremia.

■ **PREVENTION** No specific prevention is known, but older males should be encouraged to have a regular prostate examination to detect any enlargement.

Prostatitis

■ **DESCRIPTION** *Prostatitis* is inflammation of the prostate gland (refer to Fig. 9.1 to review the male reproductive system.) The condition may be acute or chronic, with the latter being more common in males older than 50 years.

■ **ETIOLOGY** Prostatitis may be either bacterial or nonbacterial in origin. Bacterial causes of the disease include *E. coli, Klebsiella, Enterobacter, Proteus, Staphylococcus, Streptococcus,* and *Pseudomonas.* Routes of infection can be either via the urethra or the bloodstream. In nonbacterial prostatitis, no infectious agent is detectable.

■ **SIGNS AND SYMPTOMS** Low back pain, myalgia, perineal fullness or pain, fever, dysuria, and urinary frequency and urgency are common symptoms of acute prostatitis. The prostate, when palpated, may be enlarged, tender, and boggy. An individual with chronic prostatitis may be asymptomatic or experience sporadic, mild forms of acute symptoms.

■ **DIAGNOSTIC PROCEDURES** Rectal examination suggests prostatitis. A firm diagnosis depends on a comparison of urine cultures of specimens obtained by the Meares and Stamey technique. Four specimens are collected: one when the client starts voiding, another midstream, another after the client stops voiding and the physician massages the prostate to produce secretions, and a final voided specimen. A significant increase in colony count in the specimens confirms prostatitis.

Abnormally high urine leukocyte counts in the absence of detectable bacteria are indicative of nonbacterial prostatitis.

■ **TREATMENT** Antibiotic and/or antimicrobial therapy is initiated, and the client may be advised to rest and increase fluid intake. Analgesics, antipyretics, and stool softeners also may be ordered. Sitz baths may be recommended. Regular ejaculation may help promote drainage of prostatic secretions. If drug therapy is not effective, TURP may be necessary.

ALTERNATIVE THERAPY: *See Benign Prostatic Hyperplasia.*

 TEACHING TIPS: Remind clients to eat nutritional meals and have adequate fluid intake. Provide individuals with information about possible complications and surgical choices as necessary.

■ **PROGNOSIS** Acute prostatitis responds well to treatment; however, chronic prostatitis does not. Complications may include epididymitis, cystitis, and urethritis. Chronic prostatitis predisposes to recurrent urinary tract infections, urethral obstruction, and acute urinary retention.

■ **PREVENTION** Early treatment of urinary tract infections is the best prevention.

Epididymitis

■ **DESCRIPTION** *Epididymitis* is inflammation of the epididymis due to infection (Fig. 9.2). The condition is typically unilateral and is one of the most common infections of the male reproductive system.

■ **ETIOLOGY** Epididymitis can occur as a result of prostatitis, a urinary tract infection, mumps, tuberculosis, or STDs such as gonorrhea and syphilis. *Chlamydia trachomatis* and *Neisseria gonorrhoeae* are the most common infectious agents that cause epididymitis in sexually active males. Other bacterial causes of this condition include *E. coli, Staphylococcus,* and *Streptococcus.* Trauma or prostatectomy can also be a cause.

■ **SIGNS AND SYMPTOMS** The epididymis may become enlarged, hard, and tender, causing pain. Scrotal and groin tenderness, fever, and malaise also may occur. Groin tenderness is the result of enlarged lymph nodes in the groin. Clients may "waddle" as they walk, trying to protect the scrotal area.

■ **DIAGNOSTIC PROCEDURES** Urinalysis and urine cultures help in the diagnosis. An increased leukocyte count is common.

■ **TREATMENT** Antibiotic and/or antimicrobial therapy appropriate for the particular causative agent will be initiated. A scrotal support and analgesics may be helpful. Bed rest may be necessary in the acute phase. Scrotal elevation and an ice bag or cold compresses to relieve pain and reduce swelling may be helpful.

ALTERNATIVE THERAPY: *No significant alternative therapy is indicated.*

TEACHING TIPS: Remind clients to take all their medications and analgesics as necessary for pain. When clients are feeling better, encourage walking and the use of an athletic supporter.

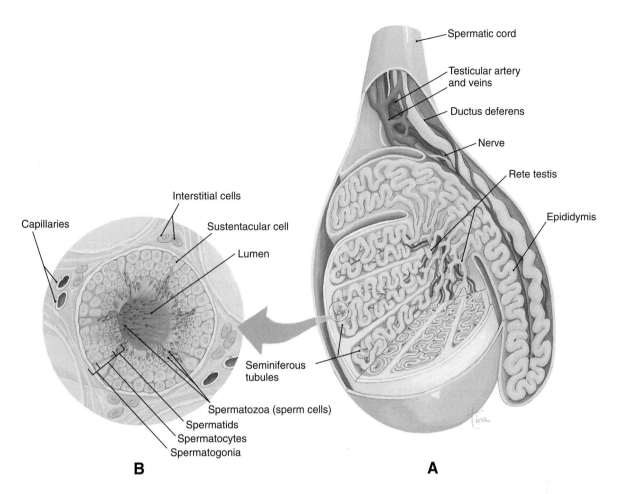

Figure 9.2 (A) Midsagittal section of portion of a testis; the epididymis is on the posterior side of the testis. (B) Cross section through a seminiferous tubule showing development of sperm. (From Scanlon, VS, and Sanders, T: Essentials of Anatomy and Physiology, ed 4. FA Davis, Philadelphia, 2003, p 439, with permission.)

■ **PROGNOSIS** The inflammation generally responds well to therapy, but portions of the epididymis may be scarred. Sterility is a threat if treatment is delayed, especially if the disease is bilateral. Orchitis may develop as a further complication. Orchitis may occur as a complication to epididymitis; it causes infection of the testicles and can lead to sterility. Any pain, swelling, and redness of the testicles should be reported immediately to the physician. Because orchitis can be the result of mumps, young males should receive the mumps vaccine.

■ **PREVENTION** Early treatment of urinary tract infection is the best prevention. The use of a condom during sexual intercourse is recommended, especially if the causitive agent was sexually transmitted.

Prostatic Cancer

■ **DESCRIPTION** *Prostatic cancer* is a malignant neoplasm of the prostate tissue. The majority of these neoplasms are classified as adenocarcinomas. Prostatic cancer is the third leading cause of cancer deaths in males (after lung and colon cancers). Prostate cancer tends to metastasize, often spreading to the bones of the spine or pelvis before it is detected. The disease is rare before the age of 50.

■ **ETIOLOGY** Four factors are suspected in this cancer:

1. Family or racial predisposition (African Americans have the highest prostate cancer rate in the world)
2. Exposure to environmental elements
3. Coexisting STDs
4. Endogenous hormonal influence

Eating fat-containing animal products has also been implicated.

■ **SIGNS AND SYMPTOMS** Most individuals with prostatic cancer are asymptomatic on diagnosis. When symptoms are present, they are typically those of urinary obstruction, such as dysuria, difficulty in voiding, urinary frequency, or urinary retention.

■ **DIAGNOSTIC PROCEDURES** A digital rectal examination will help in diagnosing the tumor. A biopsy is essential for confirmation of the diagnosis. Computed tomography (CT) or ultrasonography may be useful in localizing and gauging the extent of the tumor.

A prostate-specific antigen (PSA) blood test is used to detect prostate cancer. It detects prostatic cancer when the levels of prostatic antigens are elevated. This is a test advised for all males 50 years and over on a yearly basis.

■ **TREATMENT** The course of treatment selected will depend on the stage and grade of the disease and the client's physical condition and age. Surgery may be performed to remove the prostate and adjacent affected tissues. Various hormonal therapies also may be attempted to limit prostatic cell growth, including surgical removal of the testicle (**orchidectomy**) and estrogen therapy. Radiation therapy may be tried in some cases, and this further helps to relieve bone pain. Chemotherapy may be used in treating advanced stages of the disease.

ALTERNATIVE THERAPY: *A component of soy called* **genistein** *appears to inhibit the growth of prostate cancer. The supplement is available without a prescription and has been a popular therapy for prostate cancer in Asia for many decades. The supplement seems to work best when given before surgery, radiation therapy, or chemotherapy. A study is under way at the*

University of California at Davis using genistein. This is an example of integrative medicine at work.

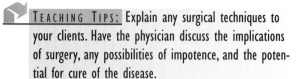

TEACHING TIPS: Explain any surgical techniques to your clients. Have the physician discuss the implications of surgery, any possibilities of impotence, and the potential for cure of the disease.

■ **PROGNOSIS** The earlier the cancer is detected, the better is the prognosis. Survival rates for all stages combined have steadily increased from 50% to 76%.

Testicular Cancer

■ **DESCRIPTION** *Testicular cancer* is a malignant neoplasm of a testis. There are various forms of the disease, classified according to the type of testicular tissue from which the malignancy originates. The disease primarily affects young to middle-aged males and is rare in males older than age 40.

■ **ETIOLOGY** The cause of cancer of the testes is essentially unknown. Predisposing factors include cryptorchidism, even after this condition has been surgically corrected, and being born to a mother who used diethylstilbestrol during pregnancy. It is rare in nonwhite males.

■ **SIGNS AND SYMPTOMS** The first sign often is a smooth, firm, painless mass of varying size in the testicles. Later symptoms may include breast enlargement and nipple tenderness.

■ **DIAGNOSTIC PROCEDURES** Diagnosis generally is through regular self-examination and palpation of the testes during a routine physical examination. Further tests such as CT or magnetic resonance imaging may be necessary to differentiate the cell type of the mass.

■ **TREATMENT** Treatment may include any combination of surgery (orchidectomy or reroperitoneal node dissection), radiation, and chemotherapy, as determined by the tumor cell type and staging.

ALTERNATIVE THERAPY: *No significant alternative therapy is indicated.*

TEACHING TIPS: Provide information on the disease and appropriate treatment methods. Reassure clients that sterility and impotence need not follow unilateral orchiectomy and that synthetic hormones can restore hormone imbalance.

■ **PROGNOSIS** The prognosis varies according to cancer type and staging. Cure rates of roughly 90% can be expected following the successful treatment of early-stage testicular cancers.

■ **PREVENTION** Although no specific prevention is known, early detection is crucial to successful treatment. Young males should be encouraged to perform monthly testicular self-examination.

Common Symptoms of Male Reproductive Diseases and Disorders

Males may present with the following common complaints, which deserve attention from health professionals:

- Any urinary complaints such as frequency, urgency, incontinence, dysuria, nocturia, etc.
- Pain in any of the reproductive organs or any unusual discharge
- Swelling or enlargement of any of the reproductive organs
- Any sexual disorder or concern

FEMALE REPRODUCTIVE DISEASES AND DISORDERS

Premenstrual Syndrome

■ **DESCRIPTION** *Premenstrual syndrome (PMS)* is a distinct cluster of physical and psychological symptoms that regularly recur 3 to 14 days before the onset of menstruation and are relieved by the onset of menses. Surveys show 30% to 40% of women experience mild to severe PMS. PMS appears more frequently in women in their 30s and 40s. (Refer to Figs. 9.3 and 9.4 to review the structure of the female reproductive system.)

■ **ETIOLOGY** The cause of PMS is not clearly understood, although it is thought to be multifactorial. Some theories suggest that the condition may be attributable to water retention, estrogen–progesterone imbalance, psychological factors, or dietary deficiencies. Some believe there is a relationship between PMS and changes in the endorphin levels.

■ **SIGNS AND SYMPTOMS** The particular assortment of symptoms and their severity vary from female to female. Symptoms associated with PMS include:

- Irritability
- Anxiety
- Sleeplessness
- Fatigue
- Depression
- Behavioral changes
- Headaches
- Vertigo
- Syncope
- Lowered resistance to infections
- Personality changes
- Nervousness
- Arthralgia
- Abdominal bloating and weight gain
- Heart palpitations
- Acne
- Swollen and tender breasts
- Easily bruised skin
- Alterations in appetite (e.g., cravings for sweet or salty foods)

The signs and symptoms may affect a female's ability to perform normal tasks and can affect relationships.

■ **DIAGNOSTIC PROCEDURES** Diagnosis depends on the timing of the symptoms rather than on the appearance of any specific set of symptoms. Consequently, the affected individual should be encouraged to keep a journal recording the onset, duration, and intensity of all symptoms for at least 3 months. Evaluation of estrogen and progesterone levels in the blood to check for imbalances should be performed. Blood tests may be done to rule out other hormonal imbalances or anemia. A history and physical examination will be done to rule out other diseases and disorders.

■ **TREATMENT** There is no one effective treatment for PMS. A reduction of salt intake for 2 weeks before menses will minimize water retention. Some-

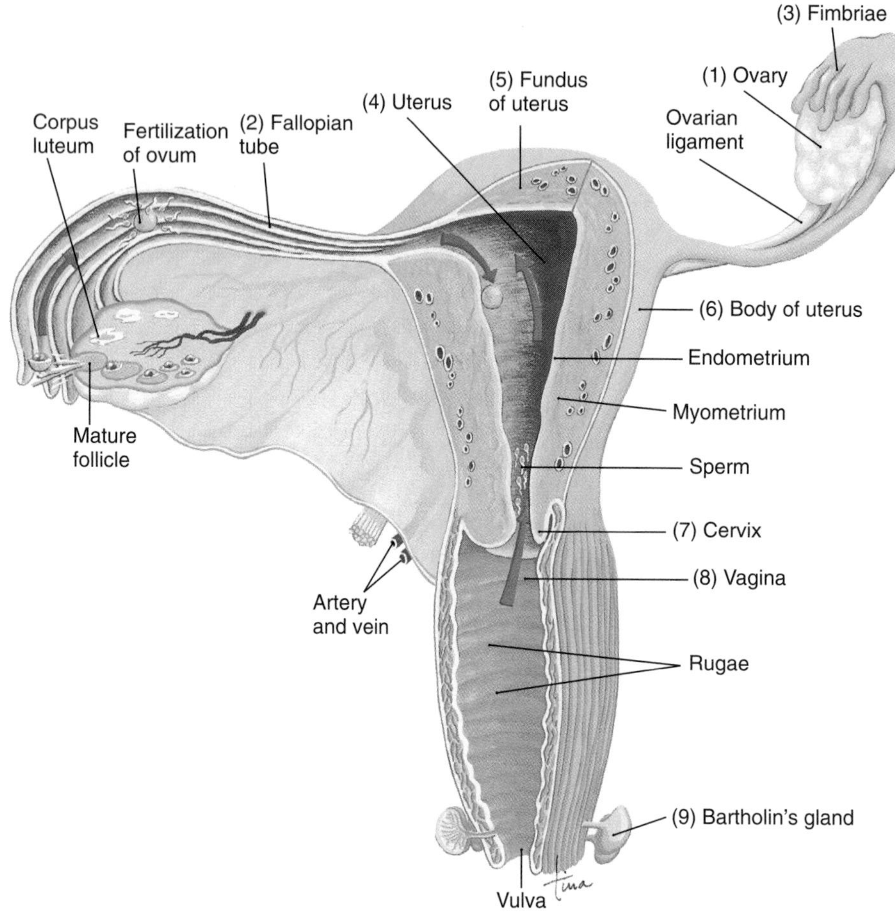

Figure 9.3 Female reproductive system (front view). (From Scanlon, VC, and Sanders, T: Essentials of Anatomy and Physiology, ed 4. FA Davis, Philadelphia, 2003, p 442, with permission.)

times diuretics and analgesics are ordered. Avoidance of stimulants (coffee, nicotine, and alcohol) and simple sugars and an increase in lean protein are suggested. Proper diet, exercise, and sufficient amounts of rest are important. Reduction in stress, relaxation techniques, and medication may be ordered to relieve the symptoms. Some physicians will recommend vitamin and mineral supplements and natural progesterone, although the latter is not well researched and is debated for use in PMS.

ALTERNATIVE THERAPY: *Continuing a daily exercise and relaxation program can improve emotional and physical symptoms. Some practitioners recommend vitamins B$_6$ and E, calcium, magne-* *sium, zinc, and oil of evening primrose capsules. Herbs and acupuncture have been used as well.*

TEACHING TIPS: Educate the client on how to keep a journal of signs and symptoms and dietary intake. Encourage support from family members, and stress the importance of following any prescribed treatment. Clients can become easily discouraged, so offer support as needed.

■ **PROGNOSIS** The prognosis is variable. The disorder is considered chronic but will cease at menopause and does not have long-term effects.

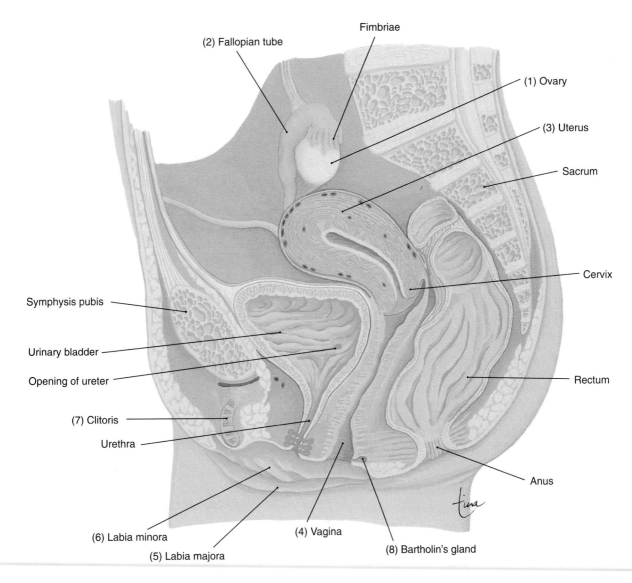

Figure 9.4 Female reproductive system (side view). (From Scanlon, VC, and Sanders, T: Essentials of Anatomy and Physiology, ed 4. FA Davis, Philadelphia, 2003, p 441, with permission.)

■ PREVENTION There is no known prevention.

Amenorrhea

■ DESCRIPTION *Amenorrhea* is the absence of **menarche**, the initial menstrual cycle, beyond age 16 (*primary* amenorrhea) or the absence of menstruation for 6 months in a female who has previously had regular, periodic menses (*secondary* amenorrhea).

■ ETIOLOGY Medically significant primary or secondary amenorrhea may be caused by a variety of hormonal imbalances capable of preventing ovulation. Primary amenorrhea is influenced by hereditary, environment, body build, physical, mental, and emotional development. Secondary amenorrhea may be caused by pregnancy, stress, or tension. Several forms of congenital anatomic defects, such as the absence of a uterus, may cause amenorrhea. The condition is also associated with endometrial problems, bulimia, anorexia, polycystic ovarian syndrome, ovarian or pituitary tumors, malnutrition, psychological stress, or too much physical exercise.

■ **SIGNS AND SYMPTOMS** A young female reporting delayed menarche or a female reporting skipped periods should be carefully assessed for amenorrhea.

■ **DIAGNOSTIC PROCEDURES** A thorough physical and pelvic examination will rule out pregnancy and anatomic abnormalities. Analysis of blood and urine samples may reveal hormonal difficulties. CT scans and laparoscopy with an endometrial biopsy may be necessary to detect tumors.

■ **TREATMENT** Treatment is dependent on the cause, if it is known. Hormone therapy usually starts the menstrual cycle, but some cases of this disorder may require more aggressive treatment, such as surgery for anatomic defects or tumor or cyst removal.

ALTERNATIVE THERAPY: *Practitioners recommend that females who exercise intensively and tend toward malnourishment eat at least an additional 500 calories a day. Whenever exercising, the client should eat an adequate and well-balanced diet to compensate for the increased metabolism and get ample rest.*

TEACHING TIPS: Encourage your clients to seek medical attention for this problem so that any underlying cause may be treated. It should not be ignored. A discussion with the physician will help to determine what steps to take to restore menstruation to a more-regular cycle.

■ **PROGNOSIS** Prognosis is good when the underlying cause can be determined and corrected. It is important that an accurate record of the menstrual cycle be kept to aid in the detection of amenorrhea.

■ **PREVENTION** Preventive measures include adequate diet and a balanced physical exercise program.

Dysmenorrhea

■ **DESCRIPTION** *Dysmenorrhea* is pain associated with menstruation. It is one of the most frequent gynecologic disorders. Dysmenorrhea is divided into *primary* and *secondary* categories. Primary dysmenorrhea is not associated with any identifiable pathologic disorder, whereas secondary dysmenorrhea accompanies some underlying disease condition.

■ **ETIOLOGY** A specific cause of primary dysmenorrhea is difficult to pinpoint. Hormonal imbalances such as increased **prostaglandin** secretions may be the cause. Prostaglandins are a class of chemically related fatty acids present in many body tissues that have the ability to stimulate smooth muscle contractions or lower blood pressure. Secondary dysmenorrhea arises as a consequence of some other problem, such as endometriosis, cervical stenosis, polycystic ovarian syndrome (PCOS), or PID. Secondary dysmenorrhea is occasionally associated with the presence of uterine polyps or benign tumors.

■ **SIGNS AND SYMPTOMS** Dull aching, spasmodic, colicky, cramping pains in the lower abdominal area are the classic symptoms. The pain may radiate to the thighs, back, and genitalia. Headache, nausea, diarrhea, fatigue, irritability, dizziness, and syncope may result. These symptoms usually start just before or immediately after menses and subside within 18 to 24 hours.

■ **DIAGNOSTIC PROCEDURES** A detailed history and pelvic examination will be performed to determine the cause. Laparoscopy and **dilation and curettage** (D&C) (a widening of the cervical opening and scraping with a curet to remove the uterine lining) may be attempted.

■ **TREATMENT** Analgesics and nonsteroidal anti-inflammatory drugs usually are sufficient for relieving the pain of this disorder. Aspirin, moreover, when taken before menses, is an inhibitor of prostaglandins. Other analgesics may be ordered. Heat applied to the abdomen may provide comfort. Sometimes sex steroid therapy (oral contraceptives) may be prescribed to relieve pain by suppressing ovulation. Uterine **leiomyomas,** a tumor of smooth muscle tissue, may require surgery.

ALTERNATIVE THERAPY: *Eating whole grains, legumes, fruit, vegetables, and nuts is recommended. The client should avoid sugars, alcohol, caffeine, dairy products, and salt. Supplements such as vitamin B, calcium, magnesium, and zinc may be ordered. Acupuncture is useful for pain reduction.*

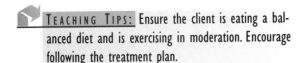

TEACHING TIPS: Ensure the client is eating a balanced diet and is exercising in moderation. Encourage following the treatment plan.

■ **PROGNOSIS** The prognosis for primary dysmenorrhea is good. Primary dysmenorrhea may disappear after a female becomes sexually active or gives birth to a child. For secondary dysmenorrhea, the prognosis is dependent on the cause.

■ **PREVENTION** Correction of any hormonal imbalance may be helpful in prevention.

Ovarian Cysts and Tumors

■ **DESCRIPTION** Benign *cysts* of the ovary are derived from ovarian follicles and the **corpus luteum**, a small, yellow structure on the ovary formed from the mass of follicle cells left behind after an ovum is released. These cysts may occur anytime from puberty to menopause. Nonneoplastic cysts (*tumors*) usually are small and produce few symptoms. True ovarian neoplasms may be benign, malignant, cystic, or solid. Dermoid or benign cystic tumors or **teratomas** also are common in the ovary. Other types of ovarian cysts include endometrioma and polycystic ovarian syndrome (PCOS). Endometrioma is a cyst-containing endometrial tissue that is attached to the ovary. PCOS is a complex endocrine disorder involving mainly females of child-bearing age. It is one of the most common endocrine diseases in females in their reproductive years. Symptoms are related to androgen excess. Irregular periods, lack of regular ovulation, hirsutism, and obesity are the usual presenting signs and symptoms. Clients with PCOS may develop insulin resistance.

■ **ETIOLOGY** The etiology of ovarian cysts and tumors is not known; however, genetics are thought to play a part, especially in PCOS. The cause may be defects in the ovary or the result of hypothalamic-pituitary dysfunction.

■ **SIGNS AND SYMPTOMS** Some cysts are asymptomatic. Large cysts may produce pelvic pain, low back pain, and dyspareunia. Cysts that are mobile and can twist may produce acute spasmodic abdominal pain. Urinary retention can result if a large fluid-filled cyst presses on the area near the bladder.

■ **DIAGNOSTIC PROCEDURES** Visualization of the ovaries through laparoscopy or ultrasonography may indicate ovarian cysts.

■ **TREATMENT** Cysts may disappear spontaneously through reabsorption or silent rupture or may require drug-induced ovulation therapy or surgical resection. Surgery may be necessary for diagnosis as well as treatment of most ovarian tumors, especially if any question exists regarding malignancy. Oral contraception may be useful to regulate periods and encourage ovulation.

ALTERNATIVE THERAPY: *An exercise program, a balanced diet, and control of weight may be useful in some types of ovarian cysts. Some recommend a vegetarian diet with organic foods. The client should avoid fried foods, coffee, tobacco, alcohol, and sugar.*

TEACHING TIPS: It is important to inform clients of their disease process so they understand the treatment plan. Offer support if needed, especially if infertility results.

■ **PROGNOSIS** Prognosis varies according to whether the diagnosis indicates nonneoplastic cysts or a true ovarian neoplasm, either benign or malignant. Some cysts may cause infertility problems. Chronic ovulation predisposes to endometrial cancer, cardiovascular disease, and hyperinsulinemia.

■ **PREVENTION** There is no known prevention.

Endometriosis

■ **DESCRIPTION** *Endometriosis* is the appearance and growth of endometrial tissue in areas outside the endometrium, the lining of the uterine cavity. The misplaced endometrial tissue generally is found within the pelvic area, but it can appear anywhere in the body (Fig. 9.5). Despite its location at an **ectopic** site (outside the uterus), the tissue still responds to the hormonal signals of the female's menstrual cycle, but the "menstruating" tissue cannot be sloughed off through the vagina. This situation gives rise to a variety of symptoms and may lead to scarring of the ectopic site. Endometriosis affects 3 to 5 million females in the United States and is a disease of females during their active reproductive years.

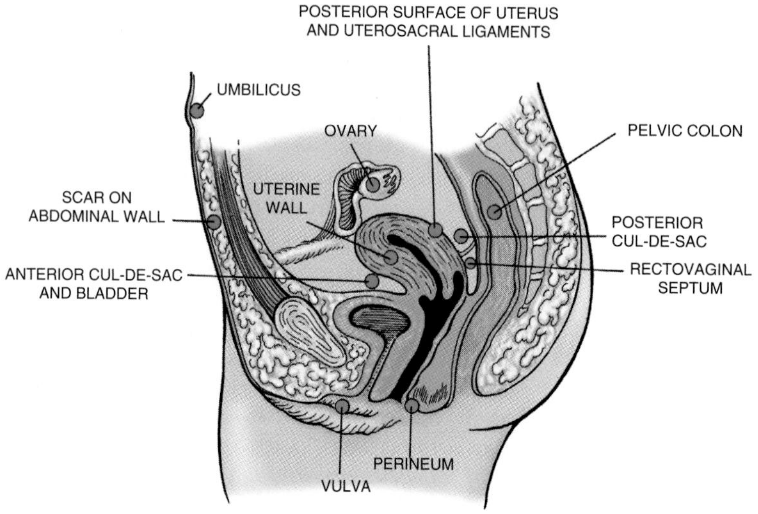

Figure 9.5 Possible sites of endometriosis. (From Venes, D and Thomas, CL [eds]: Taber's Cyclopedic Medical Dictionary, ed 19. FA Davis, Philadelphia, 2001, p 674, with permission.

■ **ETIOLOGY** The cause of endometriosis remains unknown, although various theories have been proposed, such as a familial susceptibility. Risk factors may include early menarche, regular periods with shorter cycle or heavier flow, and outflow obstruction.

■ **SIGNS AND SYMPTOMS** Dysmenorrhea occurs, with pain in the lower back and the vagina. The severity of the pain does not necessarily indicate the extent of the disease. There will be pain at the ectopic site during menses. The client may report profuse menses and infertility. She may experience dyspareunia, dysuria, and even painful defecation.

■ **DIAGNOSTIC PROCEDURES** A physical examination and a thorough health history are indicated. Diagnosis is usually made by visualizing the ectopic deposits within the pelvis through laparoscopy. Palpation may detect tender nodules or areas of the pelvis. These nodules become more tender during menses. The disease is usually staged from 1 (superficial or minor lesions) to 4 (deep involvement and dense adhesions).

■ **TREATMENT** Treatment depends on the client's symptom, her desire to have a baby, and the stage of the disease process. Hormone therapy that will completely suppress the menstrual cycle may be recommended. Birth control pills will suppress endometriosis as well. Young females may be put on androgens, which may produce a temporary remission. Laparoscopy may be used to lyse adhesions. **Panhysterosalpingo-oophorectomy**, which is surgery that can involve removal of the entire uterus, including the cervix, ovaries, and fallopian tubes, may be indicated.

ALTERNATIVE THERAPY: *The client should increase intake of essential fatty acids found in salmon, seeds, and nuts, and reduce intake of meat, eggs, and dairy products. Refer to Ovarian Cysts and Tumors for additional information.*

▶ TEACHING TIPS: It is important to dispel any myths your client may have. If infertility results, ART may be tried. Your client and her partner need support, because endometriosis can be painful.

■ **PROGNOSIS** The prognosis varies according to the location of the ectopic sites and the intensity of symptoms experienced by each affected individual. A primary complication of endometriosis is infertility. Females who have not had a child may be advised not to postpone pregnancy.

PREVENTION It may be best for females to use sanitary napkins rather than tampons to prevent displacement of the endometrial lining.

Uterine Leiomyomas

DESCRIPTION *Uterine leiomyomas* are often mislabeled as fibroids or fibroid tumors, but they are not composed of fibrous tissue. Rather, they are composed of smooth muscle tissue. These benign tumors may vary in size, number, and location within the uterine muscle. They are the most common tumors in females, but they tend to calcify after menopause.

ETIOLOGY The etiology of leiomyomas is not known, but their development is stimulated by estrogen.

SIGNS AND SYMPTOMS Frequently, leiomyomas are asymptomatic. If symptoms do occur, they may include pelvic pressure, urinary frequency, constipation, and menorrhagia. A palpable mass may be detected during a routine pelvic examination. The growths vary in size and increase during pregnancy or with oral contraceptive use.

DIAGNOSTIC PROCEDURES The client's symptoms and a thorough history and physical examination, including palpation of the tumor, are essential for diagnosis. Other possible tests are ultrasonography and D&C. These tests detect submucosal leiomyomas in the endometrial cavity, and laparoscopy, to visualize leiomyomas on the surface of the uterus.

TREATMENT Treatment is dependent on the female's age, whether she has carried a pregnancy to a point of viability or **parity**, her desire to have children, tumor status, and the severity of symptoms. If the tumors are small, no treatment may be necessary, other than periodic monitoring of the growth of the leiomyomas. A pelvic examination every 6 to 12 months may then be advised. Surgical removal of the tumors may be done, or a hysterectomy may be performed.

ALTERNATIVE THERAPY: *See Ovarian Cysts and Tumors.*

> **TEACHING TIPS:** Encourage clients to be watchful of any new signs and symptoms and report them to the physician. If infertility results, ART may be attempted.

PROGNOSIS Only a very small percentage of leiomyomas develop into a malignancy. Some tumors may outgrow their blood supply, become infected, or undergo degenerative changes. The leiomyomas may cause infertility or, if the client is pregnant, spontaneous abortion or premature labor may occur.

PREVENTION No prevention is known.

Pelvic Inflammatory Disease

DESCRIPTION *Pelvic inflammatory disease* is an acute or a subacute, or a recurrent or chronic, infection of the uterus, fallopian tubes, or ovaries. There may be inflammation of the cervix (cervicitis), uterus (endometritis), fallopian tubes (salpingitis), and ovaries (oophritis).

ETIOLOGY The causes of PID include (1) infections following **parturition,** the act of giving birth; (2) infections from *N. gonorrhoeae* or *C. trachomatis* are the most common organisms; and (3) iatrogenic causes—for instance, PID may follow the excision of cervical tissue for diagnostic testing (**conization**), cervical cauterization, or insertion of an intrauterine device (IUD) or biopsy curet. PID is most common in young nulliparous females, who have never produced a viable offspring. However, PID can also occur after childbirth, abortion, or miscarriage.

SIGNS AND SYMPTOMS This disease may exhibit both acute and chronic symptoms. Acute symptoms include sudden pelvic pain, a purulent and foul-smelling vaginal discharge, fever, sexual dysfunction, abnormal uterine bleeding (**metrorrhea**), and rebound pain. Chronic symptoms such as cervical dysplasia, the alteration in size, shape, and organization of mature cells, and laceration may go undetected for an indefinite period of time.

DIAGNOSTIC PROCEDURES Diagnosis includes taking a smear of uterine secretions for culture. Laboratory tests may include erythrocyte sedimentation rate, white blood cell count, and a measurement of C-reactive protein (CRP) in the blood. An elevated CRP level indicates an inflammation. Ultrasonography may be used to identify a uterine mass.

TREATMENT Appropriate antibiotics are the best treatment for PID. Supplemental therapy may include analgesics and bed rest. Surgery may be necessary to prevent **septicemia**, commonly called blood poisoning.

ALTERNATIVE THERAPY: *Abstinence is recommended during the infectious stage. The client must know and limit sexual partners and eat a balanced diet. If there is pain, acupuncture may be used to reduce the pain.*

> **TEACHING TIPS:** Remind the client of the importance of taking all of the antibiotic. Stress the seriousness of PID, and encourage your client to comply with the treatment plan and inform the physician of possible complications. It is necessary that partners are checked and, if necessary, treated for infection.

■ **PROGNOSIS** The prognosis of PID is good when treatment is instituted early, and few complications such as septicemia, infertility, or shock occur. If treatment is delayed, scar tissue and adhesions can form. Recurrences can occur.

■ **PREVENTION** There is no known prevention.

Menopause

I used to have Saturday night fever; now I have Saturday night hot flashes.

—MAXINE

■ **DESCRIPTION** *Menopause* (which is not a disease) is the cessation of menses and ovarian function, with a resultant decrease in estrogen levels.

■ **ETIOLOGY** Menopause occurs naturally in women between the ages of 40 and 55. It also can be surgically induced by oophorectomy, or it can result from malnutrition, severe stress, or a disease that has an adverse effect on hormone balance. Premature menopause can be idiopathic.

■ **SIGNS AND SYMPTOMS** Menstrual irregularities, a decrease in the amount of menstrual flow, and, finally, cessation of menses are the common symptoms. These occur over a period of months or years. Other changes can occur in the body systems as well, producing hot flashes, night sweats, syncope, tachycardia, loss of elasticity in the skin, reduction in size and firmness of breast tissue, some atrophy of the genitalia, and a decrease in secretion from Bartholin's glands. Some females experience transient psycho-logical symptoms such as depression, poor memory, and loss of interest in sex.

■ **DIAGNOSTIC PROCEDURES** A careful history usually suggests menopause. Blood serum levels will be checked for increased production of follicle-stimulating hormone (FSH), produced by the pituitary gland, and luteinizing hormone (LH), produced by the hypothalmus. The LH stimulates development of the corpus luteum. Radoimmunoassay testing may be done as well.

■ **TREATMENT** Some individuals need no treatment; others may require hormone replacement therapy, counseling, or both. It is recommended that a woman has a screening mammogram before hormone replacement therapy (HRT). A woman who requires HRT should be informed of the possible increased risks. See HRT on page 183.

ALTERNATIVE THERAPY: *The goal of alternative therapy is to eliminate the bothersome signs and symptoms, to prevent osteoporosis (see Chapter 15) and heart disease (see Chapter 12). The use of HRT is controversial. For hot flashes, the following foods are recommended: apples, carrots, yams, peas, red beans, brown rice, and sesame seeds. The client should increase calcium intake, and exercise in moderation is beneficial.*

> **TEACHING TIPS:** It is essential that a female understand the side effects of HRT and is given a choice of alternatives. A good understanding of menopause is essential as the signs and symptoms vary among females.

■ **PROGNOSIS** The prognosis is generally good.

■ **PREVENTION** Menopause cannot be prevented, but it is important to recognize that emotional swings may occur.

Ovarian Cancer

■ **DESCRIPTION** Ovarian cancer is the sixth most common cancer among females and the fifth-leading cause of cancer deaths in the United States. One of every 57 females will develop ovarian cancer during her lifetime. More females die of ovarian cancer than from cervical and endometrial cancer com-

Hormone Replacement Therapy (HRT)

Hormone Replacement Therapy was first prescribed in the 1940s for postmenopausal females to treat their symptoms and to prevent postmenopausal conditions such as osteoporosis. However, recently, two studies have been conducted that question whether the use of HRT outweighs its risks. The first study conducted by the National Institute of Health looked at the effect of HRT taken as combination therapy versus a placebo. The study was halted because they found that the overall risks of HRT therapy exceeded the benefits. The risks included more coronary heart disease events, more strokes, serious blood clots and invasive breast cancers. The benefits they found were fewer colorectal cancers and fewer hip fractures.

A second study completed in Britain suggests that HRT can increase the risk of dying from breast cancer in addition to raising the risk of getting the disease. The researchers also determined that stopping the HRT seemed to reduce the risk fairly quickly. It has been found that treatment for osteoporosis with ultra-low doses of estrogen appears to be safe and to increase bone density in older females.

The research seems to indicate the estrogen-only therapy would cause less breast cancer than the combination HRT. The risk of endometrial cancer with estrogen-only therapy is well documented; therefore, this type of HRT is generally only given to females who have had a hysterectomy. The Food and Drug Administration recommends that females take the lowest dose for the shortest possible duration. More research may be needed. However, the decision to use either estrogen-only or combination HRT after menopause needs to be made between a female and her physician. They need to weigh the possible risks and benefits. The latter is true also when considering estrogen therapy for the treatment of osteoporosis.

bined. Women who take oral contraceptives for at least 5 years decrease their risk of ovarian cancer by 60%. Ovarian cancer is often called the silent killer because females may be asymptomatic, delaying the diagnosis; hence, there is a poorer prognosis.

■ **ETIOLOGY** The exact cause of ovarian cancer is unknown, but contributing factors include infertility, familial tendency, irregular menses, and possible exposure to industrial pollutants.

■ **SIGNS AND SYMPTOMS** The ovarian tumor may grow to considerable size before producing any symptoms. The client may present with vague abdominal discomfort, dyspepsia, and other mild gastrointestinal symptoms. Frequency and/or urgency of urination in the absence of infection, unexplained changes in bowel habits, and ongoing fatigue may be present. Tumor rupture, infection, or torsion (twisting) may cause pain.

■ **DIAGNOSTIC PROCEDURE** Clinical evaluation, complete history, and physical examination are necessary. Transvaginal sonography, abdominal ultrasound, or CT scan may be used. Complete blood cell count and blood chemistries may be ordered. Surgical exploration is the only way to grade and stage a tumor. Histologic studies are done.

A new test is being researched for an earlier diagnosis of ovarian cancer. To detect ovarian cancer, the test uses a new biomarker, HE4, that is secreted into the blood by ovarian cancer cells. Another test used to detect ovarian cancer detects the protein CA125 and often is unreliable, so the hope is that the HE4 test will be more reliable in the earlier stages of the disease.

■ **TREATMENT** Treatment is dependent on the grading and staging of the tumor. In most cases, surgery and chemotherapy will be done and, less frequently, radiation. Surgery is used to diagnosis the cancer. Generally, it is followed by chemotherapy using such chemicals as cisplatin or platinum-containing combinations. Palliative care is needed for the client undergoing chemotherapy treatment. Other surgical procedures may include a total abdominal hysterectomy and bilateral salpingo-oophorectomy with tumor resection.

ALTERNATIVE THERAPY: *A diet consisting mainly of organically grown foods including fruits, vegetables, and whole grains is best. Organically grown* *foods are also rich in vitamin E and selenium. Increasing intake of beta carotene, vitamins B$_6$ C, D, and E, and folic acid is recommended. To help combat the side effects of chemotherapy, the Maitake mushroom is thought to banish nausea and boost energy. It is important to ensure that your client gets ample caloric intake, and whey protein is recommended. Green tea also helps nausea.*

TEACHING TIPS: Help your client understand the staging and typing of her ovarian tumor with subsequent treatment plan. If the client is young and wishes to have children, supportive care is especially needed. If chemotherapy is needed, encourage your client to report any side effects so that they can be treated. If the ovarian cancer is in the final stages, seek support of other members and of the health-care team, not only to help the family but also your client.

■ **PROGNOSIS** The prognosis is dependent on the type and stage of the cancer when it is diagnosed. If the cancer is detected early, the 5-year survival rate is approximately 95%; if the cancer has progressed, the prognosis drops to 35%.

■ **PREVENTION** The best prevention of ovarian cancer is a yearly pelvic examination. A Pap test will detect ovarian cancer only in its advanced stages. Genetic testing is available to test whether a female carries mutations of the breast cancer gene 1 (*BRCA1*) or breast cancer gene 2 (*BRCA 2*). Mutations of these genes make females at higher risk of the development of both ovarian and breast cancer.

Common Symptoms of Female Reproductive System Diseases and Disorders

Women may present with the following common symptoms, which deserve attention from health professionals:

- Premenstrual and postmenstrual complaints such as amenorrhea, dysmenorrhea, oligomenorrhea (abnormally infrequent and scanty menses), and metrorrhea; skin changes; and psychological reactions to hormonal changes
- Lower abdominal or pelvic pain

- Any abnormal vaginal discharge or itching
- Fever
- Dyspareunia or any sexual dysfunction
- Breast changes, such as unusual swelling, lumpiness, mass formation, pain, or nipple abnormalities

DISEASES AND DISORDERS OF THE BREASTS

Mammary Dysplasia or Fibrocystic Disease

■ **DESCRIPTION** *Fibrocystic disease of the breast* is a generalized diagnosis for a condition in which there are palpable lumps or cysts in the breasts that fluctuate in size with the menstrual cycle. Other benign changes in the breast epithelium include the widespread formation of warts (**papillomatosis),** fibrosis, and hyperplasia. The condition is sometimes known as *chronic cystic mastitis*. The disease is seen more frequently in women aged 30 to 55 years and rarely after menopause. It is the most common disease of the breast in premenopausal females. Refer to Figure 9.6 for a review of the structure of the breast.

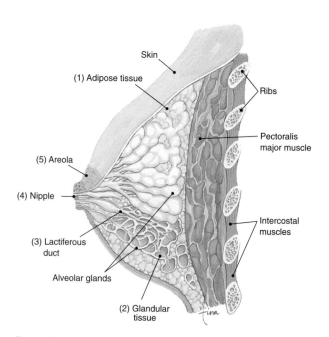

Figure 9.6 The breast. (From Scanlon, VC, and Sanders, T: Essentials of Anatomy and Physiology, ed 4. FA Davis, Philadelphia, 2003, p 445, with permission.)

■ **ETIOLOGY** The causes of fibrocystic disease are not well understood, but they are linked to the hormonal changes associated with ovarian activity. There is a tendency for the disease to run in families.

■ **SIGNS AND SYMPTOMS** The upper, outer quadrant of the breast is the most frequent segment involved. There may be widespread lumpiness or a localized mass. Pain, tenderness, and feeling of fullness are likely before menstruation.

■ **DIAGNOSTIC PROCEDURES** Monthly breast self-examinations cannot be overemphasized. Palpation is essential. A mammogram may be a useful aid, but biopsy is essential to confirm the diagnosis. The clinical picture of pain, fluctuation in size, and lumpiness helps to differentiate mammary dysplasia from breast cancer.

■ **TREATMENT** Breast pain may be alleviated with a good supportive bra. Caffeine intake may be restricted and salt intake reduced, because some studies indicate that its elimination aids in reducing dysplasia.

ALTERNATIVE THERAPY: *The client should eliminate all forms of caffeine from the diet, including chocolate. Taking vitamin E supplementation two to three times daily may be beneficial. A low-fat diet is recommended, and regular aerobic exercise is helpful.*

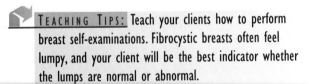

TEACHING TIPS: Teach your clients how to perform breast self-examinations. Fibrocystic breasts often feel lumpy, and your client will be the best indicator whether the lumps are normal or abnormal.

■ **PROGNOSIS** The prognosis is good, although exacerbations may continue until menopause, after which they subside. Cancer of the breast is more common in females who also have mammary dysplasia.

■ **PREVENTION** There is no known prevention. Monthly self-examination of the breast is advised, as well as regular mammography.

Benign Fibroadenoma

■ **DESCRIPTION** A *fibroadenoma* is a benign, well-circumscribed tumor of fibrous and glandular breast tissue. It is a common tumor occurring in women 20 years after puberty.

■ **ETIOLOGY** The cause is unknown.

■ **SIGNS AND SYMPTOMS** The breast mass is typically round, firm, discrete, and relatively movable. It is nontender and usually discovered by accident.

■ **DIAGNOSTIC PROCEDURES** Palpation, followed by a mammogram, is essential for diagnosis. Digital mamography is a form of mamography that allows for the transfer of images to a computer. This allows the physician to zoom in, magnify, and view the entire breast at one time. Because it uses a special software, the images can be stored and transferred for later viewing. Your client will not notice a difference when the digital mammogram is taken, and it is especially useful with more dense breast tissue. Because of its distinctive characteristics, the tumor is not difficult to diagnose, but it must be differentiated from a cyst or carcinoma through biopsy.

■ **TREATMENT** The mass is excised under local anesthesia.

ALTERNATIVE THERAPY: *No significant alternative therapy is indicated.*

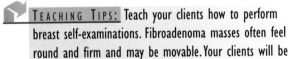

TEACHING TIPS: Teach your clients how to perform breast self-examinations. Fibroadenoma masses often feel round and firm and may be movable. Your clients will be the best indicator of any new growths.

■ **PROGNOSIS** The prognosis is good after excision of the tumor.

■ **PREVENTION** There is no known prevention.

Carcinoma of the Breast

■ **DESCRIPTION** *Breast cancer* encompasses a variety of malignant neoplasms of the breast. It is the most common site of cancer in females and until recently was the leading cause of cancer deaths among females in the United States, a position that is now occupied by lung cancer.

■ **ETIOLOGY** The exact causes of breast cancer are unknown, although hereditary patterns to the disease are likely. Women who have a family history of breast cancer have an increased risk. The risk of breast cancer increases with age and is higher in women with biopsy-confirmed atypical hyperplasia, a long menstrual history, and obesity after menopause.

Those who have not had children or who did not have children until after age 30 are also at greater risk.

■ **SIGNS AND SYMPTOMS** The earliest sign of breat cancer is an abnormality shown on a mammogram. Breast changes such as a lump, thickening, dimpling, swelling, skin irritation, distortion, retraction or scaliness of the nipple, nipple discharge, pain, or tenderness are the most common signs and symptoms. Advanced symptoms include edema, redness, nodularity or ulceration of the skin, and enlargement or shrinkage of the breast.

■ **DIAGNOSTIC PROCEDURES** The best method of early detection continues to be the monthly self-examination of the breast. Mammography and ultrasonography are also frequently used screening methods. Diagnosis, however, must be made without delay because of the possibility of metastasis. Biopsy is essential for definitive diagnosis. Diagnosed breast cancer will be staged and typed according to its pattern of growth.

■ **TREATMENT** Treatment will depend on the stage of breast cancer and the client's preferences. Curative treatment nearly always involves surgical management of the cancer. Possible surgeries are lumpectomy or mastectomy with accompanying radiation, chemotherapy, or hormone therapy. Whether lymph nodes under the arm are removed will depend on the likely spread of the disease. Radiation may be done before surgery to shrink the tumor or postoperatively to destroy any remaining malignancy. If surgery is done, breast reconstruction may follow.

The tumor tissue will be tested for the presence of hormone receptors to determine whether the tumor is estrogen or progesterone dependent. If this is the case, hormonal manipulation such as removal of the ovaries or adrenal glands and administration of testosterone may be attempted to halt tumor regrowth or to prevent its spread.

ALTERNATIVE THERAPY: *Importance will be placed on enhancing the immune system and on work-*

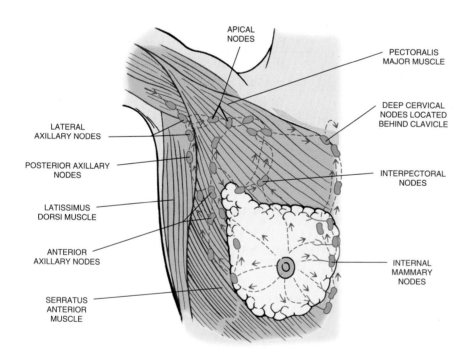

Figure 9.7 Breast cancer: possible sites of lymphatic spread. (From Thomas, CL [ed]: Taber's Cyclopedic Medical Dictionary, ed 18. FA Davis, Philadelphia, 1997, p 263, with permission.)

ing with the physician to make radiation and chemotherapy easier to handle.

 TEACHING TIPS: Information is vital so a client can make the choice appropriate for treatment. Referral to others who have been successfully treated can be beneficial.

■ **PROGNOSIS** The most reliable indicator of the prognosis is the stage of the breast cancer. In the early stages, the prognosis is good, especially if no metastasis has occurred. According to the American Cancer Society, the 5-year survival rate for localized breast cancer has risen to 97%. If the cancer has spread regionally, however, the survival rate is reduced to 77%. See Figure 9.7 for sites of lymphatic spread.

■ **PREVENTION** There is no known prevention

 Breast Reconstruction

Breast Reconstruction, *a surgical procedure, is generally used after breast cancer. The plastic surgeon rebuilds the breast contour, the nipple, and the areola. According to the American Cancer Society, the goals of reconstruction are:*

* *To provide symmetry of [the] breasts when [the woman is] wearing a bra*
* *To permanently regain [the client's] breast contour, and*
* *To give the convenience of not needing an external prosthesis*

Several surgical options are available, including the use of a breast implant, using the client's own tissue flap (section of skin, fat, and muscle, which are removed from the abdomen or other area of the client's body), or a combination of the two. The surgery can be done immediately after a mastectomy or delayed until the client completes radiation.

Two Websites to visit for more detailed information are www.cancer.org (look for breast reconstruction) or www.cancer.gov/cancerinfo (look for breast reconstruction).

of breast cancer other than breast self-examination and regular mammography for early detection.

DISEASES AND DISORDERS OF PREGNANCY AND DELIVERY

ALTERNATIVE THERAPY: *Alternative therapy in pregnancy is aimed at achieving a healthy pregnancy and preventing any difficulties. A well-balanced diet is advised, as is the avoidance of any harmful substances. These substances include caffeine, nicotine, and recreational and prescription drugs (the latter to be avoided unless specifically advised by the physician, who will seek medications that are not harmful to the unborn). Adequate rest, "mental breaks," moderate exercise, and a positive outlook are beneficial to both mother and baby.*

 TEACHING TIPS: Pregnancy is most often a happy time in a female's life. Any problem that causes difficulties during pregnancy requires special attention. Pay attention to psychological and emotional needs of those affected by the problem. Remind clients to report any signs of spotting or bleeding and cramping immediately. Prompt treatment of any pelvic infections is encouraged. Any occurrence that ends the pregnancy before delivery is traumatic; grieving occurs. Remind clients that a difficult loss in pregnancy one time does not mean that a healthy full-term pregnancy is impossible in the future.

Spontaneous Abortion

■ **DESCRIPTION** *Spontaneous abortion*, or *miscarriage*, is the expulsion of the conceptus before viability. As many as 20% to 30% of pregnancies may end in spontaneous abortion; the incidence is higher in first pregnancies.

■ **ETIOLOGY** Spontaneous abortion may be a result of (1) defective development of the embryo (chromosomal abnormalities), (2) faulty implantation of the fertilized ovum, (3) placental problems, (4) maternal infections, (5) hormonal imbalances, (6) trauma, or (7) an unknown cause.

■ **SIGNS AND SYMPTOMS** A pink or brown discharge may precede the onset of cramping and increased vaginal bleeding. The cervix will dilate, and the uterine contents will be expelled. The discharge may appear as a clotty menstrual flow. If the entire contents are expelled, bleeding and cramping stop. If any contents remain, cramping and bleeding continue.

■ **DIAGNOSTIC PROCEDURES** Evidence of the expelled uterine contents, pelvic examination, and laboratory studies will confirm the occurrence of a spontaneous abortion.

■ **TREATMENT** Bed rest may be required for as long as spotting continues. Hospitalization may be necessary to control hemorrhage. If remnants of the conceptus remain in the uterus, D&C should be performed.

■ **PROGNOSIS** The prognosis for full recovery is good, barring any complications such as hemorrhage, anemia, or infections.

■ **PREVENTION** The progression of a spontaneous abortion usually cannot be prevented.

Ectopic Pregnancy

■ **DESCRIPTION** *Ectopic pregnancy* occurs when the fertilized ovum implants and grows somewhere other than the uterine cavity. The most common ectopic site is within one of the fallopian tubes. Less frequently, ectopic implantation occurs in an ovary or in the abdominal cavity (Fig. 9.8).

■ **ETIOLOGY** Ectopic pregnancy is often due to scarring or inflammation of the fallopian tubes as a result of infection, or it may be due to congenital malformations of the tubes. Endometriosis, PID, and tumors can cause ectopic pregnancy. In general, any factor that impedes the migration of the fertilized ovum into the uterus before attachment takes place increases the likelihood of an ectopic pregnancy.

■ **SIGNS AND SYMPTOMS** Signs of early pregnancy may be present. There also may be abdominal pain and tenderness, as well as slight vaginal bleeding. A rupture of a fallopian tube due to the development of the conceptus is life threatening and will cause severe abdominal pain and intra-abdominal bleeding.

■ **DIAGNOSTIC PROCEDURES** A pelvic examination and a careful history may suggest ectopic pregnancy. A serum pregnancy test and an ultrasound examination likely will be used in this determination. Laparoscopy and exploratory laparotomy also may help in the diagnosis of this condition.

■ **TREATMENT** Laparotomy is frequently necessary. A ruptured fallopian tube may require removal. All attempts will be made to save the ovary. Transfusion of whole blood may be necessary in the event of severe intra-abdominal bleeding or hypovolemic shock.

■ **PROGNOSIS** The prognosis is good when emergency treatment is sought quickly. If rupture of the tube occurs, complications may be life threatening and include hemorrhage, shock, and peritonitis.

■ **PREVENTION** Prompt treatment of any genitourinary infection may help reduce the likelihood of ectopic pregnancy.

Pregnancy-Induced Hypertension

■ **DESCRIPTION** *Pregnancy-induced hypertension (PIH)* is a hypertensive disorder that may develop during the third trimester. Most health-care professionals prefer to use the more precise terms of *preeclampsia* and *eclampsia* to designate the condition. *Preeclampsia*, the nonconvulsive form of PIH, is the initial cluster of symptoms, characterized by hypertension, edema, and proteinuria. *Eclampsia,* the convulsive form of PIH, is the subsequent group of symptoms, characterized by convulsions and coma. Eclampsia is a medical emergency. The condition is more likely to occur in women in their first pregnancy, or **primigravidae,** who are aged 12 to 18 years or in women older than 35 who have had multiple pregnancies.

■ **ETIOLOGY** The cause of preeclampsia and eclampsia is not known, but is thought to be related to maternal nutrition. Predisposing factors include preexisting vascular and renal disease and poor nutrition during pregnancy.

■ **SIGNS AND SYMPTOMS** Hypertension, generalized edema, proteinuria, and sudden weight gain are the classic symptoms of preeclampsia. High sodium ingestion may be a contributing factor. Headache, vertigo, malaise, irritability, epigastric pain, and nausea also may occur. Eclampsia symptoms may include tonoclonic convulsions, coma, rales or rattling in the throat (**rhonchi**), rhythmic, involuntary move-

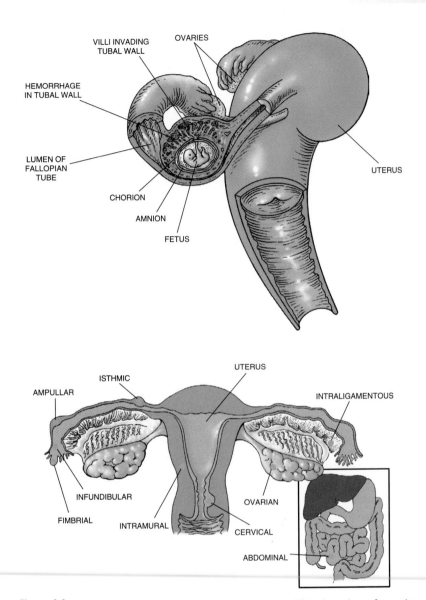

VILLI INVADING
TUBAL WALL

OVARIES

HEMORRHAGE
IN TUBAL WALL

LUMEN OF
FALLOPIAN
TUBE

UTERUS

CHORION

AMNION

FETUS

UTERUS

ISTHMIC

INTRALIGAMENTOUS

AMPULLAR

INFUNDIBULAR

OVARIAN

FIMBRIAL

INTRAMURAL

CERVICAL

ABDOMINAL

Figure 9.8 Ectopic pregnancy. (A) Actual ectopic pregnancy. (B) Various sites of ectopic pregnancy. (From Venes, D, and Thomas, CL [eds]: Taber's Cyclopedic Medical Dictionary, ed 19. FA Davis, Philadelphia, 2001, p 1663, with permission.)

ment of the eyeball (**nystagmus**), and oliguria or **anuria**. The latter is an absence of urine formation.

■ **DIAGNOSTIC PROCEDURES** Elevated—especially steadily rising—blood pressure, proteinuria, and oliguria are suggestive of preeclampsia. If the pregnant woman's urine exhibits low levels of placental growth factor and vascular endothelial growth factor, she is at high risk for PIH. Once identified, the physician can more closely monitor the pregnancy for

indications of PIH. The clinical picture of convulsions confirms a diagnosis of eclampsia.

■ **TREATMENT** In *preeclampsia*, the goal of treatment is to prevent eclampsia and to deliver a normal baby. Bed rest is advised, with sedatives prescribed. Antihypertensives may be necessary. The fetus may be delivered as soon as it is judged viable, possibly via cesarean section. With the onset of *eclampsia*, the client will be hospitalized and intensive treatment instituted. Immediate termination of the pregnancy is indicated, regardless of whether the fetus is judged viable.

■ **PROGNOSIS** The prognosis is good for preeclampsia. In eclampsia, the maternal mortality rate is about 15%.

■ **PREVENTION** Adequate nutrition, good prenatal care, and control of high blood pressure during pregnancy are important. Urinalysis to detect high levels of protein is essential. Early treatment of preeclampsia can prevent eclampsia.

Placenta Previa

■ **DESCRIPTION** In *placenta previa*, the placenta is implanted abnormally low in the uterus so that it covers all or part of the internal cervical os, or opening (Fig. 9.9). This condition is dangerous because the placenta may prematurely separate from the uterus, causing maternal hemorrhaging and interrupting oxygen flow to the fetus.

■ **ETIOLOGY** The cause is unknown, but predisposing factors include multiparity, advanced maternal age, and previous uterine surgery.

■ **SIGNS AND SYMPTOMS** A typical symptom is slight, painless bleeding, generally occurring in the third trimester, that may become more severe. The fetus may present in a variety of positions, but the situation is not critical as long as fetal heart tones remain strong. Vital signs may indicate shock.

■ **DIAGNOSTIC PROCEDURES** Ultrasonography will help in the diagnosis.

■ **TREATMENT** Hospital treatment is aimed at controlling and treating any blood loss, delivering a healthy infant, and preventing complications. A cesarean section may be necessary.

■ **PROGNOSIS** The maternal prognosis depends on the amount of bleeding; the fetal prognosis depends on gestational age, blood loss, and consequences of possible anoxia. Complications include shock and maternal or fetal death. With prompt and effective treatment, however, both mother and child usually survive.

■ **PREVENTION** There is no known prevention.

Abruptio Placentae

■ **DESCRIPTION** *Abruptio placentae* is the premature separation of a normally implanted placenta from the uterine wall about the 20th week of gestation. The condition is most common in multigravidae.

■ **ETIOLOGY** The cause is unknown, but predisposing factors include trauma, chronic hypertension, and preeclampsia or eclampsia, multiparity, smoking, and cocaine abuse.

■ **SIGNS AND SYMPTOMS** Abruptio placentae presents a wide range of symptoms depending on the separation of the placenta and the amount of blood loss. There may be mild to moderate bleeding, conti-

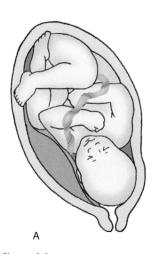 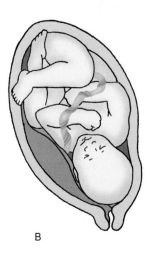 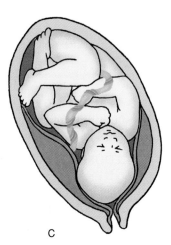

A   B   C

Figure 9.9 Placenta previa. (*A*) Low implantation. (*B*) Partial placenta previa. (*C*) Central (total) placenta previa. (From Beare, PG: Davis's NCLEX-RN Review, ed 3. FA Davis, Philadelphia, 2001, p 61, with permission.)

nous pain, or sudden, severe abdominal pain with boardlike rigidity, tenderness of the uterus, hemorrhage, and the onset of shock.

■ **DIAGNOSTIC PROCEDURES** Ultrasonography, pelvic examination, and history will help confirm the diagnosis.

■ **TREATMENT** The goals of treatment are to control the bleeding, deliver a healthy infant, and prevent complications. Hospitalization is required, and a cesarean section is typically performed. Blood replacement may be necessary.

■ **PROGNOSIS** The maternal prognosis is good if the bleeding can be controlled. The fetal prognosis depends on gestational age and the amount of blood loss. Complications include disseminated intravascular coagulation (DIC) and renal failure.

■ **PREVENTION** There is no known prevention.

Premature Labor/Premature Rupture of Membranes

■ **DESCRIPTION** *Premature rupture of membranes (PROM)* is early rupture of the amniotic sac. *Premature labor* is the early onset of rhythmic uterine contractions after fetal viability but before fetal maturity.

■ **ETIOLOGY** These conditions may be caused by "incompetent cervix," preeclampsia, multiple pregnancy, abruptio placentae, anatomic malformations, infections, or fetal death. A predisposing factor may be poor prenatal care.

■ **SIGNS AND SYMPTOMS** There may be a blood-tinged flow from the vagina, with uterine contractions and cervical dilation or **effacement**. PROM is marked by the flow of amniotic fluid from the vagina.

■ **DIAGNOSTIC PROCEDURES** Diagnosis is confirmed by prenatal history and vaginal and physical examination. Ultrasonography also may be used. Electronic fetal monitoring is used to confirm the fetal condition.

■ **TREATMENT** Attempts will be made to suppress premature labor by bed rest and appropriate drug therapy. PROM typically requires induction of labor or cesarean delivery.

■ **PROGNOSIS** The maternal prognosis is good with proper attention and care. The fetal prognosis depends on gestational age.

■ **PREVENTION** The best prevention is good prenatal care.

Common Symptoms of Diseases and Disorders of Pregnancy and Delivery

Pregnant females may present with the following common complaints, any of which deserve attention from health professionals:

- Abdominal pain, tenderness, or cramping
- Unusual discharge, pink or brown in color, or clotted
- Hypertension, rapid weight gain, edema, and malaise

Summary

Our human sexuality defines who we are. There are some diseases and disorders that are unique to either the male or the female reproductive system, yet they share numerous common factors. Because the reproductive system has the purpose of both reproduction and enhancement of caring and pleasure, any dysfunction clearly affects our sexuality and oftentimes our self-image.

 Cesarean Birth (C-Section)

A C-Section *is a surgical procedure that is performed when a vaginal birth is not possible or safe or when the health of the mother or infant is at risk. The infant is delivered through an incision is made in the abdomen and the uterus. C-section decisions may be made before labor and delivery when the baby's head or body is too large to pass through the mother's pelvis or the mother's pelvis is too small. Multiple births, placenta previa, the baby is in a horizontal or sideway position in the uterus, or a breech (buttocks) presentation also may dictate a C-section. During labor and delivery, C-sections may be necessary when there is failure of the labor to progress, when the cord is compressed, prolapsed, and when there is abruptio placentae, or fetal distress. If the C-section is an emergency, the time from incision to delivery can take 10 to 15 minutes, with the delivery of the placenta and suturing of the incision requiring an additional 45 minutes.*

CASE STUDIES

■ Case Study 1

Roberta Hills, a 15-year-old girl who has been sexually active, is informed by her boyfriend that he has gonorrhea. Roberta had noted that she has a slight vaginal discharge and some urinary difficulties, but she thought that these were just symptoms of a urinary tract infection (UTI), because she has had a UTI twice before.

Case Study Question

1. If Roberta calls the physician's office, what should she be advised to do?
2. Could Roberta's symptoms be those of a UTI? Could they be symptoms of gonorrhea? Explain.
3. Based on the assumption that the symptoms were those of a UTI, what diagnostic tests would the physician order? What action would the physician take if gonorrhea was suspected?

■ Case Study 2

LaDonna Tines, a 54-year-old woman, notices that her menstrual cycle is irregular and occurs less frequently, with decreased flow. She has hot flashes and mood swings and experiences pain from vaginal dryness during intercourse.

Case Study Question

1. What are the implications of LaDonna's age in regard to these symptoms?
2. If the physician suspects the onset of menopause, what tests would she order?
3. What might be the cause of the hot flashes?

■ Case Study 3

A 38-year-old woman, Linda Benedict, visits the physician because she has been experiencing pain in her left breast. The pain appears to be localized. In reply to the physician's question, Linda reports that she has been examining her breasts monthly and has not noted any lumps or abnormalities. After asking her to describe the pain and indicate its location, the physician examines Linda and finds no abnormalities. The physician advises Linda to return in 6 months; if the pain is still present, he tells her that he will order a mammogram.

Case Study Question

1. What are the recommendations of the American Cancer Society that apply to this situation?
2. Is pain an early symptom of cancer?

■ Case Study 4

Dean Moore is a 67-year-old man who has been diagnosed with BPH. Surgery is indicated, but Dean fears impotence and incontinence.

Case Study Question

1. How might a medical professional respond to Dean regarding his fears?

REVIEW QUESTIONS

True/False

Circle the correct answer:

T F 1. Benign cysts of the ovary are derived from ovarian follicles and the corpus luteum.

T F 2. Large ovarian cysts may produce pelvic pain and dyspareunia.

T F 3. The cause of endometriosis is bacterial in nature.

T F 4. Endometriosis most frequently occurs postmenopausally.

T F 5. Uterine leiomyomas are composed of fibrous tissue.

T F 6. Frequently leiomyomas are asymptomatic.

T F 7. Menopause is the cessation of ovarian function with an increase in estrogen.

Matching

Match each of the following definitions with its correct term:

Sexually transmitted diseases

_____ 1. Disease(s) caused by various types of papillomavirus

_____ 2. Disease(s) caused by a motile protozoan

_____ 3. Disease(s) caused by bacteria

_____ 4. Disease(s) caused by the simplex virus

a. Herpes virus type 2

b. Genital warts

c. Gonorrhea

d. Chlamydial infection

e. Syphilis

f. Trichomoniasis

Disorders of the breast

_____ 5. Breast mass that is round, firm, discrete, relatively movable, and nontender

_____ 6. Widespread lumpiness in the upper, outer quadrant of the breast

_____ 7. Breast dimpling, swelling, skin irritation, lump, nipple discharge

a. Mammary dysplasia

b. Benign fibroadenoma

c. Carcinoma of the breast

Match the following diseases or conditions with their common diagnostic procedures:

_____ 8. Pelvic examination, laboratory studies, and evidence of expelled uterine contents

_____ 9. Prenatal history, physical examination, and ultrasound

_____ 10. Pelvic examination, patient history, serum pregnancy test, and ultrasound

_____ 11. Proteinuria, oliguria, and high blood pressure.

a. Abortion

b. Toxemia

c. PROM

d. Ectopic pregnancy

Short Answer

1. List the two functions of sexuality in humans.

   a.

   b.

2. Name two inflammatory diseases of the male reproductive system and distinguish between them.

   a.

   b.

3. List two common diagnostic procedures for prostatic cancer.

   a.

   b.

4. What is the difference between amenorrhea and dysmenorrhea?

5. Spell out the following abbreviations:

   a. BPH _____.

   b. PMS _____.

   c. PID _____.

Multiple Choice

Place a checkmark next to the correct answer:

1. Diseases of the breast include

   a. Leiomyomas.

   b. Fibrocystic disease and fibroadenoma.

   c. Trichomoniasis.

   d. None of the above.

2. The most commonly known STD is

   a. Gonorrhea.

   b. Genital warts.

   c. Genital herpes.

   d. Syphilis.

3. Two reproductive diseases that go undetected and are considered silent are

   a. Prostatitis and epididymitis.

   b. Syphilis and trichomoniasis.

   c. Chlamydia and ovarian cancer.

   d. Ovarian cysts and endometriosis.

4. An effective treatment for PMS may be

   a. Reduction in salt intake.

   b. Reduction in caffeine and other stimulants.

   c. Proper diet and exercise.

   d. All of the above.

5. Pregnancy-induced hypertension

   a. Causes an implanted ovum outside the uterine cavity.

   b. Is diagnosed by ultrasonography.

   c. Results in the premature separation of the placenta from the uterine wall.

   d. Also called preeclampsia and eclampsia.

Discussion Questions/Personal Reflection

1. Discuss reasons a couple might choose ART. What are the advantages and disadvantages?

2. Discuss various complications that can occur during pregnancy. Identify any known pre-ventative measures that could be taken.

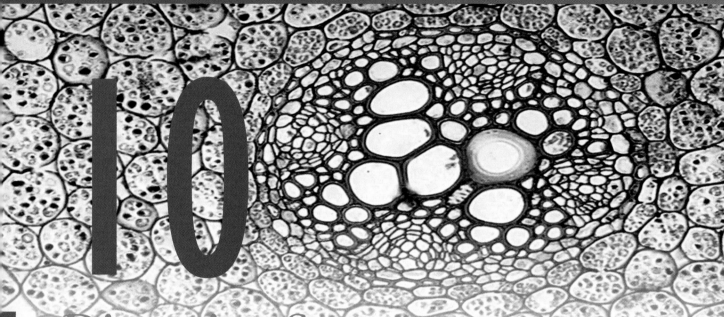

10

Digestive System Diseases and Disorders

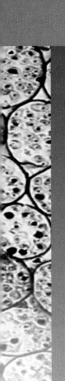

Anticholinergic (ăn•tĭ•kō•lĭn•ĕr′jĭk)
Bilirubin (bĭl•ĭ•roo′bĭn)
Bilirubinuria (bĭl•ĭ•roo•bĭn•ū′rē•ă)
Cachexia (kă•kĕks′ē•ă)
Cholestasis (kō•lē•stā′sĭs)
Colectomy (kō•lĕk′tō•mē)
Coryza (kŏ•rī′ză)
Dysphagia (dĭs•fā′jē•ă)
Enteropathy (ĕn•tĕr•ŏp′ă•thē)
Epigastric (ĕp•ĭ•găs′trĭk)
Fecalith (fē′kă•lĭth)
Fissure (fĭ′shĕr)
Fistula (fĭs′tū•lă)
Gliadin (glī′ĕ•dĕn
Hematemesis (hĕm•ăt•ĕm′ĕ•sis)
Hemolysis (hē•mŏl′ĭ•sĭs)
Hepatomegaly (hĕp•ă•tō•mĕg′ă•lē)
Hyperglycemia (hī•pĕr•glī•sē′mē•ă)
Ileostomy (ĭl•ē•ŏs′tō•mē)
Jaundice (jawn′dĭs)
Leukocytosis (loo•kō•sī•tō′sĭs)
Occult blood (ŭ•kŭlt′)
Parenteral hyperalimentation
    (păr•ĕn′tĕr•ăl hī•pĕr•ă•lĕ•mĕn•tā′shĕn)
Polyposis (pŏl•ē•pō′sĭs)
Reflux (rē′flŭks
Tetany (tĕt′ă•nē)
Varices (văr′ĭ•sēz)
Villi (vĭl′ī)

An apple a day keeps everyone away if your aim is good enough.

—MAXINE

LEARNING OBJECTIVES

Upon successful completion of this chapter, you will be able to:

• Define *stomatitis*.
• Recall the classic symptoms of gastroesophageal reflux.
• Identify at least four causes of gastritis.
• Discuss the signs and symptoms of gastroenteritis.
• List the three types of hiatal hernias.
• Define *peptic ulcers*.
• Explain the symptoms of celiac disease.
• Review causes of irritable bowel syndrome.
• Discuss the inflammatory pattern of Crohn's disease.
• List at least three predisposing factors of ulcerative colitis.
• Recall the cause and predisposing factors of diverticulitis disease.
• Describe the symptoms for appendicitis.
• Describe the condition of hemorrhoids.
• Restate the cause of, and treatment for, abdominal hernias.
• Identify populations at risk for colorectal cancer.
• Explain the implications of pancreatitis.
• Discuss the relationship between cholecystitis and cholelithiasis.
• Name two complications of cirrhosis.
• Define the different types of hepatitis.
• Recall the prognosis for pancreatic cancer.
• Recall treatment possibilities for infantile colic.
• Compare and contrast roundworm and pinworm infestations.
• List at least three common symptoms of the digestive system diseases and disorders.

The digestive system consists of the set of organs and glands associated with the ingestion and digestion of food and the absorption of nutrients (Fig. 10.1). This system also eliminates solid wastes from the body. It may be the system that is most abused. Whether a person is eating foods of little value or a well-balanced diet, the task of the digestive system is the same—to nourish the cells of the body.

The basic functions of the digestive system are to ingest, digest, and absorb the nutrients taken in. The system is composed of the alimentary canal and the accessory organs of digestion. The canal is a tube that passes from the mouth to the anus. The parts of the alimentary canal are noted in Figure 10.1 and include the mouth, teeth, tongue, salivary glands, pharynx, esophagus, stomach, small intestine, and large intestine (colon). The latter extends from the small intestine to the anus.

The accessory glands include the pancreas, liver, and gallbladder (Figs. 10.2 and 10.3). The pancreas is both an exocrine (produces digestive enzymes) and an endocrine (produces insulin and glucagons) gland. The liver, the largest organ in the abdominal cavity, produces bile and plays a central role in the metabolism of the body. The gallbladder concentrates and stores bile that is received from the liver.

The two functions of the digestive system are digestion and absorption. In *digestion,* both mechanical and chemical processes occur wherein food is broken down into simpler molecules such as amino acids, fatty acids, and simple sugars. The mechanical process involves physically breaking down food as it is chewed and swallowed. The chemical process occurs when the enzymes act on the digested food to create simpler chemical molecules. This prepares the food for absorption. In *absorption,* the simpler molecules as well as minerals, vitamins, and water move along the digestive tube across the digestive wall and into body tissue.

The various accessory organs secrete fluids into the digestive tube to help in the digestion and absorption of nutrients. These accessory organs manufacture and secrete endocrine and exocrine enzymes that are essential for digestion and absorption. The process of ingesting, digesting, and absorbing nutrients supplies the energy and chemical building blocks for growth and maintenance of the body.

UPPER GASTROINTESTINAL TRACT

Stomatitis

■ **DESCRIPTION** *Stomatitis,* or inflammation of the oral mucosa, is a common infection that occurs in two forms: *acute herpetic stomatitis* (cold sore) and *aphthous stomatitis* (canker sores). Painful blisters or ulcers characterize both.

■ **ETIOLOGY** Acute herpetic stomatitis is caused by herpes simplex type 1. The cause of aphthous stomatitis is unknown. Acute herpetic stomatitis lies dormant in nervous tissue with recurring lesions appearing throughout life. Aphthous stomatitis is activated periodically. Stress, fatigue, anxiety, and immunosuppression exacerbate both acute herpetic stomatitis and aphthous stomatitis.

■ **SIGNS AND SYMPTOMS** Acute herpetic stomatitis begins suddenly. There will be mouth pain, difficulty eating or swallowing, and fever. Gums are swollen, and mucous membrane is characterized by blisters and ulcerating inflammatory lesions that heal in less than 2 weeks. In aphthous stomatitis, there will be burning, tingling, and some swelling of mucous membrane. There will be one or more shallow ulcers with white centers and red borders. The ulcers are discrete and shallow and gradually heal in 10 to 14 days.

■ **DIAGNOSTIC PROCEDURES** Diagnosis is based on physical examination.

■ **TREATMENT** Supportive measures such as warm-water mouth rinses and topical anesthetics to relieve the pain are recommended.

ALTERNATIVE THERAPY: *A mouthwash made from steeped sage and chamomile may be helpful as a gargle. The client should avoid high-acid fruits, caffeine, alcohol, commercial mouthwashes, and smoking. Naturopaths believe that an allergy to wheat is a major cause of aphthous stomatitis.*

 TEACHING TIPS: Instruct individuals on the importance of meticulous oral hygiene and the avoidance of any irritating foods.

■ **PROGNOSIS** Both forms are self-limiting. Acute herpetic stomatitis may be severe and even life threatening in neonates.

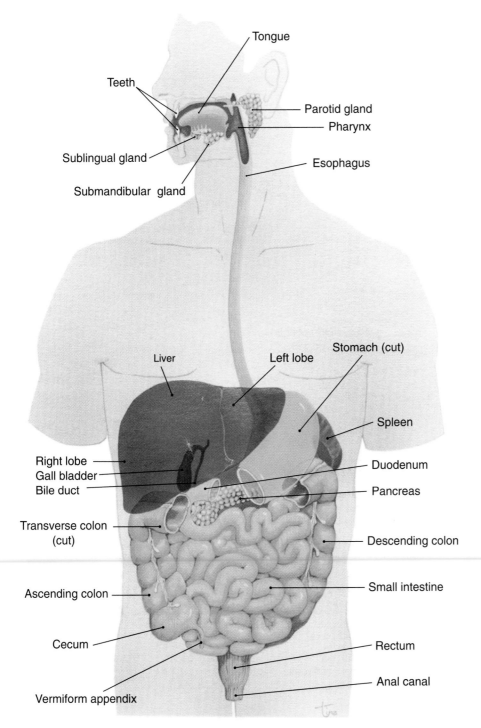

Figure 10.1 The digestive system. (Modified from Scanlon, VC, and Sanders, T: Essentials of Anatomy and Physiology, ed 4. FA Davis, Philadelphia, 2003, p 357, with permission.)

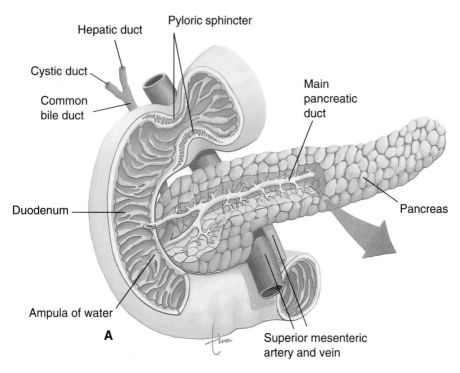

Hepatic duct

Pyloric sphincter

Cystic duct

Common bile duct

Main pancreatic duct

Duodenum

Pancreas

Ampula of water

A

Superior mesenteric artery and vein

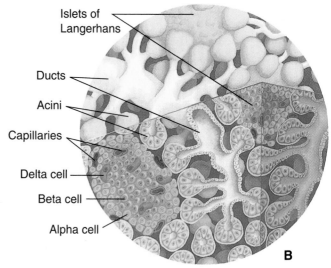

Islets of Langerhans

Ducts

Acini

Capillaries

Delta cell

Beta cell

Alpha cell

B

Figure 10.2 (A) The pancreas, sectioned to show the pancreatic ducts. The main pancreatic duct joins the bile duct. (B) Microscopic section showing acini with their ducts and several islets of Langerhans (From Scanlon, VC, and Sanders, T: Essentials of Anatomy and Physiology, ed 4. FA Davis, Philadelphia, 2003, p 363, with permission.)